THE
MASTER YOUR METABOLISM
CALORIE COUNTER

THE
MASTER YOUR
METABOLISM
CALORIE
COUNTER

Jillian Michaels

with Mariska van Aalst

THREE RIVERS PRESS
NEW YORK

The information in this work is in no way intended as medical advice or as a substitute for medical counseling. The information should be used in conjunction with the guidance and care of your physician. Consult your physician before beginning this program as you would any weight-loss or weight-maintenance program. Your physician should be aware of all medical conditions that you may have, as well as the medications and supplements you are taking. As with any weight-loss plan, the information here should not be used by patients on dialysis or by pregnant or nursing mothers.

Copyright © 2010 by Empowered Media LLC

All rights reserved.
Published in the United States by Three Rivers Press,
an imprint of the Crown Publishing Group,
a division of Random House, Inc., New York.
www.crownpublishing.com

Three Rivers Press and the Tugboat design
are registered trademarks of Random House, Inc.

Library of Congress Cataloging-in-Publication Data

Michaels, Jillian.
The master your metabolism calorie counter / Jillian Michaels
with Mariska van Aalst.—1st ed.
p.   cm.
1. Energy metabolism.   2. Food—Caloric content.
3. Weight loss.   I. Aalst, Mariska van.   II. Title.
QP176.M53 2010
612.3'9—dc22   2009053613

ISBN 978-0-307-71821-1

PRINTED IN THE UNITED STATES OF AMERICA

10 9 8 7 6 5

First Edition

ACKNOWLEDGMENTS

Many thanks to my incredible team, who work every day to bring cost-effective, accessible life solutions to the masses:

My business partner Giancarlo Chersich, all the folks at NBC, CAA, and Crown . . . thank you!

To my incredible editor, Heather Jackson; I am so lucky to have you as a friend and partner-in-crime.

Mariska van Aalst, my researcher and wordsmith extraordinaire; I couldn't have done this without you. Thank you for your genius.

CONTENTS

INTRODUCTION: Information Is Power   1

THE MASTER DIET AT-A-GLANCE   6

ANTI-NUTRIENTS, OR MASTER DISASTERS   10

HORMONE POSITIVE FOODS   13
    Mastering Estrogen   13
    Mastering Ghrelin   14
    Mastering Thyroid   15
    Mastering Insulin   16
    Mastering Cortisol   17
    Mastering Leptin   18
    Mastering DHEA   19
    Mastering Testosterone   20
    Mastering hGH   21

POWER NUTRIENT FOOD GROUPS   22
    Power Nutrient Food Group 1: Legumes   22
    Power Nutrient Food Group 2: The Allium
        Family   23
    Power Nutrient Food Group 3: Berries   23
    Power Nutrient Food Group 4: Organic Meat and
        Eggs   24

Power Nutrient Food Group 5: Colorful Fruits and
    Vegetables   25
Power Nutrient Food Group 6: Cruciferous
    Vegetables   27
Power Nutrient Food Group 7: Dark Green Leafy
    Vegetables   27
Power Nutrient Food Group 8: Nuts and Seeds   28
Power Nutrient Food Group 9: Organic Dairy   29
Power Nutrient Food Group 10: Whole Grains   29

MASTER HOME AND BODY PRODUCTS   31
Home Cleaning Products   32
Beauty and Personal Care Products   33

DECODING THE COUNTER   36

THE MASTER LIST   38
Beverages   38
Canned Foods   53
Dairy Products   67
Fresh Fruits and Vegetables   80
Frozen Foods   114
Grains, Breads, Cereals, and Pasta   130
Meat, Fish, and Eggs   149
Nuts and Seeds   162
Sauces and Dressings   169
Snacks and Sweets   176
Restaurants   195

Afterword: Use It to Lose It   321

THE
MASTER YOUR METABOLISM
CALORIE COUNTER

Introduction

....

INFORMATION IS POWER

I have people come up to me all the time to tell me that they're stuck. They just can't lose weight. "I've plateaued!" they say. "My program isn't working anymore."

I get it. When you don't see results, you get discouraged. You feel helpless and hopeless. But if you are pursuing a health and wellness goal without the proper information, it's like you're flying blind. Imagine navigating your way from Los Angeles to New York without a GPS, a road map, or a compass—you could never do it. You need the right tools to get where you want to go and to achieve the goals you set for yourself. Like the one you hold in your hands: *The Master Your Metabolism Calorie Counter*.

You already know the one universal truth that will always apply to obesity and health: Weight is an energy equation. It's calories in, calories out. We all know that; we just don't always know that there are other factors affecting this equation. That's where the Master Diet comes in.

When you find yourself stuck in your weight loss efforts, 99 times out of 100 you're simply not taking into account how much energy is going into your body and how much is going out. Without that info, your chance of getting results and maintaining them is very slim. But when you're informed, you have the ability to make educated choices, powerful choices that effect positive change.

Once you know the calories in any given food, your next question must be about its quality. The quality of your food is critical, not just for preventing disease and combating aging, but because it maximizes your calorie burn. In *Master Your Metabolism,* I shared shocking information about how low-quality foods (in addition to lifestyle factors like toxic stress and environmental toxins) have dramatically altered our endocrine systems. Those changes to our hormone levels have helped make us—and keep us—fat. If you have already read the book, you know that I didn't shy away from some of the scariest information. Yet people have told me that reading *Master Your Metabolism* changed their lives. Throughout that book, I cited dozens of scientific studies that have proven one simple fact: When you eat crappy food, it kills your metabolism, ages you, and creates disease in your body; when you eat high-quality food, you get the reverse: a boosted metabolism, stronger immunity, and a powerful weapon against aging. We now know that Hormone Positive Foods are health positive foods. I designed this book as a quick, easy-to-use reference that gives you an accessible and affordable way to stay connected to the Master Diet. With it, you can easily find those Hormone Positive, metabolism-boosting foods, every day, at every meal, no matter where you are—at home, on the road, anywhere. A health and weight-loss program has to fit *your* life—it's the only way to ensure long-term success.

In these pages, you'll find complete nutritional information for over 6,000 foods, everything from the very best organic produce to the very worst deep-fried appetizers at chain restaurants—everything you need to count calories accurately and gauge the quality of foods you encounter every day in the real world. I've included an at-a-glance guide to the Master Diet, to refresh you on the basics or, if you're new to the plan, give you a bird's-eye view of the diet.

You'll also find lists of hundreds of Hormone Positive Foods that can help increase your body's ability to burn fat and build muscle. And a woeful number of Master Disasters—horrible Anti-Nutrient foods that I wish no one would consume, ever. (Foods considered Master Disasters are included throughout the counter.)

Given that I'm basically saying, "Don't eat these, *ever*," you might wonder why I've included them at all. Again, it's about giving you power, the power to make an informed choice about what you're eating, not a mindless grab for something you don't really want and certainly don't need. If I've learned anything on the *Biggest Loser* campus, it's that people have to clearly see what exactly they have done, and what they are currently doing, that has helped create their ill health and obesity. I'll never forget when Pete Thomas from season two of the *Biggest Loser* looked at the Bloomin' Onion at the Outback Steakhouse and realized that when he routinely ate that dish by himself, he was consuming 1,560 calories and 84 grams of fat in about *10 minutes*. *That* was his true aha moment. That's when he realized, "Oh my God, this is why I am *four hundred pounds*. This is why my cholesterol is through the roof. This is why I'm diabetic."

In this toxic food environment, you need constant reminders of exactly how bad these choices are for your long-term health and well-being. Some will shock you, just like Pete was shocked. Consider the innocent tuna sandwich. Fish is good for you, right? On the Master Diet, it's a Power Nutrient. But then you're at Quiznos, you're hungry, you're thinking about ordering a large—but a quick peek in these pages tells you that a large Tuna Melt Deli Sub is actually **1,760 calories**—more than most of us should eat in *an entire day*.

While I'd prefer that you not eat at chain restaurants, I'm a realist. Okay, you're already at Quiznos—so what can you have? Scan down the list and you'll see that you can choose to have a bowl of Hearty Chili (360 calories) or a cup of Tomato Basil

Soup (125 calories) and a small Steak and Bleu Salad (230 calories) instead. By becoming aware of what's in your food and understanding which foods have previously led to diet derailment, you can cut them out and replace them with healthier choices.

I want you to bring this book with you everywhere you go. I want it to travel with you when you go out to eat and when you're at the supermarket; it should always be in your backpack, back pocket, or purse. If you use the knowledge you hold in your hands, you will get results.

It all adds up: Good choices lead to good results. Achieving results empowers and inspires you to achieve more. And these little successes will beget more success in other areas of your life.

Each one of us has the power to effect positive change within ourselves and globally—first by making the right choices for ourselves, then expanding that thinking to our families and our homes, and then bringing it to our communities. And when we do that, it all falls into place. So let's get started living a Master-full life.

THE MASTER DIET AT-A-GLANCE

So you know weight loss is all about calories in, calories out. That said, who wouldn't mind a little boost in the calories-out department? Most everyone wants to increase their metabolism, but to do this, we have to first know and understand what metabolism is.

Many folks believe that metabolism is the rate at which your body burns calories. But that's just one thing your metabolism *does*. In fact, your metabolism *is* your body's biochemistry. The way all your hormones interact, a.k.a. your endocrine system, has a major impact on your ability to lose weight. Some hormones, like DHEA and testosterone, tell our bodies to burn calories; some, like ghrelin and insulin, tell our bodies to hoard fat. Although the fundamental function of any weight-loss program is and will always be calories in and calories out, you can bolster your efforts to lose weight by optimizing the hormone levels in your body.

Unfortunately, due to the toxic levels of chronic stress, dangerously processed food (Anti-Nutrients, or what I also call Master Disasters), and endocrine-disrupting chemicals everywhere in our environment, your hormone levels and metabolism have likely been thrown off-kilter. The Master Your Metabolism plan tackles these critical threats head-on.

First, you **Remove** Anti-Nutrients, the foods your body doesn't recognize and that confuse and mess up your hormones. Next, you **Restore** Power Nutrients, the whole foods nature intended us to eat, the foods our bodies recognize, the ones that send healthy, metabolism-boosting messages to our hormones. And last, you **Rebalance** Your Energy, paying attention to when and how much you eat (which includes using this counter in your daily life—everywhere, all the time—to track the quality and the quantity of what you're taking in each day).

Follow this three-step plan and you'll reboot your entire endocrine system, so your body can get back to burning fat, building muscle, and making your metabolism work for you instead of against you. If you haven't already, read my book *Master Your Metabolism* to learn more about how our bodies are under attack and how you can fight back to protect your biochemistry with a few key lifestyle changes. In the meantime, check out this at-a-glance peek at the Master Diet. As long as you focus on its three main principles, you can't go wrong.

THE MASTER YOUR METABOLISM DIET PLAN
Step One: Remove Anti-Nutrients
- Hydrogenated fats
- Refined grains
- High fructose corn syrup
- Artificial sweeteners
- Artificial coloring and preservatives
- Nitrates and nitrites
- Glutamates
- Foods from animals treated with hormones or antibiotics
- Foods treated with pesticides

Reduce these
- Starchy vegetables
- Tropical, dried, and canned fruits
- Excess soy
- Excess alcohol
- Canned foods

Step Two: Restore Power Nutrients
- Legumes
- Alliums (garlic, onions, leeks, scallions)
- Berries
- Meat and eggs
- Colorful fruits and veggies
- Cruciferous veggies
- Dark green leafy veggies

- Nuts and seeds
- Dairy
- Whole grains

Step Three: Rebalance Energy
- Eat breakfast
- Eat every four hours
- Do not eat after 9 P.M.
- No simple carbs at night
- Eat until you're full, but not stuffed
- Eat 40 percent carbs, 30 percent fat, 30 percent protein

ANTI-NUTRIENTS, OR MASTER DISASTERS

Some foods are so bad for you, I never want you to eat them. Never. Ever. But the sad thing is, sometimes it's hard to know where they're lurking. But at least the supermarket gives you the chance to see for yourself what's in the food you're buying. When you're looking at processed foods in the store, keep your eyes peeled for these words.

Aspartame (NutraSweet)
Autolyzed yeast
Benzoic acid
Blue dye 1 and 2
Butylated hydroxyanisole (BHA)
Calcium caseinate
Enriched

Fortified
Glutamate
Glutamic acid
Green 3
High fructose corn syrup
Hydrogenated oils of any kind (palm, corn, soybean)
Hydrolyzed corn gluten
Hydrolyzed protein (wheat, milk, soy, whey—any protein that is hydrolyzed)
Monopotassium glutamate
Monosodium glutamate (MSG)
Natrium glutamate
Nitrates
Nitrites
Olestra (Olean)
Potassium benzoate
Potassium bromate
Red 3 and 40
Refined
Saccharin (Sweet'N Low)
Sodium benzoate
Sodium bisulfite
Sodium caseinate
Sodium dioxide
Sodium nitrate
Sodium nitrite
Sucralose (Splenda)
Sulfites
Textured protein

Trans fats
Yeast extract
Yeast food
Yeast nutrient
Yellow 6

....

MASTERING ESTROGEN

Our individual needs for estrogen can be very different. Some types of estrogen help us stay lean; some make us pack on fat. Perimenopausal women may find a bit of hot flash relief with phytoestrogens, while in post-menopausal women, the same foods may increase the risk of breast and uterine cancers. In men, some phytoestrogens can have a cardioprotective effect but too many can dampen testosterone and increase the risk of developing prostate cancer. And we all have to contend with harmful xenoestrogens that come from toxic substances in the environment, including our cosmetics, cleaning products, preservatives, pesticides, and plastics.

How to keep it all straight? Thankfully, these Hormone Positive Foods—remember, always organic!—can help our bodies contend with this chemical onslaught and optimize our natural levels of estrogen. Look for foods with high levels of fiber; the more fiber in your diet, the better your natural estrogen disposal system works.

Almonds
Anise
Apples
Avocadoes
Barley
Bean sprouts
Beans (black,
    garbanzo,
    kidney, navy,
    pinto)
Blackberries
Black
    raspberries
Broccoli
Brussels sprouts
Bulgur
Cabbage
Fennel
Fermented soy
    products
    (tofu, miso,
    and tempeh;
    1 serving per
    week)
Flaxseed
Green tea
Hops
Kale
Lentils
Nectarines
Oat bran
Oatmeal
Onions
Plums
Pomegranates
Prunes
Psyllium fiber
Rice bran
Rye
Sesame seeds
Sweet potatoes
Wheat germ

MASTERING GHRELIN

Ghrelin is our number one hunger hormone. When it's your normal mealtime or you smell something really delicious, ghrelin is released in your belly and travels up to trigger your brain's appetite center (and, unfortunately, simultaneously turns down your calorie burn). Keep ghrelin in check by eating slowly, and doing so every three to four hours, especially high-volume foods with lots of fiber and water—hello, vegetable soup!—because as soon as your stomach registers it's full, ghrelin levels fall again.

Apples
Artichokes
Beans (black, kidney, navy, pinto)
Beets
Blueberries
Buckwheat
Bulgur
Cabbage
Carrots
Cauliflower
Celery
Collard greens
Cranberries
Cucumber
Eggplant
Fennel
Flaxseed
Grapefruit
Green beans
High-fiber cereal

Lentils
Mustard greens
Oats
Oranges
Pistachios
Raspberries
Romaine lettuce
Shiitake mushrooms
Split peas
Strawberries
Swiss chard
Tomatoes
Turnip greens
Watermelon
Whey protein (not hydrolyzed)
Whole grains
Zucchini

....

MASTERING THYROID

Thyroid hormones help control how much oxygen your cells use, how fast your heart beats, how warm your body gets, not to mention how good your memory and mood are on any given day. Thyroid also plays a large role in the rate at which your body burns calories. Avoiding goitrogenic foods, like raw cruciferous vegetables (broccoli, cauliflower, kale), peanuts and peaches, or soy foods, like tofu or "not-dogs," is particularly important for people with thyroid issues (like me!). (These goitrogens interrupt the thyroid's uptake of iodine, the building block of thyroid hormones.) Everyone can benefit from eating more of the Hormone Positive Foods listed here, many of which are high in zinc, which helps trigger thyroid release, and selenium, a mineral that helps your body create T_4 and convert it into T_3, the metabolism-boosting thyroid hormone.

Almonds	Olive oil
Anchovies	Oysters
Asparagus	Pacific salmon
Avocadoes	Peas
Basil	Pumpkin seeds
Beef	Sardines
Brazil nuts	Sesame seeds
Brewer's yeast	Shrimp
Broccoli	Spinach
Cashews	Summer squash
Collard greens	Swiss chard
Cremini mushrooms	Thyme
Green peas	Venison
Hazelnuts	Wheat germ
Herring	Whole grains
Lamb	Yogurt
Mustard greens	

HORMONE POSITIVE FOODS

MASTERING INSULIN

When it comes to insulin, the Master plan is all about keeping it *low.* After you eat, insulin is released from the pancreas to regulate the level of sugar in your blood. But if you regularly eat foods that cause a spike in your blood sugar, like overly refined white pasta, bread, or other "fast" carbs, you can overtax your body's insulin production system and pack on the pounds—not to mention raise your risk of developing diabetes. Luckily, you can avoid this easily. Start by making sure you eat some protein at every meal and snack; protein lowers your blood sugar response and lessens your need for insulin. Also, go crazy for nonstarchy vegetables with plenty of fiber. The following foods are a good start.

Almonds	Chili peppers	Peanuts
Amaranth	Cinnamon	Pickles
Artichoke hearts	Collard greens	Psyllium
Barley	Cucumber	Radicchio
Basil	Eggs	Romaine lettuce
Beans (black,	Endive	Salmon
cannellini,	Grapefruit	Spinach
fava,	Greek yogurt	Tomatoes
garbanzo,	Green beans	Turkey breast
kidney,	Herring	Turmeric
lima, or	Kudzu	Turnip greens
pinto)	Lamb	Vinegar (apple
Bok choy	Leeks	cider,
Bran cereals	Mackerel	balsamic,
Brazil nuts	Mustard greens	red wine, or
Brewer's yeast	Oats	white)
Broccoli	Olive oil	Walnuts
Cabbage	Onions	Whole grain
Chicken	Oysters	bread

MASTERING CORTISOL

The stress hormone cortisol blocks your efforts to lose weight by slowing down your metabolism. If you're not careful to manage your stress with positive methods—yoga, meditation, exercise—high cortisol can trigger stress eating by stimulating cravings for high-fat, high-carb foods. And once you've eaten them, cortisol turns them into belly fat, the worst kind. Not good. Be sure to avoid alcohol as much as possible and limit your sodium intake to 1,500 to 2,000 mg a day (unless you are an athlete who sweats a lot—then you can go up to 3,000 mg a day). Many of these Hormone Positive Foods are high in vitamin C and fiber, nutrients that will help you keep cortisol levels where you want them: low.

Apples	Mackerel
Asparagus	Mustard and turnip greens
Barley	Oat bran
Beans	Oatmeal
Beef	Oranges
Bell peppers	Peas
Broccoli	Pork
Brown rice	Raspberries
Brussels sprouts	Rice bran
Cabbage	Snow peas
Cantaloupe	Spinach
Cauliflower	Strawberries
Celery	Sweet potatoes
Chicken	Swiss chard
Eel	Tomatoes
Grapefruit	Tuna
Herring	Turnip greens
Kale	Watermelon
Kiwi	White potatoes
Lemons	Whole grains
Limes	Zucchini

MASTERING LEPTIN

After you eat a meal, your fat cells produce leptin and send it to the hypothalamus in your brain, where it turns off hunger signals. When this satiety hormone works the way it should, not only does it help you control your appetite but it also increases your metabolism and taps into your body's long-term fat stores. Good-quality protein, especially deep sea and other foods with omega-3 fatty acids, like walnuts, can improve your body's sensitivity to leptin so you'll automatically reduce your calorie intake. Eat these foods to help your body optimize leptin levels for easier weight loss.

Beans
Beef
Broccoli
Cabbage
Cauliflower
Chicken
Edamame
Eggs
Flaxseed
Fortified breakfast
    cereal
Green beans
Ground cloves
Halibut
Herring
Mackerel
Maple syrup
Milk
Mustard seed
Nuts
Olive oil
Oregano
Oysters
Pacific wild salmon
Peas
Sardines
Scallops
Shrimp
Snapper
Sweet potatoes
Turkey
Walnuts
Whole grains
Winter squash
Yogurt

....

MASTERING DHEA

Made in your adrenal glands, DHEA is the precursor to testosterone and estrogen. Our production of this youth elixir declines as we get older, which sucks because DHEA keeps our hearts and brains strong and may even help us live longer. DHEA is especially helpful to women, as it's believed to protect against breast cancer and osteoporosis. It is tricky to increase DHEA with diet, but some preliminary studies suggest that foods with chromium, vitamin E, magnesium, and selenium, like many of these Hormone Positive Foods, can help improve your DHEA levels.

Almonds
Barley
Beans
Blueberries
Brazil nuts
Brewer's yeast
Broccoli
Button mushrooms
Canola oil
Carrots
Cod
Crab meat
Eggs
Fortified whole grain
    cereals
Garlic
Green leafy vegetables
Halibut
Herring
Kelp
Lamb
Molasses
Nuts
Oats
Olives
Onions
Oysters
Papaya
Peas
Pork
Potatoes
Pumpkin seeds
Romaine lettuce
Salmon
Sardines
Shrimp
Snapper
Spinach
Sunflower seeds
Swiss chard
Tuna
Turkey
Whole grains
Whole wheat bread
    (100%, with no HFCS!)

MASTERING TESTOSTERONE

Whether you're a girl or a guy, testosterone is your weight-loss friend. As a catabolic hormone, testosterone helps you build calorie-burning lean muscle and increases energy and strength (better for working out!). And, as we all know, testosterone increases your libido—you, too, girls. And testosterone keeps our thinking sharp. Unfortunately, our average supply of testosterone can dwindle as we get older. But luckily for us, foods with high-quality protein and zinc, such as beef, cashews, oysters, yogurt, and many other Hormone Positive Foods, will help boost our body's natural production of testosterone.

Almonds
Asparagus
Beans
Beef tenderloin
Broccoli
Canola oil
Cashews
Cheddar cheese
Chicken
Chickpeas
Coffee
Collard greens
Cremini mushrooms
Dark meat chicken and
   turkey
Dungeness crab
Eggs
Fish
Garlic
Lamb
Milk
Mustard greens
Olive oil
Onions
Oysters
Peas
Pork
Pumpkin seeds
Salmon
Sesame seeds
Spinach
Summer squash
Swiss chard
Tuna
Turkey breast
Vitamin-B fortified
   cereals
Yogurt

··

MASTERING hGH

I wish we could all have unlimited amounts of growth hormone (hGH). What doesn't this incredible hormone do? When it's produced naturally, hGH helps us build muscle, burn fat, and maintain lower levels of blood sugar as well as keep our skin smooth and increase our energy levels. Who doesn't want more of that! Sadly, it's a bit tough to naturally increase your hGH. One sure thing: Steer clear of MSG, which has been shown to suppress growth hormone levels in lab animals. And add more of the foods that contain arginine, an amino acid that supports healthy hGH levels.

Almonds	Mackerel	Shrimp
Beef	Milk	Spinach
Brazil nuts	Mung beans	Spirulina
Buckwheat	Mustard greens	Sunflower
Buffalo	Oatmeal	seeds
Cashews	Pacific cod	Tilapia
Chicken	Peanuts	Tuna
Coconut	Pecans	Turkey
Cottage cheese	Pheasant	Venison
Crab	Pine nuts	Walnuts
Egg whites	Pork	Watercress
Garbanzo	Pumpkin seeds	Wheat germ
beans	Quail	Whey protein
Haddock	Ricotta	(not
Halibut	Salmon	hydrolyzed)
Hazelnuts	Scallops	Yogurt
Lobster	Sesame seeds	

POWER NUTRIENT
FOOD GROUPS

The Master Your Metabolism plan may challenge you to try whole foods you may never have tasted before. As you get used to this new way of eating, keep an eye out for the following Power Nutrients in the grocery store or at the local farmers' market. Remember my rule: If it comes from the ground or it has a mother, you can eat it!

POWER NUTRIENT FOOD GROUP 1:
LEGUMES
Best Choice: Red Beans

Adzuki beans
Alfalfa sprouts
Anasazi beans
Black beans
Black-eyed peas
Broad (fava) beans

Cannellini (white kidney) beans
Garbanzo beans (chickpeas)
Great northern beans
Kidney beans
Lentils
Lima (butter) beans
Mung beans
Navy beans
Peas*
Pink beans
Pinto beans
Soybeans (edamame)*

* Please limit to 1 serving per week.

POWER NUTRIENT FOOD GROUP 2:
THE ALLIUM FAMILY
Best Choice: Garlic
Chives
Green onions
Leeks
Onions
Shallots

POWER NUTRIENT FOOD GROUP 3:
BERRIES
Best Choice: Blueberries
Acai berries*
Bilberries
Blackberries
Black currants
Black raspberries

Boysenberries
Cranberries
Elderberries
Goji berries*
Gooseberries
Lingonberries
Mangosteen*
Maqui berries*
Marionberries
Pomegranate*
Raspberries
Strawberries

*While not technically berries, these berry-like fruits have similar health benefits.

POWER NUTRIENT FOOD GROUP 4: ORGANIC MEAT AND EGGS

Best Choice: Alaskan Wild Salmon

Abalone
Beef tenderloin*
Bottom round*
Buffalo
Chicken breast
Eggs from free-range chickens
Extra-lean ground beef*
Eye of round*
Flank steak*
Ground turkey
Halibut
Lamb chops

Pacific cod
Pacific halibut
Pacific pollock
Pacific rockfish
Pork chops
Pork tenderloin
Round tip*
Rump roast*
Sardines
Sirloin*
Sirloin tip*
Snapper
Top loin*
Top round*
Tuna (U.S. or Canadian canned light or
    albacore)
Turkey
Venison

* All beef should be grass-fed.

POWER NUTRIENT FOOD GROUP 5: COLORFUL FRUITS AND VEGETABLES
Best Choice: Tomatoes

REDS
Pink grapefruits
Pink guavas
Watermelons

PURPLES
Cherries
Eggplants

Grapes
Olives
Plums
Prunes
Red apples
Red beets
Red pears
Red peppers

ORANGES

Acorn squash
Apricots
Cantaloupes
Carrots
Mangoes
Pumpkins
Sweet potatoes
Winter squash

YELLOWS

Honeydews
Kiwis
Lemons
Limes
Nectarines
Oranges
Papayas
Peaches
Pineapples
Tangerines
Yellow grapefruits
Yellow peppers
Zucchini

POWER NUTRIENT FOOD GROUP 6: CRUCIFEROUS VEGETABLES*

Best Choice: Broccoli

Arugula
Bok choy
Broccoli rabe
Brussels sprouts
Cabbage
Cauliflower
Chinese broccoli
Chinese cabbage
Collard greens
Kale
Kohlrabi
Rutabaga
Turnip greens
Watercress

*Cook cruciferous vegetables thoroughly to avoid negative impact on your thyroid.

POWER NUTRIENT FOOD GROUP 7: DARK GREEN LEAFY VEGETABLES

Best Choice: Spinach

Arugula
Bibb lettuce
Buttercrunch lettuce
Chicory
Collard greens
Crisphead lettuce
Dandelion greens

Endive
Escarole
Frisee
Grand Rapids leaf lettuce
Leaf lettuce
Mustard greens
Purslane
Red Salad Bowl lettuce
Romaine lettuce
Royal Oak Leaf lettuce
Ruby lettuce
Summer crisp lettuce
Swiss chard
Turnip greens

POWER NUTRIENT FOOD GROUP 8:
NUTS AND SEEDS
Best Choice: Walnuts

Almonds
Brazil nuts
Cashews
Flaxseeds
Hazelnuts
Macadamias
Pecans
Pine nuts
Pistachios
Pumpkin seeds
Sesame seeds
Sunflower seeds

POWER NUTRIENT FOOD GROUP 9:
ORGANIC DAIRY
Best Choice: Organic Low-Fat Plain Yogurt
- Cottage cheese
- Greek yogurt
- Homemade yogurt
- Kefir
- Lassi
- Part-skim mozzarella
- Part-skim ricotta
- Skim or 1% organic milk
- Sour cream

POWER NUTRIENT FOOD GROUP 10:
WHOLE GRAINS
Best Choice: Oats
- Amaranth*
- Barley
- Brown rice
- Buckwheat
- Bulgur (cracked wheat)
- Couscous
- Millet*
- Popcorn
- Quinoa*
- Sorghum
- Spelt
- Triticale
- Wheat bran
- Whole grain barley

Whole grain corn (or cornmeal)
Whole rye
Whole wheat
Wild rice

*Not technically grains, but prepared and eaten similarly.

MASTER HOME AND BODY PRODUCTS

If you've already read *Master Your Metabolism,* you know that the Master plan is not just about food—it's an entire lifestyle. The products we use in our homes and on our bodies often contain endocrine-disrupting chemicals. There's no need to put yourself at risk, because many healthier, greener options exist. That's why I've asked two of my favorite green experts to recommend their preferred home and body products. To protect you from the horrific chemicals in many home cleaning products, I've asked Caroline Howell, owner of GreenBeanie (www.greenbeanie.net), to suggest her favorite picks for natural cleaning products. Paige Padgett, my sweet makeup artist, then gives her picks for best green cosmetics and personal care products (also check out her website, paigepadgett.com).

HOME CLEANING PRODUCTS

The Basics

Baking soda

Vinegar (white)

Lemon juice

Borax

Salt

Olive oil

Hydrogen peroxide

Club soda

Essential oils (lavender, tea tree, for example)

Spray bottles (to mix your own cleaning supplies)

Cloths or rags (use fewer paper towels)

Toilet paper, napkins (recycled paper content and without bleach)

Glass storage containers (avoid plastic food storage when possible)

Cast-iron and stainless-steel cookware (not Teflon-coated)

Recommended Brands

Ecover: dishwasher tablets, laundry detergent, laundry stain remover

Simple Green: all-purpose cleaner, carpet cleaner

Shaklee: multipurpose cleaner, heavy-duty cleaning paste

Seventh Generation: dish soap, bathroom tissue, paper towels, toilet bowl cleaner

Mrs. Meyer's: powder surface scrub, liquid hand soap

Method: furniture polish, toilet cleaner

Bona: hardwood floor cleaner

Earth First: toilet paper, napkins, paper towels

Earth Friendly Products: dish soap

Skoy: cloth that replaces paper towels and sponges

BEAUTY AND PERSONAL CARE PRODUCTS

Skin Care

PAIGE'S PICKS

100% Pure: Coffee Bean Caffeine Eye Cream

Dr. Hauschka: Rose Day Cream

Nude Skin Care: Cleansing Facial Oil

COMPANIES SHE LOVES

100% Pure: www.100percentpure.com

Amala: www.amalabeauty.com

Dr. Alkatis: www.alkatis.com

Dr. Hauschka: www.drhauschka.com

Intelligent nutrients: www.intelligent nutrients.com

Nude Skin Care: www.nudeskincare.com

Suki: www.sukipure.com

Makeup

PAIGE'S PICKS

Tarte: Double-Ended Lip Gloss in Ferris and Sloane

Cargo Plant Love: Eye Liner in Bronze

RMS Beauty: "Un" Cover-Up

EcoTools: Makeup Tools

COMPANIES SHE LOVES

Cargo Plant Love: www.cargocosmetics.com/
plantlove.html

EcoTools: www.parispresents.com

Jane Iredale: www.janeiredale.com

Physician's Formula Organic Wear: www
.organicwearmakeup.com

RAW Natural Beauty: www.rawnatural
beauty.com

RMS Beauty: rmsbeauty.com

Tarte Cosmetics: www.tartecosmetics.com

Hair Care

PAIGE'S PICKS

John Masters Organics: Sea Mist

Rene Furterer: Naturia Dry Shampoo

Weleda: Rosemary Hair Oil

COMPANIES SHE LOVES

Hamadi Organics: www.hamadibeauty.com

John Masters Organics: www.john
masters.com

Rare El'Ements: www.rare-elements.com

Rene Furterer: www.renefurterer.com

Susan Henry Natural Color Process: www
.susanhenry-ncp.com

Weleda: usa.weleda.com

Body Care

PAIGE'S PICKS

Revolution Organics: All-Over Body Balm

Burt's Bees: Aloe & Witch Hazel Hand
Sanitizer

Pratima: Rose Organic Bath Oil and Salts

COMPANIES SHE LOVES

> Burt's Bees: www.burtsbees.com
> California Baby: www.californiababy.com
> Pangea Organics: pangeaorganics-store
>   .sparkart.net
> Pratima: www.pratimaskincare.com
> Ren: www.renskincare.com
> Revolution Organics: www.revolution
>   organics.com
> Soleo Organics: www.soleousa.com

Nail Care

PAIGE'S PICKS

> Butter London: 3 Free Lacquers in Aston
> Deborah Lippmann: Soul Mission Grapefruit
>   Foot Scrub
> Priti: Soy Remover

COMPANIES SHE LOVES

> Butter London: www.butterlondon.com
> Deborah Lippmann: lippmanncollection.com
> Priti: www.pritinyc.com
> Sparitual: www.sparitual.com
> Suncoat: www.suncoatproducts.com
> Zoya: www.artofbeauty.com

DECODING THE COUNTER

This food list is your bible—take it everywhere, consult it at all times, use it to hack your way through the dense jungle of misinformation that is our processed food supply right now.

I will say this until my dying day: *Organic, fresh, local whole foods are the way to go.* These foods are medicine and are the only foods that will help you truly master your metabolism. Eating this way is not only a matter of your life and death, it's about healthier soil, air, and water—the life and death of the planet. If you still need to justify this expense for yourself beyond your own health, which I really hope is enough, think of this as your investment in improving the health and safety of foods for everyone in the world. The more of us who buy our food this way, the more the prices will go down, and the more affordable and available organic food will become for everyone. This is your opportunity to vote for a healthier world with your dollars—please do it, for all of us!

Now, that said, I know these are tough economic times. If you find that buying organic meat or dairy is too expensive for every day (although I pray you don't), go with fish or seafood and limit yourself to hormone-free milk and dairy products. And by all means, the quickest, easiest, cheapest way to improve your health and help save the planet is to eat more bean-, grain-, and vegetable-based meals.

As you flip through the lists, you'll see that alongside the complete nutritional information (calories, fat, carbs, and so on) there are foods that are in **bold**. This means that these are Master Your Metabolism–Approved. I highly recommend that you fill your diet with as many of these foods as possible; these are the foods that will recalibrate your hormones and get your metabolism working *for* you, not against you. Eat away, have a blast. Obviously watch your calories, but enjoy these foods, as they will heal your body. Seriously, they're great. If it doesn't have this stamp, the food is either a Master Disaster or neutral healthwise. By now you know which foods to avoid, so I won't repeat myself here. Stay away from the disasters, and when you have to choose from the non-MYM foods—think calories. Keep this guide by your side and you'll be armed with all the information you need to navigate our insane food jungle!

Happy, healthy eating.

THE MASTER LIST

BEVERAGES

Filtered tap water. That's my favorite drink. You won't find it here, but if it were, it'd have a great big bolded thumbs-up on it. Frankly, I hope you will never even turn to this page. But if you're here, please know that it's never good to drink calories. Never. No matter what, whether it's sugary soda (big Master Disaster) or organic orange juice, drinking calories is not a good thing. Even with the OJ, your appetite doesn't register liquid calories, your blood sugar shoots up because there's no fiber to counteract the sugar, and you stay much hungrier than you would have been if you'd just eaten the orange. At the end of the day, as I've stressed before, losing weight is an energy equation, and too many calories make you fat. Don't drink 'em.

That said, I know everyone likes a cocktail once in a while. Almost all beers—light, regular, and dark—have about the same calories. When you reach for harder alcohol, don't forget to add any mixers to your calorie counts. Try to stick to clear drinks. Club soda, great. Sour mix, not so great. Cream (as in Baileys or white Russians), really bad. And try to limit yourself to one drink—the more you have, the more tempting those nachos become.

BRAND/BEVERAGE SERVING SIZE	CALORIES	FAT	CARBS	SODIUM	PROTEIN	FIBER
Juice						
Apple juice, canned or bottled, unsweetened						
1 cup	114	0	28	10	0	0
Apple juice, frozen concentrate, unsweetened, diluted						
1 cup	112	0	28	17	0	0
Apple juice, frozen concentrate, unsweetened, diluted						
1 oz	14	0	3	2	0	0
Blackberry juice, canned						
1 cup	95	2	20	3	1	0
Blend, apple and grape						
1 cup	125	0	31	18	0	0
Blend, apple, grape, and pear						
1 cup	130	0	32	12	0	1
Cranberry juice, unsweetened						
1 cup	116	0	31	5	1	0
Grape juice cocktail, frozen concentrate, diluted						
1 cup	128	0	32	5	0	0
Grape juice cocktail, frozen concentrate, diluted						
1 oz	16	0	4	1	0	0
Grape juice, canned or bottled, unsweetened						
1 cup	152	0	37	13	1	1
Grape juice, canned or bottled, unsweetened						
1 oz	19	0	5	2	0	0
Grapefruit juice, white, canned, sweetened						
1 cup	115	0	28	5	1	0
Grapefruit juice, white, canned, unsweetened						
1 cup	94	0	22	2	1	0
Grapefruit juice, white, frozen concentrate, unsweetened, diluted						
1 cup	101	0	24	2	1	0
Grapefruit juice, white, frozen concentrate, unsweetened, undiluted						
6 oz	302	1	72	6	4	1

BRAND/BEVERAGE SERVING SIZE	CALORIES	FAT	CARBS	SODIUM	PROTEIN	FIBER
Grapefruit juice, white, raw						
1 cup	96	0	23	2	1	0
Grapefruit juice, white, raw						
1 fruit yields						
	76	0	18	2	1	0
Grapefruit juice, white, raw, organic						
1 fruit yields						
	76	0	18	2	1	0
Guava nectar, canned						
1 cup	143	0	37	18	0	3
Lemon juice, canned or bottled						
1 tbsp	3	0	1	3	0	0
Mango nectar, canned						
1 cup	128	0	33	13	0	1
Orange juice, canned, unsweetened						
1 cup	117	0	27	10	2	1
Orange juice, frozen concentrate, unsweetened, diluted						
1 cup	112	0	27	2	2	1
Orange juice, raw						
1 cup	112	1	26	2	2	1
Orange juice, raw						
1 fruit yields						
	39	0	9	1	1	0
Orange juice, raw, organic						
1 fruit yields						
	39	0	9	1	1	0
Papaya nectar, canned						
1 cup	143	0	36	13	0	2
Passion-fruit juice, purple, raw						
1 cup	126	0	34	15	1	0
Passion-fruit juice, yellow, raw						
1 cup	148	0	36	15	2	0
Peach nectar, canned						
1 cup	134	0	35	17	1	1
Pear nectar, canned						
1 cup	150	0	39	10	0	2
Pomegranate juice, bottled						
1 cup	134	1	33	22	0	0
Prune juice, canned						
1 cup	182	0	45	10	2	3
Tangerine juice, canned, sweetened						
1 cup	125	0	30	2	1	0
Tangerine juice, frozen concentrate, sweetened, diluted						
1 cup	111	0	27	2	1	0
Tangerine juice, frozen concentrate, sweetened, undiluted						
6 oz	345	1	83	6	3	1
Tangerine juice, raw						
1 cup	13	0	3	0	0	0
Tangerine juice, raw, organic						
1 cup	13	0	3	0	0	0

BRAND/BEVERAGE SERVING SIZE	CALORIES	FAT	CARBS	SODIUM	PROTEIN	FIBER
Apple & Eve Naturally Cranberry						
8 oz	130	0	32	20	1	0
Bolthouse Farms 100% Carrot						
8 oz	70	0	14	150	2	4
Bolthouse Farms Amazing Mango						
8 oz	170	0	40	10	1	0
Bolthouse Farms Clementine						
8 oz	110	0	29	0	2	0
Bolthouse Farms Green Goodness						
8 oz	140	0	33	25	2	1
Bolthouse Farms Prickly Pear Cactus Lemonade						
8 oz	130	0	34	5	1	<1
Bolthouse Farms Purple Carrot						
8 oz	130	0	31	70	1	1
Campbell's Tomato Juice						
8 oz	50	0	10	680	2	2
Cascadian Farm Frozen Juice Concentrate Apple Juice						
2 oz	120	0	29	0	0	0
Cascadian Farm Frozen Juice Concentrate Cranberry						
2 oz	120	0	32	15	0	0
Cascadian Farm Frozen Juice Concentrate Grape						
2 oz	150	0	38	5	0	0
Cascadian Farm Frozen Juice Concentrate Lemonade						
1.6 oz	110	0	28	15	0	0
Cascadian Farm Frozen Juice Concentrate Orange Juice						
2 oz	110	0	27	0	1	0
Cascadian Farm Frozen Juice Concentrate Raspberry						
2 oz	130	0	31	10	0	0
Eden Foods Organic Apple Juice						
8 oz	90	0	24	0	0	0
Eden Foods Organic Cherry Juice						
8 oz	140	1	33	30	1	0
Eden Foods Organic Cherry Juice Concentrate						
1 oz	110	0	26	20	1	0
Fuze Slenderize Strawberry Melon						
8 oz	10	0	2	5	0	0
Fuze Slenderize Tropical Punch						
8 oz	5	0	1	5	0	0
Honest Tea Honest Ade Cranberry Lemonade						
8 oz	48	0	12	5	0	0
Izze Sparkling Clementine						
12 oz	120	0	30	25	0	0
Izze Sparkling Grapefruit						
12 oz	120	0	31	20	0	0
Izze Sparkling Peach						
12 oz	130	0	32	20	0	0
Izze Sparkling Pomegranate						
12 oz	120	0	31	15	0	0
Minute Maid Country Style Orange Juice						
8 oz	110	0	27	15	2	0

BRAND/BEVERAGE SERVING SIZE	CALORIES	FAT	CARBS	SODIUM	PROTEIN	FIBER
Minute Maid Cranberry Apple Raspberry Blend						
8 oz	120	0	33	25	0	0
Minute Maid Heart Wise Orange Juice						
8 oz	110	0	27	20	2	0
Minute Maid Lemonade						
8 oz	100	0	28	35	0	0
Minute Maid Light Cherry Limeade						
12 oz	10	0	3	50	0	0
Minute Maid Light Lemonade						
8 oz	5	0	1	35	0	0
Minute Maid Light Limonada-Limeade						
8 oz	15	0	4	15	0	0
Minute Maid Light Orange Juice						
8 oz	50	0	13	15	0	0
Minute Maid Light Orange Tangerine						
8 oz	15	0	4	15	0	0
Minute Maid Light Orangeade						
8 oz	5	0	2	75	0	0
Minute Maid Light Raspberry Passion						
8 oz	5	0	2	35	0	0
Minute Maid Multi-Vitamin Orange Juice						
8 oz	120	0	27	20	2	0
Minute Maid Orange Tangerine						
8 oz	110	0	27	0	0	0
Minute Maid Original Orange Juice						
8 oz	110	0	27	15	2	0
Minute Maid Pink Lemonade						
8 oz	100	0	27	35	0	0
Minute Maid Pulp Free Orange Juice						
8 oz	110	0	27	0	0	0
Minute Maid Raspberry Lemonade						
8 oz	120	0	32	15	0	0
Minute Maid Ruby Red Grapefruit						
8 oz	130	0	34	20	0	0
Newman's Own Gorilla Grape Juice						
1 cup	140	0	34	140	0	0
Newman's Own Old Fashioned Roadside Virgin Lemonade						
1 cup	110	0	27	40	0	0
Newman's Own Orange Mango Tango						
1 cup	150	0	37	5	0	0
Newman's Own Organic Virgin Lemonade						
1 cup	110	0	27	40	0	0
Newman's Own Pink Virgin Lemonade						
1 cup	110	0	27	40	0	0
Newman's Own Razz-Ma-Tazz Raspberry						
1 cup	120	0	28	5	0	0
Newman's Own Virgin Limeade						
1 cup	140	0	34	35	0	0
Ocean Spray Cran-Pomegranate Light Juice						
8 oz	40	0	10	35	0	0

BRAND/BEVERAGE SERVING SIZE	CALORIES	FAT	CARBS	SODIUM	PROTEIN	FIBER
Ocean Spray Cran-Raspberry						
8 oz	110	0	28	70	0	0
Ocean Spray Cranberry & Raspberry 100% No Sugar Added juice						
8 oz	140	0	34	35	0	0
Ocean Spray Cranberry Juice Cocktail						
8 oz	120	0	30	35	0	0
Ocean Spray Cranberry Lift Cranberry-Raspberry						
8 oz	35	0	9	50	0	0
Ocean Spray Cranberry Lift Cranergy						
8 oz	35	0	8	50	0	0
Ocean Spray Diet Cranberry juice						
8 oz	5	0	2	50	0	0
Ocean Spray Ruby Red Grapefruit						
8 oz	110	0	28	65	0	0
Ocean Spray White Cran-Peach						
8 oz	110	0	27	50	0	0
Odwalla B Monster						
8 oz	140	0	34	10	0	0
Odwalla Carrot Juice						
8 oz	70	0	15	160	2	1
Odwalla Light Lemonade						
8 oz	50	0	14	15	0	0
Odwalla Mango Tango						
8 oz	150	1	34	10	1	0
Odwalla Strawberry Banana						
8 oz	130	0	31	0	1	1
Santa Cruz Organic Apricot Mango Juice						
8 oz	120	0	29	10	0	0
Santa Cruz Concord Grape Juice						
8 oz	160	0	40	15	<1	0
Santa Cruz Cranberry Nectar Juice						
8 oz	110	0	27	25	<1	0
Santa Cruz Raspberry Lemonade						
8 oz	100	0	24	0	0	0
Snapple 100% Orange Mango Juice						
8 oz	170	0	41	15	0	0
Snapple Kiwi Strawberry Juice Drink						
8 oz	110	0	27	10	0	0
Snapple Mango Madness Juice Drink						
8 oz	100	0	26	10	0	0
V8 100% Vegetable Juice						
8 oz	50	0	10	420	2	2
V8 Splash Berry Blend						
8 oz	70	0	18	50	0	0
V8 Splash Fruit Medley						
8 oz	80	0	19	50	0	0
V8 Splash Tropical Blend						
8 oz	70	0	18	50	0	0
V8 V-Fusion Peach Mango						
8 oz	120	0	28	70	1	0

BRAND/BEVERAGE SERVING SIZE	CALORIES	FAT	CARBS	SODIUM	PROTEIN	FIBER
V8 V-Fusion Pomegranate Blueberry						
8 oz	100	0	25	60	0	0
Welch's 100% Blueberry Pomegranate Concord Grape						
8 oz	160	0	40	20	1	0
Welch's Light Concord Grape						
8 oz	50	0	13	80	0	0

Coffee and Tea

	CALORIES	FAT	CARBS	SODIUM	PROTEIN	FIBER
Coffee, brewed from grounds, prepared with tap water, organic						
8 oz	2	0	0	5	0	0
Coffee, brewed from grounds, prepared with tap water, decaffeinated, organic						
8 oz	0	0	0	5	0	0
Coffee, brewed, espresso, restaurant-prepared, organic						
1 oz	1	0	0	4	0	0
Coffee, instant, decaffeinated, powder, prepared with tap water, organic						
8 oz	5	0	1	10	0	0
Coffee, instant, regular, powder, prepared with tap water, organic						
8 oz	5	0	1	10	0	0
Tea, brewed, prepared with tap water, organic						
8 oz	2	0	1	7	0	0
Tea, brewed, prepared with tap water, decaffeinated, organic						
8 oz	2	0	1	7	0	0
Tea, herb, chamomile, brewed, organic						
8 oz	2	0	0	2	0	0
Tea, instant, sweetened with sugar, lemon-flavored						
8 oz	91	0	22	5	0	0
Tea, instant, unsweetened, powder, prepared						
8 oz	2	0	0	10	0	0
AriZona Arnold Palmer Green Tea Lemonade						
8 oz	50	0	14	25	0	0
AriZona Diet Blueberry Green Tea						
8 oz	5	0	2	20	0	0
AriZona Green Tea Ginseng & Honey						
8 oz	70	0	18	20	0	0
AriZona Mandarin Orange Green Tea						
8 oz	70	0	19	20	0	0
Bolthouse Farms Hazelnut Latte						
8 oz	199	2.5	34	115	10	0
Bolthouse Farms Mocha Cappuccino						
8 oz	178	2.5	29	106	10	0
Bolthouse Farms Vanilla Chai						
8 oz	160	3	25	60	10	0
Fuze Green Tea						
8 oz	60	0	16	0	0	0
Honest Tea Green Dragon Tea						
8 oz	30	0	8	5	0	0
Honest Tea Honey Green Tea						
8 oz	35	0	9	5	0	0

BRAND/BEVERAGE SERVING SIZE	CALORIES	FAT	CARBS	SODIUM	PROTEIN	FIBER
Honest Tea Peach Oo-La-Long Tea						
8 oz	30	0	8	5	0	0
Lipton Green Tea						
8 oz	80	0	21	75	0	0
Lipton Iced Tea, Lemon						
8 oz	60	0	16	0	0	0
Lipton Pure Leaf Iced Tea, Lemon						
8 oz	70	0	18	0	0	0
Minute Maid Lemonade Iced Tea						
8 oz	110	0	29	15	0	0
Snapple Acai Mixed Berry Red Tea						
8 oz	40	0	10	10	0	0
Snapple Diet Green Tea						
8 oz	0	0	0	5	0	0
Snapple Diet Peach Tea						
8 oz	0	0	0	5	0	0
Snapple Green Tea						
8 oz	60	0	15	5	0	0
Snapple Lemon Tea						
8 oz	80	0	21	5	0	0
SoBe Green Tea						
8 oz	100	0	25	10	0	0
Starbucks Frappucino						
1 bottle	200	3	37	100	6	0
Starbucks Vanilla Frappucino						
1 bottle	200	3	37	100	6	0
Steaz Green Tea with Lemon						
8 oz	90	0	23	35	0	0
Steaz Iced Teaz Black Tea with Lemon						
8 oz	40	0	10	10	0	0
Steaz Iced Teaz Green Tea with Blueberry Pomegranate Acai						
8 oz	40	0	10	10	0	0
Steaz Iced Teaz Green Tea with Mint						
8 oz	40	0	10	10	0	0
Steaz Iced Teaz Green Tea with Peach						
8 oz	40	0	10	10	0	0
Steaz Iced Teaz Unsweetened Green Tea with Lemon						
8 oz	0	0	2	10	0	2
Steaz Iced Teaz White Tea with Lime and Pomegranate						
8 oz	40	0	10	10	0	0
Tazo Giant Peach Green Tea						
8 oz	90	0	21	10	0	0
Tazo Lemonade Tea						
8 oz	80	0	20	5	0	0
Tazo Plum Pomegranate Green Tea						
8 oz	80	0	21	10	0	0
Tazo Tazoberry Black Tea						
8 oz	90	0	22	10	0	0
Teas' Tea Blueberry Green Tea						
8 oz	40	0	0	0	0	0

BRAND/BEVERAGE SERVING SIZE	CALORIES	FAT	CARBS	SODIUM	PROTEIN	FIBER
Teas' Tea Citrus Black Tea						
8 oz	40	0	0	0	0	0
Teas' Tea Mango Oolong Tea						
8 oz	40	0	0	0	0	0

Energy Drinks

Gatorade G Berry						
8 oz	50	0	14	110	0	0
Gatorade G Orange						
8 oz	50	0	14	110	0	0
Gatorade G2 Grape						
8 oz	25	0	7	110	0	0
Gatorade G2 Orange						
8 oz	25	0	7	110	0	0
Monster Energy Drink						
8 oz	100	0	27	180	0	0
Monster Energy Drink Assault						
8 oz	100	0	27	180	0	0
Monster Energy Drink Khaos						
8 oz	70	0	17	15	0	0
Monster Energy Drink Lo-Carb						
8 oz	10	0	3	180	0	0
Monster Java						
8 oz	100	1.5	17	340	5	0
Powerade all flavors						
8 oz	50	0	14	100	0	0
Powerade Zero Strawberry						
8 oz	3	0	0.1	55	0	0
Red Bull Energy Drink						
8 oz	110	0	28	100	<1	0
SoBe Adrenaline Rush						
8 oz	130	0	34	95	0	0
SoBe Adrenaline Rush, Sugar-Free						
8 oz	10	0	1	120	0	0
SoBe Black and Blue Berry Brew						
8 oz	120	0	31	25	0	0
SoBe Energy						
8 oz	110	0	27	15	0	0
SoBe Lean Diet Blackberry Currant						
8 oz	5	0	1	30	0	0
SoBe Lean Diet Cranberry Grapefruit						
8 oz	5	0	1	15	0	0
SoBe Lean Diet Energy						
8 oz	5	0	1	15	0	0
SoBe Lean Diet Mango Melon						
8 oz	5	0	1	15	0	0
SoBe Nirvana						
8 oz	120	0	29	15	0	0

BRAND/BEVERAGE SERVING SIZE	CALORIES	FAT	CARBS	SODIUM	PROTEIN	FIBER
SoBe Yumberry Pomegranate						
8 oz	100	0	26	20	0	0
Vitaminwater 10 Essential						
8 oz	10	0	4	0	0	0
Vitaminwater 10 Multi-V						
8 oz	10	0	4	0	0	0
Vitaminwater Energy						
8 oz	50	0	13	0	0	0
Vitaminwater Essential						
8 oz	50	0	13	0	0	0
Vitaminwater Power						
8 oz	50	0	13	0	0	0
Vitaminwater Revive						
8 oz	50	0	13	0	0	0
Vitaminwater XXX						
8 oz	50	0	13	0	0	0

Soda

Canada Dry Diet Ginger Ale						
12 oz	0	0	0	90	0	0
Canada Dry Ginger Ale						
12 oz	120	0	33	40	0	0
Coca-Cola Barq's Root Beer						
8 oz	111	0	30	48	0	0
Coca-Cola Cherry Coke						
8 oz	104	0	28	28	0	0
Coca-Cola Cherry Coke Zero						
8 oz	0.6	0	0	28	0	0
Coca-Cola Classic						
8 oz	97	0	27	33	0	0
Coca-Cola Classic, Caffeine Free						
8 oz	97	0	27	33	0	0
Coca-Cola Diet Cherry Coke						
8 oz	0.5	0	0.1	28	0	0
Coca-Cola Diet Coke						
8 oz	1	0	0.1	28	0	0
Coca-Cola Diet Coke, Caffeine Free						
8 oz	1	0	0.1	28	0	0
Coca-Cola Diet Coke with Lime						
8 oz	2	0	0.1	28	0	0
Coca-Cola Diet Coke with Splenda						
8 oz	1	0	0.1	28	0	0
Coca-Cola with Lime						
8 oz	98	0	27	25	0	0
Coca-Cola Zero						
8 oz	0.7	0	0.1	28	0	0
Coca-Cola Fresca						
8 oz	2	0	0.1	24	0	0

BRAND/BEVERAGE SERVING SIZE	CALORIES	FAT	CARBS	SODIUM	PROTEIN	FIBER
Coca-Cola Sprite						
8 oz	96	0	26	47	0	0
Coca-Cola Sprite Zero						
8 oz	2.4	0	0	24	0	0
Dr Pepper						
8 oz	100	0	27	35	0	0
Dr Pepper Diet Dr Pepper						
8 oz	0	0	0	35	0	0
Dr Pepper 7UP						
8 oz	100	0	26	25	0	0
Dr Pepper Diet 7UP						
8 oz	0	0	0	30	0	0
Hansen's Cherry Vanilla Crème Natural Cane Soda						
12 oz	160	0	43	0	0	0
Hansen's Creamy Root Beer Natural Cane Soda						
12 oz	160	0	43	0	0	0
Hansen's Diet Black Cherry Soda						
12 oz	0	0	0	0	0	0
Hansen's Diet Ginger Ale Natural Soda						
12 oz	0	0	0	0	0	0
Hansen's Diet Ginger Natural Green Tea Soda						
8 oz	0	0	0	0	0	0
Hansen's Diet Grapefruit Soda						
12 oz	0	0	0	0	0	0
Hansen's Diet Kiwi Strawberry Soda						
12 oz	0	0	0	0	0	0
Hansen's Diet Lemon Mint Natural Green Tea Soda						
8 oz	0	0	0	0	0	0
Hansen's Diet Peach Natural Soda						
12 oz	0	0	0	0	0	0
Hansen's Diet Pomegranate Natural Green Tea Soda						
8 oz	0	0	0	0	0	0
Hansen's Diet Pomegranate Soda						
12 oz	0	0	0	0	0	0
Hansen's Diet Root Beer Soda						
12 oz	0	0	0	0	0	0
Hansen's Diet Tangerine Lime Natural Soda						
12 oz	0	0	0	0	0	0
Hansen's Diet Tangerine Natural Green Tea Soda						
8 oz	0	0	0	0	0	0
Hansen's Ginger Ale Natural Cane Soda						
12 oz	170	0	44	0	0	0
Hansen's Ginger Natural Green Tea Soda						
8 oz	180	0	44	0	0	0
Hansen's Grapefruit Natural Cane Soda						
12 oz	150	0	39	0	0	0
Hansen's Key Lime Twist Natural Cane Soda						
12 oz	150	0	39	0	0	0
Hansen's Kiwi Strawberry Natural Cane Soda						
12 oz	140	0	37	0	0	0

BRAND/BEVERAGE SERVING SIZE	CALORIES	FAT	CARBS	SODIUM	PROTEIN	FIBER
Hansen's Lemon Mint Natural Green Tea Soda						
8 oz	180	0	44	0	0	0
Hansen's Mandarin Lime Natural Cane Soda						
12 oz	150	0	39	0	0	0
Hansen's Mango Orange Natural Cane Soda						
12 oz	170	0	44	0	0	0
Hansen's Pomegranate Natural Cane Soda						
12 oz	130	0	35	0	0	0
Hansen's Pomegranate Natural Green Tea Soda						
8 oz	180	0	44	0	0	0
Hansen's Raspberry Natural Cane Soda						
12 oz	140	0	37	0	0	0
Hansen's Tangerine Natural Green Tea Soda						
8 oz	180	0	44	0	0	0
Hansen's Vanilla Cola Natural Cane Soda						
12 oz	140	0	37	0	0	0
Jones Cream Soda						
12 oz	190	0	48	30	0	0
Jones Cream Soda, Sugar-Free						
12 oz	0	0	0	35	0	0
Jones Green Apple Soda						
12 oz	180	0	46	30	0	0
Jones Green Apple Soda, Sugar-Free						
12 oz	0	0	0	35	0	0
Jones Pure Cane Cola						
12 oz	160	0	40	35	0	0
Jones Root Beer						
12 oz	180	0	44	30	0	0
Jones Root Beer, Sugar-Free						
12 oz	0	0	0	30	0	0
Natural Brew Draft Root Beer						
1 bottle	180	0	44	0	0	0
Natural Brew Ginseng Cola						
1 bottle	170	0	42	20	0	0
Natural Brew Outrageous Ginger Ale						
1 bottle	170	0	42	20	0	0
Natural Brew Vanilla Crème Soda						
1 bottle	170	0	42	20	0	0
Pepsi-Cola Diet Pepsi						
8 oz	0	0	0	25	0	0
Pepsi-Cola Mountain Dew						
8 oz	110	0	31	40	0	0
Pepsi-Cola Mug Root Beer						
8 oz	100	0	29	40	0	0
Pepsi-Cola Pepsi						
8 oz	100	0	28	20	0	0
Pepsi-Cola Pepsi One						
8 oz	1	0	0	25	0	0
Santa Cruz Organic Apricot Mango Juice						
8 oz	120	0	29	10	0	0

BRAND/BEVERAGE SERVING SIZE	CALORIES	FAT	CARBS	SODIUM	PROTEIN	FIBER
Santa Cruz Organic Cherry Soda						
12 oz	140	0	34	20	0	0
Santa Cruz Organic Concord Grape Juice						
8 oz	160	0	40	15	<1	0
Santa Cruz Organic Cranberry Nectar Juice						
8 oz	110	0	27	25	<1	0
Santa Cruz Organic Ginger Ale						
12 oz	150	0	37	10	0	0
Santa Cruz Organic Lemonade Soda						
12 oz	150	0	38	0	0	0
Santa Cruz Organic Raspberry Lemonade						
8 oz	100	0	24	0	0	0
Santa Cruz Organic Root Beer						
12 oz	150	0	36	10	0	0
Santa Cruz Organic Vanilla Crème Soda						
12 oz	160	0	38	10	0	0
Steaz Cola						
8 oz	90	0	23	35	0	0
Steaz Ginger Ale						
8 oz	90	0	23	35	0	0
Steaz Grape						
8 oz	90	0	23	35	0	0
Steaz Key Lime						
8 oz	90	0	23	35	0	0
Steaz Orange						
8 oz	90	0	23	35	0	0
Steaz Raspberry						
8 oz	90	0	23	35	0	0
Steaz Root Beer						
8 oz	90	0	23	35	0	0

Alcoholic Beverages

BEER

Beer, light						
12 oz	103	0	6	14	1	0
Beer, light, organic						
12 oz	103	0	6	14	1	0
Beer, regular, all						
12 oz	153	0	13	14	2	0
Beer, regular, all, organic						
12 oz	153	0	13	14	2	0

LIQUOR

Coffee liqueur, 53 proof						
12 oz	113	0	16	3	0	0
Coffee liqueur, 63 proof						
13 oz	107	0	11	3	0	0
Creme de menthe, 72 proof						
1 oz	125	0	14	2	0	0

BRAND/BEVERAGE SERVING SIZE	CALORIES	FAT	CARBS	SODIUM	PROTEIN	FIBER
Gin, rum, vodka, whiskey 80 proof						
3 oz	64	0	0	0	0	0
Gin, rum, vodka, whiskey 86 proof						
4 oz	70	0	0	0	0	0
Gin, rum, vodka, whiskey 90 proof						
5 oz	73	0	0	0	0	0
Gin, rum, vodka, whiskey 94 proof						
6 oz	76	0	0	0	0	0
Gin, rum, vodka, whiskey 100 proof						
2 oz	82	0	0	0	0	0
Sake						
14 oz	39	0	1	1	0	0
Tequila						
1 oz	64	0	0	0	0	0
WINE						
All types						
4 oz	98	0	3	6	0	0
All types, organic						
4 oz	98	0	3	6	0	0
Dessert, dry						
4 oz	179	0	14	11	0	0
Dessert, sweet						
4 oz	189	0	16	11	0	0
RED						
All						
4 oz	100	0	3	5	0	0
Barbera						
4 oz	100	0	3	0	0	0
Burgundy						
4 oz	101	0	4	0	0	0
Cabernet Franc						
4 oz	96	0	3	0	0	0
Cabernet Sauvignon						
4 oz	96	0	3	0	0	0
Carignane						
4 oz	87	0	3	0	0	0
Claret						
4 oz	98	0	4	0	0	0
Gamay						
4 oz	92	0	3	0	0	0
Lemberger						
4 oz	94	0	3	0	0	0
Merlot						
4 oz	98	0	3	0	0	0
Mouvedre						
4 oz	103	0	3	0	0	0
Organic						
4 oz	100	0	3	5	0	0
Petite Sirah						
4 oz	100	0	3	0	0	0

BRAND/BEVERAGE SERVING SIZE	CALORIES	FAT	CARBS	SODIUM	PROTEIN	FIBER
Pinot Noir						
4 oz	96	0	3	0	0	0
Sangiovese						
4 oz	101	0	3	0	0	0
Syrah						
4 oz	98	0	3	0	0	0
Zinfandel						
4 oz	103	0	3	0	0	0
WHITE						
All						
4 oz	96	0	3	0	0	0
Chenin Blanc						
4 oz	94	0	4	0	0	0
Fume Blanc						
4 oz	96	0	3	0	0	0
Gewürztraminer						
4 oz	96	0	3	0	0	0
Late harvest						
4 oz	138	0	17	0	0	0
Muscat						
4 oz	98	0	6	0	0	0
Organic						
4 oz	96	0	3	0	0	0
Pinot Blanc						
4 oz	95	0	2	0	0	0
Pinot Gris (Grigio)						
4 oz	97	0	2	0	0	0
Riesling						
4 oz	95	0	4	0	0	0
Sauvignon Blanc						
4 oz	95	0	2	0	0	0

CANNED FOODS*

Hate to break this to you, but canned foods just suck. Almost every can in this country is lined with a plastic resin that contains bisphenol A (BPA), a chemical linked with endocrine disruption, diabetes, breast cancer, early puberty, sexual dysfunction, and a bunch of other horrible maladies. Despite some companies' efforts to have BPA-free cans, a recent *Consumer Reports* study found most cans have BPA. In fact, in 1 of every 10 servings of canned food, BPA is present in unsafe levels. If you have to eat from cans, do it sparingly. Keep an eye on calories and especially on sodium. And watch out for those glutamates!

BRAND/FOOD ITEM SERVING SIZE	CALORIES	FAT	CARBS	SODIUM	PROTEIN	FIBER
Canned Beans and Chili						
Amy's Black Bean Chili						
1 cup	200	2	31	680	13	15
Amy's Medium Chili						
1 cup	280	9	35	680	15	7
Amy's Medium Chili—Light in Sodium						
1 cup	280	9	35	340	15	7
Amy's Medium Chili with Vegetables						
1 cup	190	6	29	590	7	8
Amy's Refried Beans with Green Chiles						
½ cup	130	3	20	440	7	6
Amy's Refried Black Beans						
½ cup	140	3	21	440	8	6
Amy's Refried Black Beans—Light in Sodium						
½ cup	140	3	20	220	7	6
Amy's Southwestern Black Bean Chili						
1 cup	240	4	40	680	12	10
Amy's Spicy Chili						
1 cup	280	9	35	680	15	7

*Almost every can sold in the U.S. contains BPA, an endocrine disruptor.

BRAND/FOOD ITEM SERVING SIZE	CALORIES	FAT	CARBS	SODIUM	PROTEIN	FIBER
Amy's Spicy Chili—Light in Sodium						
1 cup	250	9	30	340	13	7
Amy's Traditional Refried Beans						
½ cup	140	3	22	390	7	6
Amy's Traditional Refried Beans—Light in Sodium						
½ cup	140	3	21	190	7	6
Amy's Vegetarian Baked Beans						
½ cup	120	0.5	24	480	6	6
Arrowhead Mills Adzuki Beans						
¼ cup	130	0	26	0	8	5
Arrowhead Mills Anasazi Beans						
¼ cup	140	1	26	10	7	6
Arrowhead Mills Chickpeas (Garbanzos)						
¼ cup	160	2.5	27	10	9	8
Arrowhead Mills Green Lentils						
¼ cup	150	1	27	5	10	7
Arrowhead Mills Green Split Peas						
¼ cup	160	1	24	10	12	4
Arrowhead Mills Pinto Beans						
¼ cup	150	0	27	0	9	10
Arrowhead Mills Red Lentils						
¼ cup	170	1	28	5	13	7
Arrowhead Mills Soybeans						
¼ cup	160	8	11	0	14	4
Campbell's Chunky Firehouse—Hot & Spicy Beef & Bean Chili						
1 cup	230	8	25	870	15	6
Campbell's Chunky Hold the Beans Chili						
1 cup	240	10	20	770	18	5
Campbell's Chunky Roadhouse Beef & Bean Chili						
1 cup	230	8	25	880	15	6
Campbell's Chunky Sizzlin' Steak—Grilled Steak Chili with Beans						
1 cup	200	3	28	870	16	5
Eden Foods Organic Adzuki Beans						
½ cup	110	0	19	10	7	5
Eden Foods Organic Baked Beans with Sorghum & Mustard						
½ cup	150	0	27	130	8	7
Eden Foods Organic Black Beans						
½ cup	110	1	18	15	7	6
Eden Foods Organic Black Beans & Quinoa Chili						
1 cup	190	1.5	35	460	10	6
Eden Foods Organic Black Eyed Peas						
½ cup	90	1	16	25	6	4
Eden Foods Organic Black Soy Beans						
½ cup	120	6	8	30	11	7
Eden Foods Organic Butter Beans						
½ cup	100	1	17	35	5	4
Eden Foods Organic Cannellini Beans						
½ cup	100	1	17	40	6	5
Eden Foods Organic Curried Rice & Lentils						
½ cup	130	1	21	200	4	1

*Almost every can sold in the U.S. contains BPA, an endocrine disruptor.

BRAND/FOOD ITEM SERVING SIZE	CALORIES	FAT	CARBS	SODIUM	PROTEIN	FIBER
Eden Foods Organic Garbanzo Beans						
½ cup	130	1	23	30	7	5
Eden Foods Organic Great Northern & Barley Chili						
1 cup	200	1	38	490	9	8
Eden Foods Organic Great Northern Beans						
½ cup	110	1	20	270	5	8
Eden Foods Organic Kidney Beans						
½ cup	100	0	18	15	8	10
Eden Foods Organic Kidney Beans & Kamut Chili						
1 cup	240	2	43	460	14	11
Eden Foods Organic Mexican Rice & Black Beans						
½ cup	110	1	22	270	5	3
Eden Foods Organic Moroccan Rice & Garbanzo Beans						
½ cup	110	1	22	230	4	3
Eden Foods Organic Navy Beans						
½ cup	110	0	20	15	7	7
Eden Foods Organic Pinto Bean & Spelt Chili						
1 cup	220	1.5	42	460	11	8
Eden Foods Organic Pinto Beans						
½ cup	110	1	18	15	6	6
Eden Foods Organic Rice and Cajun Small Red Beans						
½ cup	110	1	23	115	3	3
Eden Foods Organic Rice and Caribbean Black Beans						
½ cup	120	1	23	100	4	4
Eden Foods Organic Rice and Garbanzo Beans						
½ cup	110	1	23	135	3	2
Eden Foods Organic Rice and Kidney Beans						
½ cup	110	1	23	135	3	3
Eden Foods Organic Rice and Lentils						
½ cup	120	1	23	120	4	2
Eden Foods Organic Rice and Pinto Beans						
½ cup	120	1	24	140	4	3
Eden Foods Organic Small Red Beans						
½ cup	100	0.5	17	25	6	5
Eden Foods Organic Spanish Rice and Pinto Beans						
½ cup	120	1	22	260	4	3
Health Valley Mild Vegetarian Black Bean Chunky Chili						
1 cup	150	1	32	480	10	8
Health Valley Mild Vegetarian Chunky Chili						
1 cup	150	1	31	480	9	10
Health Valley Mild Vegetarian Three Bean Chunky Chili						
1 cup	150	1	32	480	10	10
Health Valley No Salt Added Mild Vegetarian Chunky Chili						
1 cup	150	1	31	75	9	10

Canned Fruits

APPLES

Sweetened, sliced, drained, heated

1 cup	137	1	34	6	0	4

*Almost every can sold in the U.S. contains BPA, an endocrine disruptor.

BRAND/FOOD ITEM SERVING SIZE	CALORIES	FAT	CARBS	SODIUM	PROTEIN	FIBER
Sweetened, sliced, drained, unheated						
1 cup	137	1	34	6	0	3
Applesauce, sweetened, with salt						
1 cup	194	0	51	71	0	3
Applesauce, sweetened, without salt						
1 cup	167	0	43	5	0	3
Applesauce, unsweetened						
1 cup	102	0	27	5	0	3
APRICOTS						
Nectar						
1 cup	141	0	36	8	1	2
Nectar						
1 oz	18	0	5	1	0	0
Extra-heavy syrup pack, without skin, solids and liquids						
1 cup, whole, pitted	236	0	61	32	1	4
Extra-light syrup pack, with skin, solids and liquids						
1 cup halves	121	0	31	5	1	4
Heavy syrup pack, with skin, solids and liquids						
1 cup halves	214	0	55	10	1	4
Heavy syrup pack, with skin, solids and liquids						
1 cup whole	199	0	52	10	1	4
Heavy syrup pack, with skin, solids and liquids						
1 apricot half with liquid	33	0	9	2	0	1
Heavy syrup pack, without skin, solids and liquids						
1 cup whole, pitted	214	0	55	28	1	4
Heavy syrup, drained						
1 cup halves	182	0	47	9	1	6
Heavy syrup, drained						
1 cup whole	151	0	39	7	1	5
Juice pack, with skin, solids and liquids						
1 cup halves	117	0	30	10	2	4
Juice pack, with skin, solids and liquids						
1 apricot half, with liquid	17	0	4	1	0	1
Light syrup pack, with skin, solids and liquids						
1 cup halves	159	0	42	10	1	4
Light syrup pack, with skin, solids and liquids						
1 apricot half, with liquid	25	0	7	2	0	1
Water pack, with skin, solids and liquids						
1 cup halves	66	0	16	7	2	4

*Almost every can sold in the U.S. contains BPA, an endocrine disruptor.

BRAND/FOOD ITEM SERVING SIZE	CALORIES	FAT	CARBS	SODIUM	PROTEIN	FIBER
Water pack, with skin, solids and liquids						
1 apricot half, with liquid						
10	0	2	1	0	1
Water pack, without skin, solids and liquids						
1 cup whole, pitted						
50	0	12	25	2	2

BERRIES

Blackberries, heavy syrup, solids and liquids						
1 cup	236	0	59	8	3	9
Blueberries, heavy syrup, solids and liquids						
1 cup	225	1	56	8	2	4
Blueberries, light syrup, drained						
1 cup	215	1	55	7	3	6
Blueberries, wild, heavy syrup, drained						
1 cup	341	1	90	3	2	16
Boysenberries, heavy syrup						
1 cup	225	0	57	8	3	7
Cranberry sauce, sweetened						
1 cup	418	0	108	80	1	3
Cranberry-orange relish						
1 cup	490	0	127	88	1	0
Gooseberries, light syrup pack, solids and liquids						
1 cup	184	1	47	5	2	6
Raspberries, red, heavy syrup pack, solids and liquids						
1 cup	233	0	60	8	2	8
Strawberries, heavy syrup pack, solids and liquids						
1 cup	234	1	60	10	1	4

CHERRIES

Sour, red, extra-heavy syrup pack, solids and liquids						
1 cup	298	0	76	18	2	2
Sour, red, heavy syrup pack, solids and liquids						
1 cup	233	0	60	18	2	3
Sour, red, light syrup pack, solids and liquids						
1 cup	189	0	49	18	2	2
Sweet, extra-heavy syrup pack, solids and liquids, pitted						
1 cup	266	0	68	8	2	4
Sweet, heavy syrup pack, drained, pitted						
1 cup	149	0	38	5	1	4
Sweet, heavy syrup pack, solids and liquids, pitted						
1 cup	210	0	54	8	2	4
Sweet, juice pack, solids and liquids, pitted						
1 cup	135	0	35	8	2	4
Sweet, light syrup pack, solids and liquids, pitted						
1 cup	169	0	44	8	2	4
Sweet, water pack, solids and liquids, pitted						
1 cup	114	0	29	2	2	4

GRAPEFRUIT

Sections, juice pack, solids and liquids						
1 cup	90	0	23	5	1	1

*Almost every can sold in the U.S. contains BPA, an endocrine disruptor.

BRAND/FOOD ITEM SERVING SIZE	CALORIES	FAT	CARBS	SODIUM	PROTEIN	FIBER
Sections, light syrup pack, solids and liquids						
1 cup	152	0	39	5	1	1
Sections, water pack, solids and liquids						
1 cup	88	0	22	5	1	1
GRAPES						
Thompson seedless, heavy syrup pack, solids and liquids						
1 cup	195	0	50	13	1	2
Thompson seedless, water pack, solids and liquids						
1 cup	98	0	25	15	1	1
PEACHES						
Extra-heavy syrup pack, solids and liquids						
1 cup halves or slices	252	0	68	21	1	3
Extra-light syrup, solids and liquids						
1 cup halves or slices	104	0	27	12	1	2
Heavy syrup pack, solids and liquids						
1 cup	194	0	52	16	1	3
Heavy syrup, drained						
1 cup	171	0	44	13	1	5
Juice pack, solids and liquids						
1 cup	110	0	29	10	2	3
Light syrup pack, solids and liquids						
1 cup halves or slices	136	0	37	13	1	3
Water pack, solids and liquids						
1 cup halves or slices	59	0	15	7	1	3
Water pack, solids and liquids						
1 half, with liquid	24	0	6	3	0	1
PEARS						
Extra-heavy syrup pack, solids and liquids						
1 cup halves	258	0	67	13	1	4
Extra-light syrup pack, solids and liquids						
1 cup halves	116	0	30	5	1	4
Heavy syrup pack, solids and liquids						
1 cup	197	0	51	13	1	4
Heavy syrup, drained						
1 cup	149	0	38	10	0	5
Juice pack, solids and liquids						
1 cup halves	124	0	32	10	1	4
Light syrup pack, solids and liquids						
1 cup halves	143	0	38	13	0	4
Water pack, solids and liquids						
1 cup halves	71	0	19	5	0	4

*Almost every can sold in the U.S. contains BPA, an endocrine disruptor.

BRAND/FOOD ITEM SERVING SIZE	CALORIES	FAT	CARBS	SODIUM	PROTEIN	FIBER
PLUMS						
Heavy syrup, drained						
1 cup, with pits	163	0	42	35	1	3
Purple, extra-heavy syrup pack, solids and liquids						
1 cup, pitted	264	0	69	50	1	3
Purple, heavy syrup pack, solids and liquids						
1 cup, pitted	230	0	60	49	1	2
Purple, juice pack, solids and liquids						
1 cup, pitted	146	0	38	3	1	2
Purple, light syrup pack, solids and liquids						
1 cup, pitted	159	0	41	50	1	2
Purple, water pack, solids and liquids						
1 cup, pitted	102	0	27	2	1	2
TANGERINES (MANDARIN ORANGES)						
Juice pack						
1 cup	92	0	24	12	2	2
Juice pack, drained						
1 cup	72	0	18	9	1	2
Light syrup pack						
1 cup	154	0	41	15	1	2

Canned Soup

BRAND/FOOD ITEM SERVING SIZE	CALORIES	FAT	CARBS	SODIUM	PROTEIN	FIBER
Amy's Alphabet Soup						
1 cup	80	0	16	580	3	2
Amy's Black Bean Vegetable Soup						
1 cup	130	1.5	25	430	6	5
Amy's Butternut Squash Soup, Light in Sodium						
1 cup	100	2.5	20	290	2	2
Amy's Chunky Tomato Bisque						
1 cup	120	3.5	21	680	2	2
Amy's Chunky Tomato Bisque Soup, Light in Sodium						
1 cup	120	3.5	21	340	2	2
Amy's Chunky Vegetable Soup						
1 cup	60	0	13	680	3	3
Amy's Cream of Mushroom Soup						
¾ cup	150	9	13	590	3	2
Amy's Cream of Tomato Soup						
1 cup	100	2	17	690	2	3
Amy's Cream of Tomato Soup, Light in Sodium						
1 cup	100	2.5	17	340	2	3
Amy's Curried Lentil Soup						
1 cup	230	8	30	680	9	11

*Almost every can sold in the U.S. contains BPA, an endocrine disruptor.

BRAND/FOOD ITEM SERVING SIZE	CALORIES	FAT	CARBS	SODIUM	PROTEIN	FIBER
Amy's Fire Roasted Southwestern Vegetable Soup						
1 cup	140	4	21	680	4	4
Amy's Lentil Soup						
1 cup	180	5	25	590	8	6
Amy's Lentil Soup, Light in Sodium						
1 cup	180	5	25	290	8	6
Amy's Lentil Vegetable Soup						
1 cup	150	4	23	680	7	6
Amy's Lentil Vegetable Soup, Light in Sodium						
1 cup	160	4	24	340	7	8
Amy's Minestrone Soup						
1 cup	90	1.5	17	580	3	3
Amy's Minestrone Soup, Light in Sodium						
1 cup	90	2	17	290	3	3
Amy's No Chicken Noodle Soup						
1 cup	100	3	13	540	5	2
Amy's Pasta & 3 Bean Soup						
1 cup	150	4	22	680	5	4
Amy's Split Pea Soup						
1 cup	100	0	19	670	7	3
Amy's Split Pea Soup, Light in Sodium						
1 cup	100	0	19	280	7	4
Amy's Summer Corn & Vegetable Soup						
1 cup	150	6	23	680	4	3
Amy's Thai Coconut Soup						
½ cup	140	10	9	580	4	2
Amy's Tuscan Bean & Rice Soup						
1 cup	160	4.5	25	680	5	5
Amy's Vegetable Barley Soup						
1 cup	70	1	13	580	2	3
Campbell's Chunky Baked Potato with Cheddar & Bacon Bits Soup						
1 cup	190	9	23	790	5	2
Campbell's Chunky Baked Potato with Steak & Cheese Soup						
1 cup	200	9	21	840	8	3
Campbell's Chunky Beef and Dumplings with Hearty Vegetables Soup						
1 cup	130	2	20	800	8	2
Campbell's Chunky Beef Rib Roast with Potatoes & Herbs Soup						
1 cup	110	1	17	890	7	2
Campbell's Chunky Beef with Country Vegetables Soup						
1 cup	130	3	18	920	8	3
Campbell's Chunky Beef with White & Wild Rice Soup						
1 cup	140	1.5	24	890	8	2
Campbell's Chunky Chicken Broccoli Cheese & Potato Soup						
1 cup	210	11	20	880	7	3
Campbell's Chunky Chicken Corn Chowder						
1 cup	200	10	20	860	7	2
Campbell's Chunky Classic Chicken Noodle Soup						
1 cup	120	3	14	790	8	2
Campbell's Chunky Creamy Chicken & Dumplings Soup						
1 cup	180	8	19	890	8	3
Campbell's Chunky Fajita Chicken with Rice & Beans Soup						
1 cup	130	1.5	23	850	7	2

*Almost every can sold in the U.S. contains BPA, an endocrine disruptor.

BRAND/FOOD ITEM SERVING SIZE	CALORIES	FAT	CARBS	SODIUM	PROTEIN	FIBER
Campbell's Chunky Grilled Chicken & Sausage Gumbo Soup						
1 cup	140	3	21	850	7	2
Campbell's Chunky Grilled Chicken with Vegetables & Pasta Soup						
1 cup	100	2.5	14	880	6	2
Campbell's Chunky Grilled Sirloin Steak with Hearty Vegetables Soup						
1 cup	130	2	19	890	8	3
Campbell's Chunky Hearty Bean 'N' Ham Soup						
1 cup	180	2	30	780	11	8
Campbell's Chunky Hearty Beef Barley Soup						
1 cup	160	2	26	790	9	4
Campbell's Chunky Hearty Chicken with Vegetables Soup						
1 cup	110	2	17	710	6	3
Campbell's Chunky Manhattan Clam Chowder						
1 cup	130	3.5	19	830	5	3
Campbell's Chunky New England Clam Chowder						
1 cup	230	13	20	890	7	3
Campbell's Chunky Old Fashioned Potato Ham Chowder						
1 cup	190	11	17	800	6	3
Campbell's Chunky Old Fashioned Vegetable Beef Soup						
1 cup	120	2.5	17	890	8	3
Campbell's Chunky Roasted Beef Tips with Vegetables Soup						
1 cup	130	1.5	20	800	8	2
Campbell's Chunky Salisbury Steak with Mushrooms & Onions Soup						
1 cup	140	4.5	19	800	7	2
Campbell's Chunky Savory Chicken with White and Wild Rice Soup						
1 cup	110	2	18	810	7	2
Campbell's Chunky Savory Pot Roast Soup						
1 cup	120	1	20	790	7	2
Campbell's Chunky Savory Vegetable Soup						
1 cup	110	1	22	770	3	4
Campbell's Chunky Sirloin Burger with Country Vegetables Soup						
1 cup	130	2.5	18	800	8	3
Campbell's Chunky Slow Roasted Beef with Mushrooms Soup						
1 cup	120	1.5	18	830	8	3
Campbell's Chunky Split Pea & Ham Soup						
1 cup	190	2.5	30	780	12	5
Campbell's Chunky Steak & Potato Soup						
1 cup	120	2	18	920	8	3
Campbell's Condensed Beef Broth						
½ cup	10	0	1	860	2	0
Campbell's Condensed Chicken Noodle Soup						
½ cup	60	2	8	890	3	1
Campbell's Condensed Vegetable Soup						
½ cup	100	0.5	20	890	4	3
Health Valley Beef Broth, No Salt Added, Fat-Free						
1 cup	10	0	0	120	3	0
Health Valley Chicken Broth, Fat-Free						
1 cup	20	0	0	390	5	0
Health Valley Vegetable Broth, Fat-Free						
1 cup	20	0	5	330	0	0
Health Valley Organic Black Bean Soup, No Salt Added						
1 cup	130	1	25	25	7	5

*Almost every can sold in the U.S. contains BPA, an endocrine disruptor.

BRAND/FOOD ITEM SERVING SIZE	CALORIES	FAT	CARBS	SODIUM	PROTEIN	FIBER
Health Valley Organic Lentil Soup, No Salt Added						
1 cup	100	1	21	25	8	8
Health Valley Organic Minestrone Soup, No Salt Added						
1 cup	70	0	17	45	3	3
Health Valley Organic Mushroom Barley Soup, No Salt Added						
1 cup	70	0	17	25	2	3
Health Valley Organic Potato Leek Soup, No Salt Added						
1 cup	70	0	15	35	4	3
Health Valley Organic Split Pea Soup, No Salt Added						
1 cup	110	0	23	115	10	8
Health Valley Organic Tomato Soup, No Salt Added						
1 cup	80	0	18	35	3	1
Health Valley Organic Vegetable Soup, No Salt Added						
1 cup	90	2	16	70	3	4
Health Valley Organic 14 Garden Vegetable Soup						
1 cup	80	0	18	480	3	4
Health Valley Organic 5 Bean Vegetable Soup						
1 cup	100	0	23	480	5	6
Health Valley Organic Black Bean & Vegetable Soup						
1 cup	110	0	25	480	5	5
Health Valley Organic Chicken Noodle Soup						
1 cup	80	2	11	480	4	1
Health Valley Organic Chicken Rice Soup						
1 cup	90	29	14	480	4	1
Health Valley Organic Corn and Vegetable Soup						
1 cup	100	0	22	460	3	4
Health Valley Organic Cream of Celery Soup						
1 cup	90	5	11	680	2	0
Health Valley Organic Cream of Chicken Soup						
1 cup	110	6	11	650	3	0
Health Valley Organic Cream of Mushroom Soup						
1 cup	100	5	11	680	2	1
Health Valley Organic Italian Minestrone Soup						
1 cup	110	0	26	470	6	7
Health Valley Organic Lentil & Carrots Soup						
1 cup	110	0	24	450	8	8
Health Valley Organic Split Pea & Carrots Soup						
1 cup	120	0	26	480	7	7
Health Valley Organic Tomato Vegetable Soup						
1 cup	70	0	17	470	3	5
Health Valley Organic Vegetable Barley Soup						
1 cup	80	0	20	480	3	4
Muir Glen Beef & Vegetable Soup						
1 cup	90	1	15	880	6	2
Muir Glen Beef Barley Soup						
1 cup	100	1.5	18	880	6	3
Muir Glen Cajun Style Chicken Gumbo Soup						
1 cup	80	1	14	790	5	1
Muir Glen Chicken & Wild Rice Soup						
1 cup	80	1.5	12	800	5	1
Muir Glen Chicken Noodle Soup						
1 cup	80	1.5	10	880	6	1

*Almost every can sold in the U.S. contains BPA, an endocrine disruptor.

BRAND/FOOD ITEM SERVING SIZE	CALORIES	FAT	CARBS	SODIUM	PROTEIN	FIBER
Muir Glen Chicken Tortilla Soup						
1 cup	130	2	21	860	7	3
Muir Glen Classic Minestrone Soup						
1 cup	110	1.5	22	860	6	5
Muir Glen Creamy Tomato Bisque Soup						
1 cup	150	4	25	820	4	2
Muir Glen Garden Vegetable Soup						
1 cup	90	0.5	18	890	4	3
Muir Glen Hearty Tomato Soup						
1 cup	130	1.5	25	880	5	2
Muir Glen Homestyle Split Pea Soup						
1 cup	130	0.5	23	890	8	4
Muir Glen Reduced Sodium Chicken Noodle Soup						
1 cup	90	2	11	480	7	1
Muir Glen Reduced Sodium Garden Vegetable Soup						
1 cup	100	0.5	20	480	3	3
Muir Glen Savory Lentil Soup						
1 cup	130	1.5	23	880	7	4
Muir Glen Southwest Black Bean Soup						
1 cup	140	0.5	27	650	8	7
Muir Glen Tomato Basil Soup						
1 cup	90	1	18	740	2	2
Progresso High Fiber Chicken Tuscany Soup						
1 cup	130	3	20	690	8	7
Progresso High Fiber Creamy Tomato Basil Soup						
1 cup	130	4	26	690	3	7
Progresso High Fiber Hearty Vegetable and Noodles Soup						
1 cup	90	1.5	18	690	4	7
Progresso High Fiber Homestyle Minestrone Soup						
1 cup	110	2	24	690	5	7
Progresso Light Beef Pot Roast Soup						
1 cup	80	1	12	660	7	2
Progresso Light Chicken & Dumpling Soup						
1 cup	80	1.5	12	690	6	2
Progresso Light Chicken Noodle Soup						
1 cup	70	1.5	10	680	5	2
Progresso Light Chicken Vegetable Rotini Soup						
1 cup	70	1	11	660	5	2
Progresso Light Homestyle Vegetable and Rice Soup						
1 cup	60	0	14	690	2	4
Progresso Light Italian-Style Meatball Soup						
1 cup	80	2	13	480	3	2
Progresso Light Italian-Style Vegetable Soup						
1 cup	60	0	14	690	2	4
Progresso Light Roasted Chicken & Vegetable Soup						
1 cup	70	1	10	460	5	3
Progresso Light Santa Fe Style Chicken Soup						
1 cup	80	1	12	670	5	2
Progresso Light Savory Vegetable Barley Soup						
1 cup	60	0	14	690	2	4
Progresso Light Southwestern-Style Vegetable Soup						
1 cup	60	0.5	12	690	3	4

*Almost every can sold in the U.S. contains BPA, an endocrine disruptor.

BRAND/FOOD ITEM SERVING SIZE	CALORIES	FAT	CARBS	SODIUM	PROTEIN	FIBER
Progresso Light Vegetable and Noodle Soup						
1 cup	60	0.5	13	690	2	4
Progresso Light Vegetable Soup						
1 cup	60	0	14	470	2	4
Progresso Microwaveable Bowl Beef Vegetable Soup						
1 package	110	1.5	16	690	8	2
Progresso Microwaveable Bowl Chicken & Wild Rice Soup						
1 package	120	1.5	22	680	6	2
Progresso Microwaveable Bowl Chicken Noodle Soup						
1 package	90	2.5	10	690	6	1
Progresso Microwaveable Bowl Italian-Style Wedding Soup with Meatballs						
1 package	120	4.5	13	690	6	1
Progresso Microwaveable Bowl Light Vegetable and Noodle Soup						
1 package	60	0.5	12	690	2	4
Progresso Microwaveable Bowl Minestrone Soup						
1 package	90	1.5	17	690	4	4
Progresso Microwaveable Bowl Vegetable Soup						
1 package	80	0.5	15	690	3	2
Swanson Organic Beef Broth						
1 cup	15	0.5	1	550	2	0
Swanson Organic Chicken Broth						
1 cup	15	0.5	1	550	1	0
Swanson Organic Vegetable Broth						
1 cup	15	0	3	550	0	0

Canned Vegetables

	CALORIES	FAT	CARBS	SODIUM	PROTEIN	FIBER
Beets						
1 cup	74	0	18	352	2	3
Beets, drained						
1 beet	7	0	2	47	0	0
Beets, Harvard						
1 cup sliced	180	0	45	399	2	6
Beets, no salt added						
1 cup	69	0	16	52	2	3
Beets, pickled						
1 cup sliced	148	0	37	599	2	6
Carrot juice						
1 cup	94	0	22	68	2	2

*Almost every can sold in the U.S. contains BPA, an endocrine disruptor.

BRAND/FOOD ITEM SERVING SIZE	CALORIES	FAT	CARBS	SODIUM	PROTEIN	FIBER
Carrots						
½ cup sliced	28	0	7	295	1	2
Carrots, drained						
1 cup sliced	37	0	8	353	1	2
Carrots, no salt added						
½ cup sliced	28	0	7	42	1	2
Carrots, no salt added, drained						
1 cup sliced	37	0	8	61	1	2
Corn, sweet, yellow, brine pack						
½ cup	82	1	20	273	2.5	2
Corn, sweet, yellow, cream style, no salt added						
1 cup	184	1	46	8	4	3
Corn, sweet, yellow, whole kernel, drained						
1 cup	133	1.5	31	489	4	3
Green snap beans, drained						
1 cup	35	0	7	401	2	3.5
Mushrooms, drained						
1 cup	39	0	8	663	3	4
Onions						
½ cup chopped or diced	21	0	5	416	1	1
Peas, green						
½ cup	66	0	12	310	4	4
Peas and carrots						
1 cup	97	1	22	663	5.5	5
Spinach						
1 cup	44	1	7	746	5	4
Spinach, drained						
1 cup	49	1	7	58	6	5
Spinach, no salt added						
1 cup	44	1	7	176	5	5
Squash, summer, crookneck and straightneck, drained, solid						
1 cup diced	42	1	9	0	2	3
Squash, summer, crookneck and straightneck, drained, solid						
1 cup mashed	48	1	10	0	2	3
Squash, summer, zucchini, Italian style						
1 cup	66	0	16	849	2	0
Tomato products, paste, with salt added						
½ cup	107	1	25	1035	6	5
Tomato products, paste, without salt added						
1 tbsp	13	0	3	16	1	1
Tomato products, puree, with salt added						
1 cup	95	1	22	998	4	5

*Almost every can sold in the U.S. contains BPA, an endocrine disruptor.

BRAND/FOOD ITEM SERVING SIZE	CALORIES	FAT	CARBS	SODIUM	PROTEIN	FIBER
Tomato products, puree, without salt added						
1 cup	95	1	22	70	4	5
Eden Foods Organic Crushed Tomatoes						
¼ cup	20	0	3	0	1	1
Eden Foods Organic Crushed Tomatoes with Basil						
¼ cup	20	0	3	0	1	1
Eden Foods Organic Crushed Tomatoes with Onion & Garlic						
¼ cup	20	0	3	0	1	1
Eden Foods Organic Diced Tomatoes						
½ cup	30	0	6	5	1	2
Eden Foods Organic Diced Tomatoes with Basil						
½ cup	30	0	6	5	1	2
Eden Foods Organic Diced Tomatoes with Green Chilies						
½ cup	30	0	5	35	2	2
Eden Foods Organic Diced Tomatoes with Roasted Onion						
½ cup	30	0	6	5	1	2
Eden Foods Organic Whole Roma Tomatoes						
½ cup	30	0	4	10	1	1
Eden Foods Organic Whole Roma Tomatoes with Basil						
½ cup	30	0	4	10	1	1
Muir Glen Crushed Tomatoes with Basil						
¼ cup	25	0	5	190	1	1
Muir Glen Diced Tomatoes						
½ cup	30	0	6	290	1	1
Muir Glen Diced Tomatoes No Salt Added						
½ cup	30	0	6	15	1	1
Muir Glen Diced Tomatoes with Basil and Garlic						
½ cup	30	0	6	290	1	1
Muir Glen Diced Tomatoes with Garlic and Onion						
½ cup	30	0	6	220	1	1
Muir Glen Diced Tomatoes with Italian Herbs						
½ cup	30	0	6	250	1	1
Muir Glen Fire Roasted Crushed Tomatoes						
¼ cup	20	0	5	160	1	1
Muir Glen Fire Roasted Diced Tomatoes						
½ cup	30	0	6	290	1	1
Muir Glen Fire Roasted Diced Tomatoes with Green Chilies						
½ cup	25	0	5	55	1	1
Muir Glen Fire Roasted Whole Tomatoes						
½ cup	25	0	5	290	1	1
Muir Glen Ground Peeled Tomatoes						
¼ cup	20	0	4	190	<1	<1
Muir Glen Stewed Tomatoes						
½ cup	30	0	6	290	1	1
Muir Glen Whole Peeled Plum Tomatoes						
½ cup	25	0	5	260	1	1
Muir Glen Whole Peeled Tomatoes						
½ cup	25	0	5	260	1	1
Muir Glen Whole Peeled Tomatoes with Basil						
½ cup	25	0	5	260	1	1

*Almost every can sold in the U.S. contains BPA, an endocrine disruptor.

DAIRY PRODUCTS*

As with meat and eggs, dairy is an area where I consider organic to be absolutely mandatory. Do not even consider drinking nonorganic milk—it's like drinking liquid hormones. Even Walmart sells organic milk and yogurt, so no excuses now. I'll admit it—organic cheese can be pricey, so use this opportunity to cut down on fatty, processed cheeses. Instead, seek out artisanal cheeses from dairies or goat farms in your area. Another option is to look for "dairy" products made from almonds or coconuts, such as coconut milk or yogurt or almond cheese. You'll be amazed at how delicious they are.

BRAND/ DAIRY PRODUCT SERVING SIZE	CALORIES	FAT	CARBS	SODIUM	PROTEIN	FIBER
Butter						
Salted 1 cup	1628	184	0	1308	2	0
Salted 1 tbsp	102	12	0	82	0	0
Salted 1 pat	36	4	0	29	0	0
Salted 1 stick	810	92	0	651	1	0
Whipped, with salt 1 cup	1083	122	0	1249	1	0
Whipped, with salt 1 tbsp	67	8	0	78	0	0
Whipped, with salt 1 pat	27	3	0	31	0	0
Whipped, with salt 1 stick	545	62	0	629	1	0

*All nonorganic dairy products are Master Disasters.

BRAND/ DAIRY PRODUCT SERVING SIZE	CALORIES	FAT	CARBS	SODIUM	PROTEIN	FIBER
Without salt						
1 cup	1628	184	0	25	2	0
Without salt						
1 tbsp	102	12	0	2	0	0
Without salt						
1 pat	36	4	0	1	0	0
Without salt						
1 stick	810	92	0	12	1	0
Without salt, organic						
1 cup	1628	184	0	25	2	0
Without salt, organic						
1 tbsp	102	12	0	2	0	0
Without salt, organic						
1 pat	36	4	0	1	0	0
Without salt, organic						
1 stick	810	92	0	12	1	0
Horizon Salted						
1 tbsp	100	11	0	115	0	0
Horizon Unsalted						
1 tbsp	100	11	0	0	0	0

Cheese

	CALORIES	FAT	CARBS	SODIUM	PROTEIN	FIBER
American cheddar, imitation cheese						
1 cup	535	31	26	3013	37	0
American cheddar, imitation cheese						
1 slice	50	3	2	282	4	0
American cheese spread						
1 oz	82	6	2	461	5	0
American processed cheese, low fat						
1 cup diced	252	10	5	2002	34	0
American processed cheese, low fat, organic						
1 cup diced	252	10	5	2002	34	0
Bleu cheese						
1 oz	100	8	1	395	6	0
Bleu cheese						
1 cup crumbled	477	39	3	1883	29	0
Brick cheese						
1 oz	105	8	1	159	7	0
Brick cheese						
1 cup diced	490	39	4	739	31	0
Brie cheese						
1 oz	95	8	0	178	6	0
Brie cheese						
1 cup melted	802	66	1	1510	50	0

*All nonorganic dairy products are Master Disasters.

BRAND/ DAIRY PRODUCT SERVING SIZE	CALORIES	FAT	CARBS	SODIUM	PROTEIN	FIBER
Camembert cheese						
1 oz	85	7	0	239	6	0
Camembert cheese						
1 wedge	114	9	0	320	8	0
Caraway cheese						
1 oz	107	8	1	196	7	0
Cheddar cheese						
1 cup diced						
	532	44	2	820	33	0
Cheddar cheese						
1 oz	113	9	0	174	7	0
Cheddar cheese						
1 cup melted						
	983	81	3	1515	61	0
Cheddar cheese						
1 cup shredded						
	455	37	1	702	28	0
Cheddar, low-fat cheese						
1 oz	49	2	1	174	7	0
Cheddar, low-fat cheese						
1 cup shredded						
	195	8	2	692	28	0
Cheddar, low-sodium cheese						
1 cup shredded						
	450	37	2	24	28	0
Cheddar, low-sodium cheese						
1 oz	113	9	1	6	7	0
Cheese food, American, cold pack						
1 oz	94	7	2	274	6	0
Cheese food, American, pasteurized process						
1 oz	93	7	2	452	6	0
Cheese food, Swiss						
1 oz	92	7	1	440	6	0
Cheshire cheese						
1 oz	110	9	1	198	7	0
Colby cheese						
1 cup diced						
	520	42	3	797	31	0
Colby cheese						
1 cup shredded						
	445	36	3	683	27	0
Colby cheese						
1 oz	110	9	1	169	7	0
Cottage cheese, creamed, large curd						
1 cup	206	9	7	764	23	0
Cottage cheese, creamed, small curd						
1 cup	221	10	8	819	25	0
Cottage cheese, creamed, with fruit						
1 cup	219	9	10	777	24	0
Cottage cheese, low fat, 1% milkfat						
1 cup	163	2	6	918	28	0

*All nonorganic dairy products are Master Disasters.

BRAND/ DAIRY PRODUCT SERVING SIZE	CALORIES	FAT	CARBS	SODIUM	PROTEIN	FIBER
Cottage cheese, low fat, 1% milkfat, lactose reduced						
1 cup	168	2	7	499	28	1
Cottage cheese, low fat, 1% milkfat, lactose reduced, organic						
1 cup	**168**	**2**	**7**	**499**	**28**	**1**
Cottage cheese, low fat, 1% milkfat, no sodium added						
1 cup	163	2	6	29	28	0
Cottage cheese, low fat, 1% milkfat, no sodium added, organic						
1 cup	**163**	**2**	**6**	**29**	**28**	**0**
Cottage cheese, low fat, 1% milkfat, organic						
1 cup	**163**	**2**	**6**	**918**	**28**	**0**
Cottage cheese, low fat, 1% milkfat, with vegetables						
1 cup	151	2	7	911	25	0
Cottage cheese, low fat, 1% milkfat, with vegetables, organic						
1 cup	**151**	**2**	**7**	**911**	**25**	**0**
Cottage cheese, low fat, 2% milkfat						
1 cup	194	6	8	746	27	0
Cottage cheese, low fat, 2% milkfat, organic						
1 cup	**194**	**6**	**8**	**746**	**27**	**0**
Cottage cheese, nonfat, uncreamed, dry, large or small curd						
1 cup	104	0	10	479	15	0
Cottage cheese, nonfat, uncreamed, dry, large or small curd, organic						
1 cup	**104**	**0**	**10**	**479**	**15**	**0**
Cottage cheese, with vegetables						
1 cup	215	9	7	911	25	0
Cream cheese						
1 tbsp	50	5	1	47	1	0
Cream cheese						
1 tbsp whipped						
	34	3	0	32	1	0
Cream cheese, fat free						
100 g	105	1	8	702	16	0
Cream cheese, fat free, organic						
100 g	**105**	**1**	**8**	**702**	**16**	**0**
Cream cheese, low fat						
1 tbsp	30	2	1	71	1	0
Cream cheese, low fat						
1 tbsp whipped						
	20	2	1	47	1	0
Cream cheese, low fat, organic						
1 tbsp	**30**	**2**	**1**	**71**	**1**	**0**
Cream cheese, low fat, organic						
1 tbsp whipped						
	20	**2**	**1**	**47**	**1**	**0**
Edam cheese						
1 oz	101	8	0	274	7	0
Feta cheese						
1 oz	75	6	1	316	4	0
Feta cheese						
1 cup crumbled						
	396	32	6	1674	21	0

*All nonorganic dairy products are Master Disasters.

BRAND/ DAIRY PRODUCT SERVING SIZE	CALORIES	FAT	CARBS	SODIUM	PROTEIN	FIBER
Fondue cheese						
½ cup	247	15	4	143	15	0
Fontina cheese						
1 cup shredded	420	34	2	864	28	0
Gjetost cheese						
1 oz	132	8	12	170	3	0
Goat cheese, hard						
1 oz	128	10	1	98	9	0
Goat cheese, semisoft						
1 oz	103	8	1	146	6	0
Goat cheese, soft						
1 oz	76	6	0	104	5	0
Gouda cheese						
1 oz	101	8	1	232	7	0
Gruyère cheese						
1 oz	117	9	0	95	8	0
Gruyère cheese						
1 cup diced	545	43	0	444	39	0
Limburger cheese						
1 oz	93	8	0	227	6	0
Monterey cheese						
1 oz	104	8	0	150	7	0
Monterey cheese						
1 cup shredded	421	34	1	606	28	0
Monterey cheese, low fat						
1 oz	88	6	0	158	8	0
Monterey cheese, low fat						
1 cup shredded	354	24	1	637	32	0
Monterey cheese, low fat, organic						
1 oz	**88**	**6**	**0**	**158**	**8**	**0**
Monterey cheese, low fat, organic						
1 cup shredded	**354**	**24**	**1**	**637**	**32**	**0**
Mozzarella cheese, low sodium						
1 cup diced	370	23	4	21	36	0
Mozzarella cheese, low sodium						
1 cup shredded	316	19	4	18	31	0
Mozzarella cheese, low sodium						
1 oz	78	5	1	4	8	0
Mozzarella cheese, nonfat						
1 cup shredded	168	0	4	840	36	2
Mozzarella cheese, nonfat, organic						
1 cup shredded	**168**	**0**	**4**	**840**	**36**	**2**

*All nonorganic dairy products are Master Disasters.

BRAND/ DAIRY PRODUCT SERVING SIZE	CALORIES	FAT	CARBS	SODIUM	PROTEIN	FIBER
Mozzarella cheese, part skim milk						
1 oz	72	5	1	175	7	0
Mozzarella cheese, part skim milk, low moisture						
1 oz	86	6	1	150	7	0
Mozzarella cheese, part skim milk, low moisture						
1 cup shredded						
	341	23	4	597	29	0
Mozzarella cheese, part skim milk, low moisture, organic						
1 oz	**86**	**6**	**1**	**150**	**7**	**0**
Mozzarella cheese, part skim milk, low moisture, organic						
1 cup shredded						
	341	**23**	**4**	**597**	**29**	**0**
Mozzarella cheese, part skim milk, organic						
1 oz	**72**	**5**	**1**	**175**	**7**	**0**
Mozzarella cheese, whole milk						
1 cup shredded						
	336	25	2	702	25	0
Mozzarella cheese, whole milk						
1 oz	85	6	1	178	6	0
Mozzarella cheese, whole milk, low moisture						
1 oz	90	7	1	118	6	0
Mozzarella, cheese substitute						
1 cup shredded						
	280	14	27	774	13	0
Mozzarella, cheese substitute						
1 oz	69	3	7	192	3	0
Muenster cheese						
1 oz	104	9	0	178	7	0
Muenster cheese						
1 slice (approx 1 oz)						
	103	8	0	176	7	0
Muenster cheese						
1 cup diced						
	486	40	1	829	31	0
Muenster cheese						
1 cup shredded						
	416	34	1	710	26	0
Neufchâtel cheese						
1 oz	72	6	1	95	3	0
Parmesan cheese, dry grated, reduced fat						
1 cup	265	20	1	1529	20	0
Parmesan cheese, dry grated, reduced fat						
1 tbsp	13	1	0	76	1	0
Parmesan cheese, grated						
1 cup	431	29	4	1529	38	0
Parmesan cheese, grated						
1 tbsp	22	1	0	76	2	0
Parmesan cheese, hard						
1 oz	111	7	1	454	10	0
Parmesan cheese, low sodium						
1 tbsp	23	1	0	3	2	0

*All nonorganic dairy products are Master Disasters.

BRAND/ DAIRY PRODUCT SERVING SIZE	CALORIES	FAT	CARBS	SODIUM	PROTEIN	FIBER
Parmesan cheese, shredded						
1 tbsp	21	1	0	85	2	0
Pimento processed cheese						
1 cup diced	525	44	2	1999	31	0
Port-Salut cheese						
1 slice	99	8	0	150	7	0
Provolone cheese						
1 slice	98	7	1	245	7	0
Provolone cheese						
1 cup diced	463	35	3	1156	34	0
Ricotta cheese, part skim milk						
1 oz	39	2	1	35	3	0
Ricotta cheese, part skim milk						
½ cup	171	10	6	155	14	0
Ricotta cheese, part skim milk, organic						
1 oz	**39**	**2**	**1**	**35**	**3**	**0**
Ricotta cheese, part skim milk, organic						
½ cup	**171**	**10**	**6**	**155**	**14**	**0**
Ricotta cheese, whole milk						
½ cup	216	16	4	104	14	0
Romano cheese						
1 oz	110	8	1	340	9	0
Roquefort cheese						
1 oz	105	9	1	513	6	0
Swiss cheese						
1 cup diced	502	37	7	253	36	0
Swiss cheese						
1 cup melted	927	68	13	468	66	0
Swiss cheese						
1 oz	106	8	2	54	8	0
Swiss cheese, low fat						
1 cup shredded	193	6	4	281	31	0
Swiss cheese, low fat						
1 oz	50	1	1	73	8	0
Swiss cheese, low fat, organic						
1 cup shredded	**193**	**6**	**4**	**281**	**31**	**0**
Swiss cheese, low fat, organic						
1 oz	**50**	**1**	**1**	**73**	**8**	**0**
Swiss cheese, low sodium						
1 cup diced	496	36	4	18	37	0
Swiss cheese, low sodium						
1 cup shredded	406	30	4	15	31	0

*All nonorganic dairy products are Master Disasters.

BRAND/ DAIRY PRODUCT SERVING SIZE	CALORIES	FAT	CARBS	SODIUM	PROTEIN	FIBER
Horizon Organic American Singles Cheese Slices						
1 slice	60	5	1	250	4	0
Horizon Organic Cheddar Cheese, Shredded						
¼ cup	110	9	30	180	7	0
Horizon Organic Cheddar Cheese Slices						
1 slice	80	7	0	135	5	0
Horizon Organic Colby Cheese Sticks						
1 stick	110	9	<1	180	7	0
Horizon Organic Cottage Cheese						
½ cup	120	5	4	390	13	0
Horizon Organic Cottage Cheese, Low-Fat						
½ cup	**100**	**3**	**4**	**390**	**13**	**0**
Horizon Organic Cream Cheese						
2 tbsp	110	10	<1	90	2	0
Horizon Organic Cream Cheese, Reduced Fat						
2 tbsp	**70**	**7**	**2**	**100**	**2**	**0**
Horizon Organic Mexican Blend Cheese, Shredded						
¼ cup	110	9	<1	180	7	0
Horizon Organic Monterey Jack Cheese, Shredded						
¼ cup	100	8	0	170	7	0
Horizon Organic Mozzarella Cheese, Shredded						
¼ cup	**80**	**5**	**<1**	**170**	**8**	**0**
Horizon Organic Mozzarella Cheese Sticks						
1 stick	**80**	**5**	**<1**	**170**	**8**	**0**
Horizon Organic Provolone Cheese Slices						
1 slice	70	6	0	140	5	0

Milk

	CALORIES	FAT	CARBS	SODIUM	PROTEIN	FIBER
Half and half						
1 cup	315	28	10	99	7	0
Half and half						
1 tbsp	20	2	1	6	0	0
Half and half						
1 oz	39	3	1	12	1	0
Heavy whipping cream						
1 tbsp	52	6	0	6	0	0
Heavy whipping cream						
1 cup whipped	414	44	3	46	2	0
Hot cocoa, homemade						
1 cup	192	6	27	110	9	0
Hot cocoa, homemade						
1 oz	24	1	3	14	1	0
Light cream (coffee cream or table cream)						
1 tbsp	29	3	1	6	0	0
Light whipping cream						
1 tbsp	44	5	0	5	0	0
Lowfat/1% milk						
1 cup	102	2	12	107	8	0

*All nonorganic dairy products are Master Disasters.

BRAND/ DAIRY PRODUCT SERVING SIZE	CALORIES	FAT	CARBS	SODIUM	PROTEIN	FIBER
Lowfat/1% milk						
1 oz	13	0	2	13	1	0
Lowfat/1% milk, organic						
1 cup	102	2	12	107	8	0
Lowfat/1% milk, organic						
1 oz	13	0	2	13	1	0
Nonfat, fat free, or skim milk						
1 cup	86	0	12	128	8	0
Nonfat, fat free, or skim milk						
1 oz	11	0	2	16	1	0
Nonfat, fat free, or skim milk, organic						
1 cup	86	0	12	128	8	0
Nonfat, fat free, or skim milk, organic						
1 oz	11	0	2	16	1	0
Reduced fat/2% milk						
1 cup	122	5	12	115	8	0
Reduced fat/2% milk						
1 oz	15	1	1	14	1	0
Whole/3.25% milk						
1 cup	149	8	12	105	8	0
Whole/3.25% milk						
1 oz	19	1	1	13	1	0
Eden Foods Organic Edensoy Carob						
8 oz	170	4	28	95	7	<1
Eden Foods Organic Edensoy Chocolate						
8 oz	180	4	28	105	8	<1
Eden Foods Organic Edensoy Extra Original						
8 oz	130	4	13	100	11	<1
Eden Foods Organic Edensoy Extra Vanilla						
8 oz	150	3	23	90	7	<1
Eden Foods Organic Edensoy Light Original						
8 oz	100	2	15	90	5	0
Eden Foods Organic Edensoy Light Vanilla						
8 oz	110	1	22	110	4	0
Eden Foods Organic Edensoy Original						
8 oz	140	5	14	105	11	<1
Eden Foods Organic Edensoy Unsweetened						
8 oz	120	6	5	5	12	<1
Eden Foods Organic Edensoy Vanilla						
8 oz	150	3	24	85	7	<1
Horizon Organic Chocolate Milk						
1 cup	170	3	27	140	8	<1
Horizon Organic Fat-Free Milk						
1 cup	90	0	12	130	9	0
Horizon Organic Lowfat Milk						
1 cup	100	3	12	125	8	0
Horizon Organic Reduced Fat Milk						
1 cup	120	5	12	125	8	0
Horizon Organic Whole Milk						
1 cup	150	8	12	125	8	0

*All nonorganic dairy products are Master Disasters.

BRAND/ DAIRY PRODUCT SERVING SIZE	CALORIES	FAT	CARBS	SODIUM	PROTEIN	FIBER
Horizon Organic Whole Milk Plus DHA Omega-3						
1 cup	150	8	12	125	8	0
Stonyfield Farm Organic Fat Free Milk						
1 cup	80	0	13	125	8	0
Stonyfield Farm Organic Lowfat/1% Milk						
1 cup	110	3	13	125	8	0
Stonyfield Farm Organic Reduced Fat/2% Milk						
1 cup	130	5	13	125	8	0
Stonyfield Farm Organic Whole Milk						
1 cup	150	8	12	125	8	0

Yogurt

	CALORIES	FAT	CARBS	SODIUM	PROTEIN	FIBER
Activia Blueberry Yogurt						
4 oz	110	2	19	65	4	0
Activia Cherry Yogurt						
4 oz	110	2	19	75	5	0
Activia Mixed Berry Yogurt						
4 oz	110	2	19	65	5	0
Activia Peach Yogurt						
4 oz	110	2	19	70	5	0
Activia Plain Yogurt						
8 oz	170	5	20	170	11	0
Activia Prune Yogurt						
4 oz	110	2	19	75	5	0
Activia Strawberry Yogurt						
4 oz	110	2	19	75	5	0
Activia Vanilla Yogurt						
8 oz	220	4	37	140	10	0
Activia Vanilla Yogurt						
4 oz	110	2	19	70	5	0
Dannon All Natural Strawberry Yogurt						
3.3 oz	120	1	21	70	5	0
Dannon DanActive Blueberry						
3.3 oz	80	2	14	40	3	0
Dannon DanActive Peach						
3.3 oz	80	2	14	40	3	0
Dannon DanActive Strawberry						
3.3 oz	80	2	13	40	3	0
Dannon DanActive Vanilla						
3.3 oz	80	2	14	40	3	0
Dannon Fruit Blends Banana Yogurt						
6 oz	160	2	30	100	6	0
Dannon Fruit Blends Peach Yogurt						
6 oz	170	2	33	125	6	0
Dannon Fruit Blends Strawberry Yogurt						
6 oz	170	2	33	125	6	0
Dannon Fruit on the Bottom Apple Cinnamon Yogurt						
6 oz	150	2	28	130	6	<1

*All nonorganic dairy products are Master Disasters.

BRAND/ DAIRY PRODUCT SERVING SIZE	CALORIES	FAT	CARBS	SODIUM	PROTEIN	FIBER
Dannon Fruit on the Bottom Blueberry Yogurt						
6 oz	140	2	26	130	6	<1
Dannon Fruit on the Bottom Boysenberry Yogurt						
6 oz	150	2	27	110	6	<1
Dannon Fruit on the Bottom Cherry Yogurt						
6 oz	140	2	26	280	6	0
Dannon Fruit on the Bottom Mixed Berries Yogurt						
6 oz	150	2	27	120	6	<1
Dannon Fruit on the Bottom Peach Yogurt						
6 oz	150	2	28	95	6	0
Dannon Fruit on the Bottom Pineapple Yogurt						
6 oz	150	2	28	125	6	0
Dannon Fruit on the Bottom Raspberry Yogurt						
6 oz	150	2	28	115	6	<1
Dannon Fruit on the Bottom Strawberry Banana Yogurt						
6 oz	150	2	26	95	6	<1
Dannon Fruit on the Bottom Strawberry Yogurt						
6 oz	150	2	28	110	6	<1
Dannon Light & Fit Blackberry Yogurt						
6 oz	80	0	16	75	5	0
Dannon Light & Fit Blueberry Yogurt						
6 oz	80	0	16	75	5	0
Dannon Light & Fit Cherry Vanilla Yogurt						
6 oz	80	0	16	80	5	0
Dannon Light & Fit Cherry Yogurt						
6 oz	80	0	16	75	5	0
Dannon Light & Fit Key Lime Yogurt						
6 oz	80	0	16	95	5	0
Dannon Light & Fit Lemon Chiffon Yogurt						
6 oz	80	0	15	80	5	0
Dannon Light & Fit Mixed Berry Yogurt						
6 oz	80	0	15	85	5	0
Dannon Light & Fit Orange Mango Yogurt						
6 oz	80	0	16	75	5	0
Dannon Light & Fit Peach Yogurt						
6 oz	80	0	16	75	5	0
Dannon Light & Fit Raspberry Yogurt						
6 oz	80	0	16	75	5	0
Dannon Light & Fit Strawberry Banana Yogurt						
6 oz	80	0	16	75	5	0
Dannon Light & Fit Strawberry Kiwi Yogurt						
6 oz	80	0	16	75	5	0
Dannon Light & Fit Strawberry Yogurt						
6 oz	80	0	16	80	5	0
Dannon Light & Fit Vanilla Yogurt						
6 oz	80	0	16	75	5	0
Dannon Light & Fit White Chocolate Raspberry Yogurt						
6 oz	80	0	16	75	5	0
Horizon Organic Blackberry Lowfat Blended Yogurt						
6 oz	150	2	28	115	7	2

*All nonorganic dairy products are Master Disasters.

BRAND/ DAIRY PRODUCT SERVING SIZE	CALORIES	FAT	CARBS	SODIUM	PROTEIN	FIBER
Horizon Organic Blueberry Fruit-on-the-Bottom Yogurt						
6 oz	140	0	27	105	7	1
Horizon Organic Blueberry Lowfat Blended Yogurt						
6 oz	150	2	27	110	7	2
Horizon Organic Lemon Lowfat Blended Yogurt						
6 oz	150	2	28	110	7	2
Horizon Organic Peach Lowfat Blended Yogurt						
6 oz	150	2	27	110	7	2
Horizon Organic Plain Yogurt						
6 oz	**80**	**0**	**12**	**120**	**8**	**1**
Horizon Organic Raspberry Fruit-on-the-Bottom Yogurt						
6 oz	140	0	27	105	7	2
Horizon Organic Raspberry Lowfat Blended Yogurt						
6 oz	150	2	28	110	7	2
Horizon Organic Strawberry Fruit-on-the-Bottom Yogurt						
6 oz	140	0	28	105	7	1
Horizon Organic Strawberry Lemonade Squeeze/Sour Apple Spray Tuberz						
2 oz	60	1	11	40	2	0
Horizon Organic Strawberry Lowfat Blended Yogurt						
6 oz	150	2	28	110	7	2
Horizon Organic Strawberry-Banana Lowfat Blended Yogurt						
6 oz	150	2	27	110	7	2
Horizon Organic Surfin' Strawberry Tuberz						
2 oz	60	1	11	40	2	0
Horizon Organic Surfin' Strawberry/Blueberry Wave Tuberz						
2 oz	60	1	11	40	2	0
Horizon Organic Vanilla Bean Lowfat Blended Yogurt						
6 oz	150	2	26	110	7	1
Horizon Organic Vanilla Fruit-on-the-Bottom Yogurt						
6 oz	80	0	25	105	7	1
Oikos Organic Blueberry Greek Yogurt						
4 oz	90	0	12	40	10	0
Oikos Organic Honey Greek Yogurt						
4 oz	90	0	13	40	10	0
Oikos Organic Plain Greek Yogurt						
4 oz	**70**	**0**	**5**	**45**	**12**	**0**
Oikos Organic Strawberry Greek Yogurt						
4 oz	90	0	12	60	10	0
Oikos Organic Vanilla Greek Yogurt						
4 oz	80	0	9	45	11	0
Stonyfield Farm Organic Yogurt, French Vanilla, Fat Free						
6 oz	130	0	25	110	7	0
Stonyfield Farm Organic Yogurt, Key Lime, Fat Free						
6 oz	130	0	25	120	7	0
Stonyfield Farm Organic Yogurt, Lemon, Fat Free						
6 oz	130	0	26	115	7	0
Stonyfield Farm Organic Yogurt, Peach, Fat Free						
6 oz	130	0	25	110	7	0
Stonyfield Farm Organic Yogurt, Plain, Fat Free						
6 oz	**80**	**0**	**11**	**120**	**8**	**0**

*All nonorganic dairy products are Master Disasters.

BRAND/ DAIRY PRODUCT SERVING SIZE	CALORIES	FAT	CARBS	SODIUM	PROTEIN	FIBER
Stonyfield Farm Organic Yogurt, Pomegranate Berry, Fat Free						
6 oz	130	0	25	115	7	0
Stonyfield Farm Organic Yogurt, Smoothie Peach						
10 oz	230	3	41	140	10	<1
Stonyfield Farm Organic Yogurt, Smoothie Raspberry						
10 oz	230	3	39	150	10	<1
Stonyfield Farm Organic Yogurt, Smoothie Strawberry						
10 oz	230	3	39	150	10	<1
Stonyfield Farm Organic Yogurt, Smoothie Strawberry Banana						
10 oz	230	3	40	150	10	<1
Stonyfield Farm Organic Yogurt, Smoothie Vanilla						
10 oz	240	3	40	140	10	<1
Stonyfield Farm Organic Yogurt, Smoothie Wild Berry						
10 oz	230	3	39	150	10	<1
Stonyfield Farm Organic Yogurt, Strawberry, Fat Free						
6 oz	110	0	22	125	6	<1
Yoplait Light Thick & Creamy Yogurt						
6 oz	100	0	20	90	5	0
Yoplait Light Yogurt, fruit flavors						
6 oz	100	0	19	85	5	0
Yoplait Original Yogurt, fruit flavors						
6 oz	170	2	33	80	5	0
Yoplait Thick & Creamy Yogurt, fruit flavors						
6 oz	190	4	32	100	7	0
Yoplait Whips! Yogurt, fruit flavors						
4 oz	140	3	25	75	5	0
Yoplait Yo-Plus Light Yogurt, fruit flavors						
4 oz	70	0	15	65	4	3
Yoplait Yo-Plus Yogurt, all flavors						
4 oz	110	2	21	70	4	3

FRESH FRUITS AND VEGETABLES

I wish I could have music playing as you open this page. This is the list of the food gods—these are the foods that will make your body sing. Please, please eat as many organic vegetables as you possibly can, every single day. Packed with antioxidants, fiber, vitamins, and minerals, organic fresh fruits are also some of the healthiest foods on the planet. Keep your calories in mind, of course, but when you're in the mood for sweets, I hope you come here first.

You'll notice throughout the list that the organic options are in bold, but the nonorganic options are not. When it comes to thin-skinned fruits, if you don't eat organic, they become Master Disasters. The risk of pesticides from these fruits is too great—if you don't pick organic for these varieties, I'd rather you not eat them at all. However, thick-skinned fruits (such as avocados, pineapples, mangos, kiwi, and watermelon) and vegetables (such as onion, cabbage, asparagus, sweet peas, and eggplant) are much less risky. But again, whenever possible, reach for the organic. Your body will love you for it.

FOOD ITEM / SERVING SIZE	CALORIES	FAT	CARBS	SODIUM	PROTEIN	FIBER
Fruit						
APPLES						
Dehydrated, stewed						
1 cup	143	0	38	50	1	5
Dehydrated, uncooked						
1 cup	208	0	56	74	1	7

FOOD ITEM / SERVING SIZE	CALORIES	FAT	CARBS	SODIUM	PROTEIN	FIBER
Dried, stewed, with added sugar						
1 cup	232	0	58	53	1	5
Dried, stewed, without added sugar						
1 cup	145	0	39	51	1	5
Dried, uncooked						
1 cup	209	0	57	75	1	7
Dried, uncooked						
1 slice	16	0	4	6	0	1
With skin						
1 cup quartered or chopped						
	65	0	17	1	0	3
With skin						
1 cup sliced						
	57	0	15	1	0	3
With skin						
1 large	116	0	31	2	1	5
With skin						
1 medium						
	95	0	25	2	0	4
With skin						
1 small	77	0	21	1	0	4
With skin, organic						
1 cup quartered or chopped						
	65	0	17	1	0	3
With skin, organic						
1 cup sliced						
	57	0	15	1	0	3
With skin, organic						
1 large	116	0	31	2	1	5
With skin, organic						
1 medium						
	95	0	25	2	0	4
With skin, organic						
1 small	77	0	21	1	0	4
Without skin						
1 cup sliced						
	53	0	14	0	0	1
Without skin						
1 large	104	0	28	0	1	3
Without skin						
1 medium						
	77	0	21	0	0	2
Without skin						
1 small	63	0	17	0	0	2
Without skin, organic						
1 cup sliced						
	53	0	14	0	0	1
Without skin, organic						
1 large	104	0	28	0	1	3
Without skin, organic						
1 medium						
	77	0	21	0	0	2
Without skin, organic						
1 small	63	0	17	0	0	2

FOOD ITEM SERVING SIZE	CALORIES	FAT	CARBS	SODIUM	PROTEIN	FIBER
Without skin, cooked, boiled						
1 cup sliced	91	1	23	2	0	4
Without skin, cooked, boiled, organic						
1 cup sliced	**91**	**1**	**23**	**2**	**0**	**4**
Without skin, cooked, microwave						
1 cup sliced	95	1	24	2	0	5
Without skin, cooked, microwave, organic						
1 cup sliced	**95**	**1**	**24**	**2**	**0**	**5**
APRICOTS						
Plain						
1 cup halves	74	1	17	2	2	3
Plain						
1 cup sliced	79	1	18	2	2	3
Plain						
1 medium	17	0	4	0	0	1
Dehydrated (low-moisture), stewed						
1 cup	314	1	81	12	5	0
Dehydrated (low-moisture), uncooked						
1 cup	381	1	99	15	6	0
Dried, stewed, with added sugar						
1 cup halves	305	0	79	8	3	11
Dried, stewed, without added sugar						
1 cup halves	213	0	55	10	3	6
Dried, uncooked						
1 cup halves	313	1	81	13	4	9
Dried, uncooked						
1 half	8	0	2	0	0	0
Organic						
1 cup halves	**74**	**1**	**17**	**2**	**2**	**3**
Organic						
1 cup sliced	**79**	**1**	**18**	**2**	**2**	**3**
Organic						
1 apricot	**17**	**0**	**4**	**0**	**0**	**1**
BANANAS						
Banana chips						
1 oz	147	10	17	2	1	2
Plain						
1 cup mashed	200	1	51	2	2	6

FOOD ITEM	SERVING SIZE	CALORIES	FAT	CARBS	SODIUM	PROTEIN	FIBER
Plain	1 cup sliced	134	0	34	2	2	4
Plain	1 small	90	0	23	1	1	3
Plain	1 medium	105	0	27	1	1	3
Plain	1 large	121	0	31	1	1	4
Organic	1 cup mashed	200	1	51	2	2	6
Organic	1 cup sliced	134	0	34	2	2	4
Organic	1 small	90	0	23	1	1	3
Organic	1 medium	105	0	27	1	1	3
Organic	1 large	121	0	31	1	1	4
BLACKBERRIES							
Plain	1 cup	62	1	14	1	2	8
Organic	1 cup	62	1	14	1	2	8
BLUEBERRIES							
Plain	1 cup	84	0	21	1	1	4
Organic	1 cup	84	0	21	1	1	4
CHERRIES							
Sour, red	1 cup, pitted	78	0	19	5	2	2
Sour, red	1 cup, with pits	52	0	13	3	1	2
Sour, red, organic	1 cup, pitted	78	0	19	5	2	2
Sour, red, organic	1 cup, with pits	52	0	13	3	1	2
Sweet	1 cup, pitted	97	0	25	0	2	3
Sweet	1 cup, with pits	87	0	22	0	1	3

FOOD ITEM / SERVING SIZE	CALORIES	FAT	CARBS	SODIUM	PROTEIN	FIBER
Sweet						
1 cherry	5	0	1	0	0	0
Sweet, organic						
1 cup, pitted	97	0	25	0	2	3
Sweet, organic						
1 cup, with pits	87	0	22	0	1	3
Sweet, organic						
1 cherry	5	0	1	0	0	0
CRANBERRIES						
Plain						
1 cup chopped	51	0	13	2	0	5
Plain						
1 cup whole	46	0	12	2	0	5
Dried, sweetened						
⅓ cup	123	1	33	1	0	2
Organic						
1 cup chopped	51	0	13	2	0	5
Organic						
1 cup whole	46	0	12	2	0	5
ELDERBERRIES						
Plain						
1 cup	106	1	27	9	1	10
Organic						
1 cup	106	1	27	9	1	10
GOOSEBERRIES						
Plain						
1 cup	66	1	15	2	1	6
Organic						
1 cup	66	1	15	2	1	6
GRAPEFRUIT						
Pink and red, California and Arizona						
1 cup sections, with juice	85	0	22	2	1	0
Pink and red, California and Arizona						
½ medium	46	0	12	1	1	0
Pink and red, California and Arizona, organic						
1 cup sections, with juice	85	0	22	2	1	0
Pink and red, California and Arizona, organic						
½ medium	46	0	12	1	1	0
Pink and red, Florida						
1 cup sections, with juice	69	0	17	0	1	3

FOOD ITEM SERVING SIZE	CALORIES	FAT	CARBS	SODIUM	PROTEIN	FIBER
Pink and red, Florida						
½ medium	37	0	9	0	1	1
Pink and red, Florida, organic						
1 cup sections, with juice	**69**	**0**	**17**	**0**	**1**	**3**
Pink and red, Florida, organic						
½ medium	37	0	9	0	1	1
White, California						
1 cup sections, with juice	85	0	21	0	2	0
White, California						
½ medium	44	0	11	0	1	0
White, California, organic						
1 cup sections, with juice	**85**	**0**	**21**	**0**	**2**	**0**
White, California, organic						
½ medium	**44**	**0**	**11**	**0**	**1**	**0**
White, Florida						
1 cup sections, with juice	74	0	19	0	1	0
White, Florida						
½ medium	38	0	10	0	1	0
White, Florida, organic						
1 cup sections, with juice	**74**	**0**	**19**	**0**	**1**	**0**
White, Florida, organic						
½ medium	**38**	**0**	**10**	**0**	**1**	**0**
GRAPES						
Plain						
1 cup	62	0	16	2	1	1
Plain						
1 grape	2	0	0	0	0	0
Organic						
1 cup	**62**	**0**	**16**	**2**	**1**	**1**
Organic						
1 grape	**2**	**0**	**0**	**0**	**0**	**0**
Red or green (European type, such as Thompson seedless)						
1 cup	104	0	27	3	1	1
Red or green (European type, such as Thompson seedless)						
10 grapes	34	0	9	1	0	0
Red or green (European type, such as Thompson seedless), organic						
1 cup	**104**	**0**	**27**	**3**	**1**	**1**
Red or green (European type, such as Thompson seedless), organic						
10 grapes	**34**	**0**	**9**	**1**	**0**	**0**

FOOD ITEM SERVING SIZE	CALORIES	FAT	CARBS	SODIUM	PROTEIN	FIBER
GUAVAS						
Plain						
1 cup	112	2	24	3	4	9
Plain						
1 medium	37	1	8	1	1	3
Organic						
1 cup	**112**	**2**	**24**	**3**	**4**	**9**
Organic						
1 medium	**37**	**1**	**8**	**1**	**1**	**3**
Strawberry						
1 cup	168	1	42	90	1	13
Strawberry, organic						
1 cup	**168**	**1**	**42**	**90**	**1**	**13**
KIWIFRUIT						
Plain						
1 cup sliced	110	1	26	5	2	5
Plain						
1 medium	76	1	18	3	1	4
Organic						
1 cup sliced	**110**	**1**	**26**	**5**	**2**	**5**
Organic						
1 medium	**76**	**1**	**18**	**3**	**1**	**4**
LEMONS						
Lemon juice						
1 wedge	1	0	1	0	0	0
Lemon juice						
1 lemon	12	0	4	0	0	0
Lemon juice, organic						
1 wedge	**1**	**0**	**1**	**0**	**0**	**0**
Lemon juice, organic						
1 lemon	**12**	**0**	**4**	**0**	**0**	**0**
Lemon peel						
1 tbsp	3	0	1	0	0	1
Lemon peel						
1 tsp	1	0	0	0	0	0
Lemon peel, organic						
1 tbsp	**3**	**0**	**1**	**0**	**0**	**1**
Lemon peel, organic						
1 tsp	**1**	**0**	**0**	**0**	**0**	**0**
Raw without peel						
1 wedge	2	0	1	0	0	0

FOOD ITEM SERVING SIZE	CALORIES	FAT	CARBS	SODIUM	PROTEIN	FIBER
Raw without peel, organic						
1 wedge 2		0	1	0	0	0
MANGOS						
Plain						
1 cup sliced						
	107	0	28	3	1	3
Plain						
1 medium						
	135	1	35	4	1	4
Organic						
1 cup sliced						
	107	0	28	3	1	3
Organic						
1 medium						
	135	1	35	4	1	4
MELONS						
Cantaloupe						
1 cup balls						
	60	0	14	28	1	2
Cantaloupe						
1 cup diced						
	53	0	13	25	1	1
Cantaloupe						
1 large 277		2	66	130	7	7
Cantaloupe						
1 large wedge						
	35	0	8	16	1	1
Cantaloupe						
1 small 150		1	36	71	4	4
Cantaloupe						
1 small wedge						
	19	0	4	9	0	0
Cantaloupe						
10 balls 47		0	11	22	1	1
Cantaloupe, organic						
1 cup balls						
	60	0	14	28	1	2
Cantaloupe, organic						
1 cup diced						
	53	0	13	25	1	1
Cantaloupe, organic						
1 large 277		2	66	130	7	7
Cantaloupe, organic						
1 large wedge						
	35	0	8	16	1	1
Cantaloupe, organic						
1 small 150		1	36	71	4	4
Cantaloupe, organic						
1 small wedge						
	19	0	4	9	0	0
Cantaloupe, organic						
10 balls 47		0	11	22	1	1

FOOD ITEM / SERVING SIZE	CALORIES	FAT	CARBS	SODIUM	PROTEIN	FIBER
Casaba 1 cup cubes	48	0	11	15	2	2
Casaba 1 medium	459	2	108	148	18	15
Casaba ½ melon	229	1	54	74	9	7
Casaba, organic 1 cup cubes	48	0	11	15	2	2
Casaba, organic 1 medium	459	2	108	148	18	15
Casaba, organic ½ medium	46	0	11	15	2	1
Honeydew 1 cup balls	64	0	16	32	1	1
Honeydew 1 cup diced	61	0	15	31	1	1
Honeydew 1 medium	360	1	91	180	5	8
Honeydew 1 wedge	45	0	11	23	1	1
Honeydew 10 balls	50	0	13	25	1	1
Honeydew, organic 1 cup balls	64	0	16	32	1	1
Honeydew, organic 1 cup diced	61	0	15	31	1	1
Honeydew, organic 1 medium	360	1	91	180	5	8
Honeydew, organic 1 wedge	45	0	11	23	1	1
Honeydew, organic 10 balls	50	0	13	25	1	1
NECTARINES Plain 1 cup sliced	63	0	15	0	2	2
Plain 1 medium	62	0	15	0	2	2

FOOD ITEM / SERVING SIZE	CALORIES	FAT	CARBS	SODIUM	PROTEIN	FIBER
Organic						
1 cup slices	63	0	15	0	2	2
Organic						
1 medium	62	0	15	0	2	2
ORANGES						
All varieties						
1 cup sections	85	0	21	0	2	4
All varieties						
1 large	62	0	15	0	1	3
All varieties						
1 medium	47	0	12	0	1	2
All varieties, organic						
1 cup sections	85	0	21	0	2	4
All varieties, organic						
1 large	62	0	15	0	1	3
All varieties, organic						
1 medium	47	0	12	0	1	2
California, Valencias						
1 cup sections	88	1	21	0	2	5
California, Valencias						
1 medium	59	0	14	0	1	3
California, Valencias, organic						
1 cup sections	88	1	21	0	2	5
California, Valencias, organic						
1 medium	59	0	14	0	1	3
Florida						
1 cup sections	85	0	21	0	1	4
Florida						
1 medium	65	0	16	0	1	3
Florida, organic						
1 cup sections	85	0	21	0	1	4
Florida, organic						
1 medium	65	0	16	0	1	3
Navels						
1 cup sections	81	0	21	2	2	4

FOOD ITEM / SERVING SIZE	CALORIES	FAT	CARBS	SODIUM	PROTEIN	FIBER
Navels						
1 medium	69	0	18	1	1	3
Navels, organic						
1 cup sections	81	0	21	2	2	4
Navels, organic						
1 medium	69	0	18	1	1	3
Tangerines (Mandarin oranges)						
1 cup sections	103	1	26	4	2	4
Tangerines (Mandarin oranges)						
1 medium	47	0	12	2	1	2
Tangerines (Mandarin oranges)						
1 large	64	0	16	2	1	2
Tangerines (Mandarin oranges), raw						
1 small	40	0	10	2	1	1
Tangerines (Mandarin oranges), organic						
1 cup sections	103	1	26	4	2	4
Tangerines (Mandarin oranges), organic						
1 small	40	0	10	2	1	1
Tangerines (Mandarin oranges), organic						
1 medium	47	0	12	2	1	2
Tangerines (Mandarin oranges), organic						
1 large	64	0	16	2	1	2
PAPAYAS						
Plain						
1 cup cubes	55	0	14	4	1	3
Plain						
1 cup mashed	90	0	23	7	1	4
Plain						
1 small	59	0	15	5	1	3
Plain						
1 medium	119	0	30	9	2	5
Organic						
1 cup cubes	55	0	14	4	1	3
Organic						
1 cup mashed	90	0	23	7	1	4
Organic						
1 small	59	0	15	5	1	3
Organic						
1 medium	119	0	30	9	2	5

FOOD ITEM SERVING SIZE	CALORIES	FAT	CARBS	SODIUM	PROTEIN	FIBER
PASSION FRUIT						
Purple						
1 cup	229	2	55	66	5	25
Purple						
1 medium	17	0	4	5	0	2
PEACHES						
Plain						
1 cup sliced	60	0	15	0	1	2
Plain						
1 small	51	0	12	0	1	2
Plain						
1 medium	59	0	14	0	1	2
Dried, stewed, with added sugar						
1 cup	278	1	72	5	3	6
Dried, stewed, without added sugar						
1 cup	199	1	51	5	3	7
Dried, uncooked						
1 cup	382	1	98	11	6	13
Organic						
1 cup sliced	60	0	15	0	1	2
Organic						
1 small	51	0	12	0	1	2
Organic						
1 medium	59	0	14	0	1	2
PEARS						
Plain						
1 small	86	0	23	1	1	5
Plain						
1 medium	103	0	28	2	1	6
Plain						
1 cup sliced	81	0	22	1	1	4
Plain						
1 cup cubes	93	0	25	2	1	5
Asian						
1 medium	51	0	13	0	1	4
Asian, organic						
1 medium	51	0	13	0	1	4
Dried, stewed, with added sugar						
1 cup halves	392	1	104	8	2	16
Dried, stewed, without added sugar						
1 cup halves	324	1	86	8	2	16

FOOD ITEM / SERVING SIZE	CALORIES	FAT	CARBS	SODIUM	PROTEIN	FIBER
Dried, uncooked						
1 cup halves	472	1	125	11	3	14
Organic						
1 small	86	0	23	1	1	5
Organic						
1 medium	103	0	28	2	1	6
Organic						
1 cup sliced	81	0	22	1	1	4
Organic						
1 cup cubes	93	0	25	2	1	5
PLUMS						
Plain						
1 cup sliced	76	0	19	0	1	2
Plain						
1 medium	30	0	8	0	0	1
Dried (prunes), stewed, with added sugar						
1 cup, pitted	308	1	82	5	3	9
Dried (prunes), stewed, without added sugar						
1 cup, pitted	265	0	70	2	2	8
Dried (prunes), uncooked						
1 cup, pitted	418	1	111	3	4	12
Dried (prunes), uncooked						
1 medium, pitted	23	0	6	0	0	1
Organic						
1 cup sliced	76	0	19	0	1	2
Organic						
1 medium	30	0	8	0	0	1
POMEGRANATES						
Plain						
½ cup seeds	72	1	16	3	1	3
Plain						
1 medium	234	3	53	8	5	11
Organic						
½ cup seeds	72	1	16	3	1	3
Organic						
1 medium	234	3	53	8	5	11

FOOD ITEM	SERVING SIZE	CALORIES	FAT	CARBS	SODIUM	PROTEIN	FIBER
RASPBERRIES							
Plain	1 cup	64	1	15	1	1	8
Plain	10 berries	10	1	2	0	0	1
Plain	1 pint	162	2	37	3	4	20
Organic	1 cup	64	1	15	1	1	8
Organic	10 berries	10	1	2	0	0	1
Organic	1 pint	162	2	37	3	4	20
RHUBARB							
Plain	1 cup sliced	26	0	6	5	1	2
Plain	1 stalk	11	0	2	2	0	1
Organic	1 cup sliced	26	0	6	5	1	2
Organic	1 stalk	11	0	2	2	0	1
STRAWBERRIES							
Plain	1 cup halves	49	0	12	2	1	3
Plain	1 cup pureed	74	1	18	2	2	5
Plain	1 cup sliced	53	0	13	2	1	3
Plain	1 cup whole	46	0	11	1	1	3
Plain	1 large	6	0	1	0	0	0
Plain	1 pint	114	1	27	4	2	7
Organic	1 cup halves	49	0	12	2	1	3
Organic	1 cup pureed	74	1	18	2	2	5
Organic	1 cup sliced	53	0	13	2	1	3

FOOD ITEM / SERVING SIZE	CALORIES	FAT	CARBS	SODIUM	PROTEIN	FIBER
Organic						
1 cup whole	46	0	11	1	1	3
Organic						
1 large	6	0	1	0	0	0
Organic						
1 pint	114	1	27	4	2	7
Eden Foods Dried Montmorency Cherries						
⅓ cup	140	0	36	15	1	3
Eden Foods Organic Dried Cranberries						
⅓ cup	140	1	33	115	0	2
Eden Foods Organic Dried Wild Blueberries						
¼ cup	150	0	35	15	<1	5

Vegetables

ARUGULA

FOOD ITEM / SERVING SIZE	CALORIES	FAT	CARBS	SODIUM	PROTEIN	FIBER
Raw						
1 leaf	1	0	0	1	0	0
Raw						
½ cup	3	0	0	3	0	0
Raw, organic						
1 leaf	1	0	0	1	0	0
Raw, organic						
½ cup	3	0	0	3	0	0

BEETS

FOOD ITEM / SERVING SIZE	CALORIES	FAT	CARBS	SODIUM	PROTEIN	FIBER
Beet greens, cooked, boiled, drained, with salt						
1 cup	39	0	8	687	4	4
Beet greens, cooked, boiled, drained, with salt, organic						
1 cup	39	0	8	687	4	4
Beet greens, cooked, boiled, drained, without salt						
1 cup	39	0	8	347	4	4
Beet greens, cooked, boiled, drained, without salt, organic						
1 cup	39	0	8	347	4	4
Beet greens, raw						
1 cup	8	0	2	86	1	1
Beet greens, raw, organic						
1 cup	8	0	2	86	1	1
Boiled, drained						
½ cup sliced	37	0	8	65	1	2
Boiled, drained						
2 beets	44	0	10	77	2	2
Boiled, drained, organic						
½ cup sliced	37	0	8	65	1	2
Boiled, drained, organic						
2 beets	44	0	10	77	2	2
Boiled. drained, with salt						
½ cup sliced	37	0	8	242	1	2

FOOD ITEM SERVING SIZE	CALORIES	FAT	CARBS	SODIUM	PROTEIN	FIBER
Boiled, drained, with salt						
2 beets	44	0	10	285	2	2
Boiled, drained, with salt, organic						
½ cup sliced						
	37	**0**	**8**	**242**	**1**	**2**
Boiled, drained, with salt, organic						
2 beets	**44**	**0**	**10**	**285**	**2**	**2**
Raw						
1 cup	58	0	13	106	2	4
Raw						
1 beet	35	0	8	64	1	2
Raw, organic						
1 cup	**58**	**0**	**13**	**106**	**2**	**4**
Raw, organic						
1 beet	**35**	**0**	**8**	**64**	**1**	**2**
BROCCOLI						
Boiled, drained, with salt						
1 stalk	63	1	13	472	4	6
Boiled, drained, with salt						
½ cup chopped						
	27	0	6	204	2	3
Boiled, drained, with salt, organic						
1 stalk	**63**	**1**	**13**	**472**	**4**	**6**
Boiled, drained, with salt, organic						
½ cup chopped						
	27	**0**	**6**	**204**	**2**	**3**
Boiled, drained, without salt						
1 stalk	63	1	13	74	4	6
Boiled, drained, without salt						
½ cup chopped						
	27	0	6	32	2	3
Boiled, drained, without salt, organic						
1 stalk	**63**	**1**	**13**	**74**	**4**	**6**
Boiled, drained, without salt, organic						
½ cup chopped						
	27	**0**	**6**	**32**	**2**	**3**
Chinese, cooked						
1 cup	19	1	3	6	1	2
Chinese, cooked, organic						
1 cup	**19**	**1**	**3**	**6**	**1**	**2**
Raw						
1 spear	11	0	2	10	1	1
Raw						
1 cup chopped						
	31	0	6	30	3	2
Raw						
1 bunch	207	2	40	201	17	16
Raw, organic						
1 spear	**11**	**0**	**2**	**10**	**1**	**1**

FOOD ITEM SERVING SIZE	CALORIES	FAT	CARBS	SODIUM	PROTEIN	FIBER
Raw, organic						
1 cup chopped						
	31	0	6	30	3	2
Raw, organic						
1 bunch	**207**	**2**	**40**	**201**	**17**	**16**
Stalks, raw						
1 stalk	32	0	6	31	3	0
Stalks, raw, organic						
1 stalk	**32**	**0**	**6**	**31**	**3**	**0**
BROCCOLI RABE						
Cooked						
1 bunch	144	2	14	245	17	12
Cooked, organic						
1 bunch	**144**	**2**	**14**	**245**	**17**	**12**
Raw						
1 cup chopped						
	9	0	1	13	1	1
Raw						
1 stalk	4	0	1	6	1	1
Raw, organic						
1 cup chopped						
	9	0	1	13	1	1
Raw, organic						
1 stalk	**4**	**0**	**1**	**6**	**1**	**1**
CABBAGE						
Chinese (pak-choi), boiled, drained, with salt						
1 cup shredded						
	20	0	3	459	3	2
Chinese (pak-choi), boiled, drained, with salt, organic						
1 cup shredded						
	20	**0**	**3**	**459**	**3**	**2**
Chinese (pak-choi), boiled, drained, without salt						
1 cup shredded						
	20	0	3	58	3	2
Chinese (pak-choi), boiled, drained, without salt, organic						
1 cup shredded						
	20	**0**	**3**	**58**	**3**	**2**
Chinese (pak-choi), raw						
1 cup shredded						
	9	0	2	46	1	1
Chinese (pak-choi), raw						
1 head	109	2	18	546	13	8
Chinese (pak-choi), raw						
1 leaf	2	0	0	9	0	0
Chinese (pak-choi), raw, organic						
1 cup shredded						
	9	**0**	**2**	**46**	**1**	**1**
Chinese (pak-choi), raw, organic						
1 head	**109**	**2**	**18**	**546**	**13**	**8**
Chinese (pak-choi), raw, organic						
1 leaf	**2**	**0**	**0**	**9**	**0**	**0**

FOOD ITEM / SERVING SIZE	CALORIES	FAT	CARBS	SODIUM	PROTEIN	FIBER
Chinese (pe-tsai), boiled, drained, with salt						
1 cup shredded	17	0	3	292	2	2
Chinese (pe-tsai), boiled, drained, with salt, organic						
1 cup shredded	**17**	**0**	**3**	**292**	**2**	**2**
Chinese (pe-tsai), boiled, drained, without salt						
1 cup shredded	17	0	3	11	2	2
Chinese (pe-tsai), boiled, drained, without salt, organic						
1 cup shredded	**17**	**0**	**3**	**11**	**2**	**2**
Chinese (pe-tsai), raw						
1 cup shredded	19	0	4	11	1	1
Chinese (pe-tsai), raw						
1 leaf	2	0	0	1	0	0
Chinese (pe-tsai), raw, organic						
1 cup shredded	**19**	**0**	**4**	**11**	**1**	**1**
Chinese (pe-tsai), raw, organic						
1 leaf	**2**	**0**	**0**	**1**	**0**	**0**
Green, boiled, drained, without salt						
1 head	290	1	70	101	16	24
Green, boiled, drained, without salt						
½ cup shredded	17	0	4	6	1	1
Green, boiled, drained, without salt, organic						
1 head	**290**	**1**	**70**	**101**	**16**	**24**
Green, boiled, drained, without salt, organic						
½ cup shredded	**17**	**0**	**4**	**6**	**1**	**1**
Green, raw						
1 cup chopped	22	0	5	16	1	2
Green, raw						
1 cup shredded	18	0	4	13	1	2
Green, raw						
1 head	227	1	53	163	12	23
Green, raw, organic						
1 cup chopped	**22**	**0**	**5**	**16**	**1**	**2**
Green, raw, organic						
1 cup shredded	**18**	**0**	**4**	**13**	**1**	**2**
Green, raw, organic						
1 head	**227**	**1**	**53**	**163**	**12**	**23**
Japanese style, fresh, pickled						
1 cup	45	0	9	416	2	5
Japanese style, fresh, pickled, organic						
1 cup	**45**	**0**	**9**	**416**	**2**	**5**

FOOD ITEM / SERVING SIZE	CALORIES	FAT	CARBS	SODIUM	PROTEIN	FIBER
Mustard, salted						
1 cup	36	0	7	918	1	4
Mustard, salted, organic						
1 cup	**36**	**0**	**7**	**918**	**1**	**4**
Red, boiled, drained, with salt						
1 leaf	6	0	2	54	0	1
Red, boiled, drained, with salt						
½ cup shredded						
	22	0	5	183	1	2
Red, boiled, drained, with salt, organic						
1 leaf	**6**	**0**	**2**	**54**	**0**	**1**
Red, boiled, drained, with salt, organic						
½ cup shredded						
	22	**0**	**5**	**183**	**1**	**2**
Red, boiled, drained, without salt						
1 leaf	6	0	2	6	0	1
Red, boiled, drained, without salt						
½ cup shredded						
	22	0	5	21	1	2
Red, boiled, drained, without salt, organic						
1 leaf	**6**	**0**	**2**	**6**	**0**	**1**
Red, boiled, drained, without salt, organic						
½ cup shredded						
	22	**0**	**5**	**21**	**1**	**2**
Red, raw						
1 cup chopped						
	28	0	7	24	1	2
Red, raw						
1 cup shredded						
	22	0	5	19	1	1
Red, raw						
1 head	260	1	62	227	12	18
Red, raw						
1 leaf	7	0	2	6	0	0
Red, raw, organic						
1 cup chopped						
	28	**0**	**7**	**24**	**1**	**2**
Red, raw, organic						
1 cup shredded						
	22	**0**	**5**	**19**	**1**	**1**
Red, raw, organic						
1 head	**260**	**1**	**62**	**227**	**12**	**18**
Red, raw, organic						
1 leaf	**7**	**0**	**2**	**6**	**0**	**0**
Savoy, boiled, drained, with salt						
1 cup shredded						
	35	0	8	377	3	4
Savoy, boiled, drained, with salt, organic						
1 cup shredded						
	35	**0**	**8**	**377**	**3**	**4**

FOOD ITEM SERVING SIZE	CALORIES	FAT	CARBS	SODIUM	PROTEIN	FIBER
Savoy, boiled, drained, without salt						
1 cup shredded						
	35	0	8	35	3	4
Savoy, boiled, drained, without salt, organic						
1 cup shredded						
	35	**0**	**8**	**35**	**3**	**4**
Savoy, raw						
1 cup shredded						
	19	0	4	20	1	2
Savoy, raw, organic						
1 cup shredded						
	19	**0**	**4**	**20**	**1**	**2**
CARROTS						
Baby, raw						
1 carrot	4	0	1	8	0	0
Baby, raw, organic						
1 carrot	**4**	**0**	**1**	**8**	**0**	**0**
Boiled, drained, with salt						
½ cup sliced						
	27	0	6	236	1	2
Boiled, drained, with salt, organic						
½ cup sliced						
	27	**0**	**6**	**236**	**1**	**2**
Boiled, drained, without salt						
½ cup sliced						
	27	0	6	45	1	2
Boiled, drained, without salt, organic						
½ cup sliced						
	27	**0**	**6**	**45**	**1**	**2**
Raw						
1 cup chopped						
	52	0	12	88	1	4
Raw						
1 cup grated						
	45	0	11	76	1	3
Raw						
1 cup strips or slices						
	50	0	12	84	1	3
Raw						
1 carrot	25	0	6	42	1	2
Raw, organic						
1 cup chopped						
	52	**0**	**12**	**88**	**1**	**4**
Raw, organic						
1 cup grated						
	45	**0**	**11**	**76**	**1**	**3**
Raw, organic						
1 cup strips or slices						
	50	**0**	**12**	**84**	**1**	**3**
Raw, organic						
1 carrot	**25**	**0**	**6**	**42**	**1**	**2**

FOOD ITEM / SERVING SIZE	CALORIES	FAT	CARBS	SODIUM	PROTEIN	FIBER
CAULIFLOWER						
Boiled, drained, with salt						
½ cup	14	0	3	150	1	1
Boiled, drained, with salt, organic						
½ cup	**14**	**0**	**3**	**150**	**1**	**1**
Boiled, drained, without salt						
½ cup	14	0	3	9	1	1
Boiled, drained, without salt, organic						
½ cup	**14**	**0**	**3**	**9**	**1**	**1**
Green, no salt added						
½ head	29	0	6	21	3	3
Green, no salt added, organic						
½ head	**29**	**0**	**6**	**21**	**3**	**3**
Green, raw						
1 cup	20	0	4	15	2	2
Green, raw, organic						
1 cup	**20**	**0**	**4**	**15**	**2**	**2**
Raw						
1 cup chopped	27	0	6	32	2	3
Raw						
1 floret	3	0	1	4	0	0
Raw						
1 head	147	1	31	176	12	15
Raw, organic						
1 cup chopped	**27**	**0**	**6**	**32**	**2**	**3**
Raw, organic						
1 floret	**3**	**0**	**1**	**4**	**0**	**0**
Raw, organic						
1 head	**147**	**1**	**31**	**176**	**12**	**15**
CHARD						
Swiss, boiled, drained, with salt						
1 cup chopped	35	0	7	726	3	4
Swiss, boiled, drained, with salt, organic						
1 cup chopped	**35**	**0**	**7**	**726**	**3**	**4**
Swiss, boiled, drained, without salt						
1 cup chopped	35	0	7	313	3	4
Swiss, boiled, drained, without salt, organic						
1 cup chopped	**35**	**0**	**7**	**313**	**3**	**4**
Swiss, raw						
1 cup	7	0	1	77	1	1
Swiss, raw						
1 leaf	9	0	2	102	1	1
Swiss, raw, organic						
1 cup	**7**	**0**	**1**	**77**	**1**	**1**

FOOD ITEM / SERVING SIZE	CALORIES	FAT	CARBS	SODIUM	PROTEIN	FIBER
Swiss, raw, organic						
1 leaf	9	0	2	102	1	1
GARLIC						
Powder						
1 tsp	10	0	2	1	1	0
Powder, organic						
1 tsp	10	0	2	1	1	0
Raw						
1 cup	203	1	45	23	9	3
Raw						
1 tsp	4	0	1	0	0	0
Raw						
1 clove	4	0	1	1	0	0
Raw, organic						
1 cup	203	1	45	23	9	3
Raw, organic						
1 tsp	4	0	1	0	0	0
Raw, organic						
1 clove	4	0	1	1	0	0
KALE						
Boiled, drained, with salt						
1 cup chopped	36	1	7	337	2	3
Boiled, drained, with salt, organic						
1 cup chopped	36	1	7	337	2	3
Boiled, drained, without salt						
1 cup chopped	36	1	7	30	2	3
Boiled, drained, without salt, organic						
1 cup chopped	36	1	7	30	2	3
Raw						
1 cup chopped	34	0	7	29	2	1
Raw, organic						
1 cup chopped	34	0	7	29	2	1
Scotch, boiled, drained, with salt						
1 cup chopped	36	1	7	365	2	2
Scotch, boiled, drained, with salt, organic						
1 cup chopped	36	1	7	365	2	2
Scotch, boiled, drained, without salt						
1 cup chopped	36	1	7	59	2	2
Scotch, boiled, drained, without salt, organic						
1 cup chopped	36	1	7	59	2	2

FOOD ITEM SERVING SIZE	CALORIES	FAT	CARBS	SODIUM	PROTEIN	FIBER
Scotch, raw						
1 cup chopped	28	0	6	47	2	1
Scotch, raw, organic						
1 cup chopped	**28**	**0**	**6**	**47**	**2**	**1**
KOHLRABI						
Boiled, drained, with salt						
1 cup sliced	48	0	11	424	3	2
Boiled, drained, with salt, organic						
1 cup sliced	**48**	**0**	**11**	**424**	**3**	**2**
Boiled, drained, without salt						
1 cup sliced	48	0	11	35	3	2
Boiled, drained, without salt, organic						
1 cup sliced	**48**	**0**	**11**	**35**	**3**	**2**
Raw						
1 cup	36	0	8	27	2	5
Raw, organic						
1 cup	**36**	**0**	**8**	**27**	**2**	**5**
LEEKS (BULB AND LOWER LEAF-PORTION)						
Boiled, drained, with salt						
1 leek	38	0	9	305	1	1
Boiled, drained, with salt						
¼ cup chopped	8	0	2	64	0	0
Boiled, drained, with salt, organic						
1 leek	**38**	**0**	**9**	**305**	**1**	**1**
Boiled, drained, with salt, organic						
¼ cup chopped	**8**	**0**	**2**	**64**	**0**	**0**
Boiled, drained, without salt						
1 leek	38	0	9	12	1	1
Boiled, drained, without salt						
¼ cup chopped	8	0	2	3	0	0
Boiled, drained, without salt, organic						
1 leek	**38**	**0**	**9**	**12**	**1**	**1**
Boiled, drained, without salt, organic						
¼ cup chopped	**8**	**0**	**2**	**3**	**0**	**0**
Raw						
1 cup	54	0	13	18	1	2
Raw						
1 leek	54	0	13	18	1	2
Raw, organic						
1 cup	**54**	**0**	**13**	**18**	**1**	**2**

FOOD ITEM / SERVING SIZE	CALORIES	FAT	CARBS	SODIUM	PROTEIN	FIBER
Raw, organic						
1 leek	54	0	13	18	1	2
LETTUCE						
Butterhead (includes Boston and Bibb types), raw						
1 cup chopped	7	0	1	3	1	1
Butterhead (includes Boston and Bibb types), raw						
1 head	21	0	4	8	2	2
Butterhead (includes Boston and Bibb types), raw						
1 leaf	1	0	0	0	0	0
Butterhead (includes Boston and Bibb types), raw, organic						
1 cup chopped	7	0	1	3	1	1
Butterhead (includes Boston and Bibb types), raw, organic						
1 head	21	0	4	8	2	2
Butterhead (includes Boston and Bibb types), raw, organic						
1 leaf	1	0	0	0	0	0
Cos or romaine, raw						
1 cup shredded	8	0	2	4	1	1
Cos or romaine, raw						
1 head	106	2	21	50	8	13
Cos or romaine, raw						
1 leaf	1	0	0	0	0	0
Cos or romaine, raw, organic						
1 cup shredded	8	0	2	4	1	1
Cos or romaine, raw, organic						
1 head	106	2	21	50	8	13
Cos or romaine, raw, organic						
1 leaf	1	0	0	0	0	0
Green leaf, raw						
1 cup shredded	5	0	1	10	0	0
Green leaf, raw						
1 head	54	1	10	101	5	5
Green leaf, raw						
1 leaf	1	0	0	1	0	0
Green leaf, raw, organic						
1 cup shredded	5	0	1	10	0	0
Green leaf, raw, organic						
1 head	54	1	10	101	5	5
Green leaf, raw, organic						
1 leaf	1	0	0	1	0	0
Iceberg						
1 cup shredded	10	0	2	7	1	1
Iceberg						
1 cup chopped	8	0	2	6	1	1

FOOD ITEM SERVING SIZE	CALORIES	FAT	CARBS	SODIUM	PROTEIN	FIBER
Iceberg						
1 head	75	1	16	54	5	6
Iceberg						
1 leaf	1	0	0	1	0	0
Iceberg, organic						
1 cup shredded						
	10	0	2	7	1	1
Iceberg, organic						
1 cup chopped						
	8	0	2	6	1	1
Iceberg, organic						
1 head	75	1	16	54	5	6
Iceberg, organic						
1 leaf	1	0	0	1	0	0
Red leaf, raw						
1 cup shredded						
	4	0	1	7	0	0
Red leaf, raw						
1 head	49	1	7	77	4	3
Red leaf, raw						
1 leaf	0	0	0	1	0	0
Red leaf, raw, organic						
1 cup shredded						
	4	0	1	7	0	0
Red leaf, raw, organic						
1 head	49	1	7	77	4	3
Red leaf, raw, organic						
1 leaf	0	0	0	1	0	0
MUSTARD GREENS						
Boiled, drained, with salt						
1 cup chopped						
	21	0	3	353	3	3
Boiled, drained, with salt, organic						
1 cup chopped						
	21	0	3	353	3	3
Boiled, drained, without salt						
1 cup chopped						
	21	0	3	22	3	3
Boiled, drained, without salt, organic						
1 cup chopped						
	21	0	3	22	3	3
Raw						
1 cup chopped						
	15	0	3	14	2	2
Raw, organic						
1 cup chopped						
	15	0	3	14	2	2
MUSTARD SPINACH						
Boiled, drained, with salt						
1 cup chopped						
	29	0	5	450	3	4

FOOD ITEM SERVING SIZE	CALORIES	FAT	CARBS	SODIUM	PROTEIN	FIBER
Boiled, drained, with salt, organic						
1 cup chopped	**29**	**0**	**5**	**450**	**3**	**4**
Boiled, drained, without salt						
1 cup chopped	29	0	5	25	3	4
Boiled, drained, without salt, organic						
1 cup chopped	**29**	**0**	**5**	**25**	**3**	**4**
Raw						
1 cup chopped	33	0	6	32	3	4
Raw, organic						
1 cup chopped	**33**	**0**	**6**	**32**	**3**	**4**
ONIONS						
Boiled, drained, with salt						
1 cup	88	0	20	502	3	3
Boiled, drained, with salt						
1 tbsp chopped	6	0	1	36	0	0
Boiled, drained, with salt						
1 slice	5	0	1	29	0	0
Boiled, drained, with salt, organic						
1 cup	**88**	**0**	**20**	**502**	**3**	**3**
Boiled, drained, with salt, organic						
1 tbsp chopped	**6**	**0**	**1**	**36**	**0**	**0**
Boiled, drained, with salt, organic						
1 slice	**5**	**0**	**1**	**29**	**0**	**0**
Boiled, drained, without salt						
1 cup	92	0	21	6	3	3
Boiled, drained, without salt						
1 tbsp chopped	7	0	2	0	0	0
Boiled, drained, without salt						
1 slice	5	0	1	0	0	0
Boiled, drained, without salt, organic						
1 cup	**92**	**0**	**21**	**6**	**3**	**3**
Boiled, drained, without salt, organic						
1 tbsp chopped	**7**	**0**	**2**	**0**	**0**	**0**
Boiled, drained, without salt, organic						
1 slice	**5**	**0**	**1**	**0**	**0**	**0**
Dehydrated flakes						
1 tbsp	17	0	4	1	0	0
Dehydrated flakes, organic						
1 tbsp	**17**	**0**	**4**	**1**	**0**	**0**
Raw						
1 cup chopped	64	0	15	6	2	3

FOOD ITEM / SERVING SIZE	CALORIES	FAT	CARBS	SODIUM	PROTEIN	FIBER
Raw						
1 cup sliced	46	0	11	5	1	2
Raw						
1 tbsp chopped	4	0	1	0	0	0
Raw						
1 onion	44	0	10	4	1	2
Raw						
1 slice	6	0	1	1	0	0
Raw, organic						
1 cup chopped	64	0	15	6	2	3
Raw, organic						
1 cup sliced	46	0	11	5	1	2
Raw, organic						
1 tbsp chopped	4	0	1	0	0	0
Raw, organic						
1 onion	44	0	10	4	1	2
Raw, organic						
1 slice	6	0	1	1	0	0
Spring or scallions (includes tops and bulb), raw						
1 cup chopped	32	0	7	16	2	3
Spring or scallions (includes tops and bulb), raw						
1 tbsp chopped	2	0	0	1	0	0
Spring or scallions (includes tops and bulb), raw						
1 onion	5	0	1	2	0	0
Spring or scallions (includes tops and bulb), raw, organic						
1 cup chopped	32	0	7	16	2	3
Spring or scallions (includes tops and bulb), raw, organic						
1 tbsp chopped	2	0	0	1	0	0
Spring or scallions (includes tops and bulb), raw, organic						
1 onion	5	0	1	2	0	0
Sweet, raw						
1 onion	106	0	25	26	3	3
Sweet, raw, organic						
1 onion	106	0	25	26	3	3
Yellow, sautéed						
1 cup chopped	115	9	7	10	1	1
Yellow, sautéed, organic						
1 cup chopped	115	9	7	10	1	1
Young green, tops only						
1 tbsp	2	0	0	0	0	0

FOOD ITEM / SERVING SIZE	CALORIES	FAT	CARBS	SODIUM	PROTEIN	FIBER
Young green, tops only, organic						
1 tbsp	**2**	**0**	**0**	**0**	**0**	**0**
RUTABAGAS						
Boiled, drained, with salt						
½ cup mashed	47	0	10	305	2	2
Boiled, drained, with salt, organic						
½ cup mashed	**47**	**0**	**10**	**305**	**2**	**2**
Boiled, drained, without salt						
1 cup mashed	94	1	21	48	3	4
Boiled, drained, without salt, organic						
1 cup mashed	**94**	**1**	**21**	**48**	**3**	**4**
Raw						
1 cup cubes	50	0	11	28	2	4
Raw						
1 rutabaga	139	1	31	77	5	10
Raw, organic						
1 cup cubes	**50**	**0**	**11**	**28**	**2**	**4**
Raw, organic						
1 rutabaga	**139**	**1**	**31**	**77**	**5**	**10**
SHALLOTS						
Raw						
1 tbsp chopped	7	0	2	1	0	0
Raw, organic						
1 tbsp chopped	**7**	**0**	**2**	**1**	**0**	**0**
SPINACH						
Boiled, drained, with salt						
1 cup	41	0	7	551	5	4
Boiled, drained, with salt, organic						
1 cup	**41**	**0**	**7**	**551**	**5**	**4**
Boiled, drained, without salt						
1 cup	41	0	7	126	5	4
Boiled, drained, without salt, organic						
1 cup	**41**	**0**	**7**	**126**	**5**	**4**
Raw						
1 cup	7	0	1	24	1	1
Raw						
1 bunch	78	1	12	269	10	7
Raw						
1 leaf	2	0	0	8	0	0
Raw, organic						
1 cup	**7**	**0**	**1**	**24**	**1**	**1**

FOOD ITEM SERVING SIZE	CALORIES	FAT	CARBS	SODIUM	PROTEIN	FIBER
Raw, organic						
1 bunch	78	1	12	269	10	7
Raw, organic						
1 leaf	2	0	0	8	0	0
SQUASH						
Summer, all varieties, boiled, drained, with salt						
1 cup sliced	36	1	8	427	2	3
Summer, all varieties, boiled, drained, with salt, organic						
1 cup sliced	36	1	8	427	2	3
Summer, all varieties, boiled, drained, without salt						
1 cup sliced	36	1	8	2	2	3
Summer, all varieties, boiled, drained, without salt, organic						
1 cup sliced	36	1	8	2	2	3
Summer, all varieties, raw						
1 cup sliced	18	0	4	2	1	1
Summer, all varieties, raw						
1 medium	31	0	7	4	2	2
Summer, all varieties, raw						
1 slice	2	0	0	0	0	0
Summer, all varieties, raw, organic						
1 cup sliced	18	0	4	2	1	1
Summer, all varieties, raw, organic						
1 squash	31	0	7	4	2	2
Summer, all varieties, raw, organic						
1 slice	2	0	0	0	0	0
Summer, crookneck and straightneck, raw						
1 cup sliced	24	0	5	3	1	2
Summer, crookneck and straightneck, raw, organic						
1 cup sliced	24	0	5	3	1	2
Summer, scallop, boiled, drained, with salt						
½ cup sliced	14	0	3	213	1	2
Summer, scallop, boiled, drained, with salt, organic						
½ cup sliced	14	0	3	213	1	2
Summer, zucchini, includes skin, boiled, drained, with salt						
½ cup sliced	14	0	4	215	1	1
Summer, zucchini, includes skin, boiled, drained, with salt, organic						
½ cup sliced	14	0	4	215	1	1

FOOD ITEM / SERVING SIZE	CALORIES	FAT	CARBS	SODIUM	PROTEIN	FIBER
Summer, zucchini, includes skin, boiled, drained, without salt						
1 cup sliced	29	0	7	5	1	3
Summer, zucchini, includes skin, boiled, drained, without salt, organic						
1 cup sliced	**29**	**0**	**7**	**5**	**1**	**3**
Summer, zucchini, includes skin, raw						
1 cup chopped	20	0	4	12	2	1
Summer, zucchini, includes skin, raw						
1 cup sliced	18	0	4	11	1	1
Summer, zucchini, includes skin, raw						
1 small	19	0	4	12	1	1
Summer, zucchini, includes skin, raw						
1 medium	31	0	7	20	2	2
Summer, zucchini, includes skin, raw						
1 large	52	1	11	32	4	4
Summer, zucchini, includes skin, raw						
1 slice	2	0	0	1	0	0
Summer, zucchini, includes skin, raw, organic						
1 cup chopped	**20**	**0**	**4**	**12**	**2**	**1**
Summer, zucchini, includes skin, raw, organic						
1 cup sliced	**18**	**0**	**4**	**11**	**1**	**1**
Summer, zucchini, includes skin, raw, organic						
1 small	**19**	**0**	**4**	**12**	**1**	**1**
Summer, zucchini, includes skin, raw, organic						
1 medium	**31**	**0**	**7**	**20**	**2**	**2**
Summer, zucchini, includes skin, raw, organic						
1 large	**52**	**1**	**11**	**32**	**4**	**4**
Summer, zucchini, includes skin, raw, organic						
1 slice	**2**	**0**	**0**	**1**	**0**	**0**
Winter, acorn, baked, with salt						
1 cup cubed	115	0	30	492	2	9
Winter, acorn, baked, with salt, organic						
1 cup cubed	**115**	**0**	**30**	**492**	**2**	**9**
Winter, acorn, baked, without salt						
1 cup cubed	115	0	30	8	2	9
Winter, acorn, baked, without salt, organic						
1 cup cubed	**115**	**0**	**30**	**8**	**2**	**9**

FOOD ITEM SERVING SIZE	CALORIES	FAT	CARBS	SODIUM	PROTEIN	FIBER
Winter, acorn, boiled, mashed, with salt						
1 cup	83	0	22	586	2	6
Winter, acorn, boiled, mashed, with salt, organic						
1 cup	**83**	**0**	**22**	**586**	**2**	**6**
Winter, acorn, boiled, mashed, without salt						
1 cup	83	0	22	7	2	6
Winter, acorn, boiled, mashed, without salt, organic						
1 cup	**83**	**0**	**22**	**7**	**2**	**6**
Winter, acorn, raw						
1 cup cubed	56	0	15	4	1	2
Winter, acorn, raw						
1 medium	172	0	45	13	3	6
Winter, acorn, raw, organic						
1 cup cubed	**56**	**0**	**15**	**4**	**1**	**2**
Winter, acorn, raw, organic						
1 medium	**172**	**0**	**45**	**13**	**3**	**6**
Winter, all varieties, baked, with salt						
1 cup cubed	80	1	18	486	2	6
Winter, all varieties, baked, with salt, organic						
1 cup cubed	**80**	**1**	**18**	**486**	**2**	**6**
Winter, all varieties, baked, without salt						
1 cup cubed	76	1	18	2	2	6
Winter, all varieties, baked, without salt, organic						
1 cup cubed	**76**	**1**	**18**	**2**	**2**	**6**
Winter, all varieties, raw						
1 cup cubed	39	0	10	5	1	2
Winter, all varieties, raw, organic						
1 cup cubed	**39**	**0**	**10**	**5**	**1**	**2**
Winter, butternut, baked, with salt						
1 cup cubed	82	0	22	492	2	n/a
Winter, butternut, baked, with salt, organic						
1 cup cubed	**82**	**0**	**22**	**492**	**2**	**n/a**
Winter, butternut, baked, without salt						
1 cup cubed	82	0	22	8	2	n/a
Winter, butternut, baked, without salt, organic						
1 cup cubed	**82**	**0**	**22**	**8**	**2**	**n/a**

FOOD ITEM SERVING SIZE	CALORIES	FAT	CARBS	SODIUM	PROTEIN	FIBER
Winter, butternut, raw						
1 cup cubed	63	0	16	6	1	3
Winter, butternut, raw, organic						
1 cup cubed	**63**	**0**	**16**	**6**	**1**	**3**
Winter, hubbard, baked, with salt						
1 cup cubed	103	1	22	500	5	n/a
Winter, hubbard, baked, with salt, organic						
1 cup cubed	**103**	**1**	**22**	**500**	**5**	**n/a**
Winter, hubbard, baked, without salt						
1 cup cubed	103	1	22	16	5	n/a
Winter, hubbard, baked, without salt, organic						
1 cup cubed	**103**	**1**	**22**	**16**	**5**	**n/a**
Winter, hubbard, boiled, mashed, with salt						
1 cup	71	1	15	569	3	7
Winter, hubbard, boiled, mashed, with salt, organic						
1 cup	**71**	**1**	**15**	**569**	**3**	**7**
Winter, hubbard, boiled, mashed, without salt						
1 cup	71	1	15	12	3	7
Winter, hubbard, boiled, mashed, without salt, organic						
1 cup	**71**	**1**	**15**	**12**	**3**	**7**
Winter, hubbard, raw						
1 cup cubed	46	1	10	8	2	5
Winter, hubbard, raw, organic						
1 cup, cubed	**46**	**1**	**10**	**8**	**2**	**5**
Winter, spaghetti, boiled, drained, or baked, with salt						
1 cup	42	0	10	394	1	2
Winter, spaghetti, boiled, drained, or baked, with salt, organic						
1 cup	**42**	**0**	**10**	**394**	**1**	**2**
Winter, spaghetti, boiled, drained, or baked, without salt						
1 cup	42	0	10	28	1	2
Winter, spaghetti, boiled, drained, or baked, without salt, organic						
1 cup	**42**	**0**	**10**	**28**	**1**	**2**
Winter, spaghetti, raw						
1 cup cubed	31	1	7	17	1	n/a
Winter, spaghetti, raw, organic						
1 cup cubed	**31**	**1**	**7**	**17**	**1**	**n/a**
Zucchini, baby, raw						
1 medium	2	0	0	0	0	0

FOOD ITEM SERVING SIZE	CALORIES	FAT	CARBS	SODIUM	PROTEIN	FIBER
Zucchini, baby, raw						
1 large	3	0	0	0	0	0
Zucchini, baby, raw, organic						
1 medium	2	0	0	0	0	0
Zucchini, baby, raw, organic						
1 large	3	0	0	0	0	0
TOMATOES						
Sauce, no salt added						
1 cup	103	0	21	27	3	4
Green, raw						
1 slice	5	0	1	3	0	0
Green, raw, organic						
1 slice	5	0	1	3	0	0
Orange, raw						
1 tomato	18	0	4	47	1	1
Orange, raw, organic						
1 tomato	18	0	4	47	1	1
Red, ripe, cooked						
1 cup	43	0	10	26	2	2
Red, ripe, cooked, organic						
1 cup	43	0	10	26	2	2
Red, ripe, stewed						
1 cup	80	3	13	460	2	2
Red, ripe, stewed, organic						
1 cup	80	3	13	460	2	2
Red, ripe, cooked, with salt						
1 cup	43	0	10	593	2	2
Red, ripe, cooked, with salt, organic						
1 cup	43	0	10	593	2	2
Sun-dried						
1 cup	139	2	30	1131	8	7
Sun-dried						
1 piece	5	0	1	42	0	0
Sun-dried, organic						
1 cup	139	2	30	1131	8	7
Sun-dried, organic						
1 piece	5	0	1	42	0	0
Sun-dried, packed in oil, drained						
1 piece	6	0	1	8	0	0
Sun-dried, packed in oil, drained						
1 cup	234	15	26	293	6	6
Sun-dried, packed in oil, drained, organic						
1 piece	6	0	1	8	0	0
Sun-dried, packed in oil, drained, organic						
1 cup	234	15	26	293	6	6
Yellow, raw						
1 tomato	32	1	6	49	2	1

FOOD ITEM SERVING SIZE	CALORIES	FAT	CARBS	SODIUM	PROTEIN	FIBER
Yellow, raw						
1 cup chopped	21	0	4	32	1	1
Yellow, raw, organic						
1 tomato	**32**	**1**	**6**	**49**	**2**	**1**
Yellow, raw, organic						
1 cup chopped	21	0	4	32	1	1
TURNIP GREENS						
Boiled, drained, with salt						
1 cup chopped	29	0	6	382	2	5
Boiled, drained, with salt, organic						
1 cup chopped	29	0	6	382	2	5
Boiled, drained, without salt						
1 cup chopped	29	0	6	42	2	5
Boiled, drained, without salt, organic						
1 cup chopped	29	0	6	42	2	5
Raw						
1 cup chopped	18	0	4	22	1	2
Raw, organic						
1 cup chopped	18	0	4	22	1	2
TURNIPS						
Boiled, drained, with salt						
1 cup cubed	34	0	8	446	1	3
Boiled, drained, with salt						
1 cup mashed	51	0	12	658	2	5
Boiled, drained, with salt, organic						
1 cup cubed	**34**	**0**	**8**	**446**	**1**	**3**
Boiled, drained, with salt, organic						
1 cup mashed	51	0	12	658	2	5

FROZEN FOODS

The vast majority of frozen meals are packed with yucky oils and preservatives. Stick to Amy's, Kashi, and Newman's Own—while they're still processed (often nonorganic) foods, at least the raw ingredients they start with are somewhat more decent. Frozen fruits and vegetables follow the same guidelines as fresh—if they're organic, they get a big thumbs up. If they're nonorganic or have added sugars, soy, or other Anti-Nutrients, they don't.

When it comes to frozen desserts, beware—many of the thaw-and-eat cakes feature the same Anti-Nutrients found in frozen meals. But if you need the ice cream, have the ice cream—just have one serving of ice cream, not the whole pint. Look for products with no high-fructose corn syrup or hydrogenated oils; in fact, ice cream should not have oil at all. While the real ice cream is full of calories, those calories are bound to satisfy your sweet tooth way more than some icky frozen cake with lots of added oil and sugar (or worse, artificial sweeteners).

BRAND/FOOD ITEM SERVING SIZE	CALORIES	FAT	CARBS	SODIUM	PROTEIN	FIBER

Frozen Meals

BRAND/FOOD ITEM SERVING SIZE	CALORIES	FAT	CARBS	SODIUM	PROTEIN	FIBER
Amy's 3 Cheese Pizza with Cornmeal Crust						
⅓ pizza	370	19	41	580	10	2
Amy's All American Veggie Burger						
1 patty	120	3	15	390	10	3
Amy's Apple Toaster Pops						
1 piece	150	3.5	27	110	3	1
Amy's Asian Noodle Stir-Fry						
1 box	290	7	50	630	9	4
Amy's Baked Ziti Bowl						
1 box	390	12	62	590	9	6
Amy's Bean & Cheese Burrito						
1 burrito	300	9	43	580	11	6
Amy's Bean & Rice Burrito—Non Dairy						
1 burrito	280	6	48	550	9	5
Amy's Bistro Burger						
1 patty	110	2.5	16	370	5	2
Amy's Black Bean Enchilada Whole Meal						
1 meal	330	8	53	740	9	9
Amy's Black Bean Tamale Verde						
1 meal	330	10	55	780	7	8
Amy's Black Bean Vegetable Burrito						
1 burrito	280	8	44	580	9	4
Amy's Black Bean Vegetable Enchilada						
½ box	180	6	26	390	5	3
Amy's Breakfast Burrito						
1 burrito	250	7	38	540	9	5
Amy's Breakfast Scramble Wrap						
1 burrito	380	19	30	490	21	4
Amy's Broccoli and Cheese in a Pocket Sandwich						
1 piece	270	10	37	560	8	3
Amy's Broccoli Pot Pie						
1 pie	430	22	46	630	11	4
Amy's Brown Rice & Vegetables Bowl						
1 box	260	9	36	550	9	5
Amy's Brown Rice, Black-Eyed Peas & Veggies Bowl						
1 box	290	11	38	580	11	8
Amy's Burrito Especial						
1 burrito	270	6	45	620	9	4
Amy's California Veggie Burger						
1 patty	140	5	19	430	6	4
Amy's Cheddar Veggie Burger						
1 patty	160	5	20	430	8	3
Amy's Cheese & Pesto Pizza with Whole Wheat Crust						
⅓ pizza	360	18	37	680	13	4
Amy's Cheese Enchilada						
½ box	240	14	18	440	10	2
Amy's Cheese Enchilada Whole Meal						
1 meal	350	15	38	680	15	6

BRAND/FOOD ITEM SERVING SIZE	CALORIES	FAT	CARBS	SODIUM	PROTEIN	FIBER
Amy's Cheese Pizza						
⅓ pizza	290	12	33	590	12	2
Amy's Cheese Pizza in a Pocket Sandwich						
1 piece	310	10	42	450	14	4
Amy's Cheese Pizza Snacks						
5 pieces	190	7	22	390	9	2
Amy's Cheese Pizza Toaster Pops						
5 pops	160	6	21	220	5	1
Amy's Cheese Tamale Verde						
1 meal	360	16	45	780	10	5
Amy's Chili & Cornbread Whole Meal						
1 meal	340	6	59	680	11	1
Amy's Country Cheddar Bowl						
1 box	400	19	41	690	15	4
Amy's Garden Vegetable Lasagna						
1 box	290	9	41	720	13	5
Amy's Indian Mattar Paneer						
1 box	320	8	54	780	11	6
Amy's Indian Mattar Paneer—Light in Sodium						
1 box	320	8	54	390	11	6
Amy's Indian Mattar Tofu						
1 box	260	8	40	680	12	5
Amy's Indian Palak Paneer						
1 box	270	9	38	680	10	5
Amy's Indian Paneer Tikka						
1 box	320	18	36	550	8	5
Amy's Indian Samosa Wrap						
1 burrito	250	9	35	680	8	4
Amy's Indian Spinach Tofu Wrap						
1 burrito	310	14	35	690	11	7
Amy's Indian Vegetable Korma						
1 box	310	12	41	680	9	7
Amy's Light in Sodium Veggie Loaf Whole Meal						
1 meal	290	8	47	340	9	10
Amy's Macaroni & Cheese						
1 box (9 oz)						
	410	16	47	590	16	3
Amy's Macaroni & Soy Cheeze						
1 box	370	15	42	500	16	4
Amy's Margherita Pizza						
⅓ pizza	250	12	32	550	11	2
Amy's Mexican Casserole Bowl						
1 box	470	16	70	780	11	7
Amy's Mexican Tamale Pie						
1 pie	150	3	27	590	5	4
Amy's Mexican Tofu Scramble						
1 box	400	18	40	680	20	8
Amy's Mushroom and Olive Pizza						
⅓ pizza	250	9	33	560	10	2
Amy's Nacho Snacks						
5 pieces	210	8	26	460	9	<1

BRAND/FOOD ITEM SERVING SIZE	CALORIES	FAT	CARBS	SODIUM	PROTEIN	FIBER
Amy's Non Dairy Vegetable Pot Pie						
1 pie	360	13	50	640	10	4
Amy's Pesto Pizza						
⅓ pizza	310	12	39	480	12	2
Amy's Pesto Tortellini Bowl						
1 box	430	19	45	640	20	3
Amy's Quarter Pound Veggie Burger						
1 patty	200	3.5	23	600	21	6
Amy's Ravioli Bowl						
1 box	380	12	55	680	14	4
Amy's Rice Crust Cheese Pizza						
⅓ pizza	320	16	34	590	10	2
Amy's Rice Crust Spinach Pizza						
⅓ pizza	350	20	34	580	8	4
Amy's Rice Mac & Cheese						
1 box	400	16	47	590	16	1
Amy's Roasted Vegetable Lasagna						
1 box	350	11	47	680	16	4
Amy's Roasted Vegetable Pizza						
⅓ pizza	270	9	42	490	6	2
Amy's Roasted Vegetable Tamale						
1 meal	280	7	46	680	9	8
Amy's Santa Fe Enchilada Bowl						
1 box	350	11	47	780	16	9
Amy's Shepherd's Pie						
1 pie	160	4	27	590	5	5
Amy's Shepherd's Pie—Light in Sodium						
1 pie	160	4	27	290	5	5
Amy's Single Serve Cheese Pizza						
1 box	420	17	49	720	18	3
Amy's Single Serve Margherita Pizza						
1 box	400	17	47	720	16	3
Amy's Single Serve Mushroom & Olive Pizza						
1 box	450	19	56	780	18	3
Amy's Single Serve Non-Dairy Rice Crust Cheeze Pizza						
1 box	460	28	46	680	10	4
Amy's Single Serve Pesto Pizza						
1 box	440	19	39	780	12	2
Amy's Single Serve Roasted Vegetable Pizza						
1 box	410	14	62	780	11	5
Amy's Single Serve Spinach Pizza						
1 box	440	18	54	780	19	3
Amy's Single Serve Spinach Pizza—Light in Sodium						
1 box	440	18	54	390	19	3
Amy's Southern Dinner						
1 meal	310	7	51	720	11	8
Amy's Southwestern Burrito						
1 burrito	300	10	43	680	12	6
Amy's Soy Cheeze Pizza						
⅓ pizza	290	11	37	590	12	2
Amy's Spinach Feta in a Pocket Sandwich						
1 piece	260	9	34	590	11	3

BRAND/FOOD ITEM SERVING SIZE	CALORIES	FAT	CARBS	SODIUM	PROTEIN	FIBER
Amy's Spinach Pizza						
⅓ pizza	310	12	38	590	12	2
Amy's Spinach Pizza in a Pocket Sandwich						
1 piece	280	9	37	460	13	3
Amy's Spinach Pizza Snack						
5 pieces	200	7	26	420	8	1
Amy's Strawberry Toaster Pops						
1 piece	150	3.5	27	110	3	1
Amy's Stuffed Pasta Shells Bowl						
1 box	310	13	30	740	19	5
Amy's Teriyaki Bowl						
1 box	290	4.5	52	780	10	4
Amy's Teriyaki Wrap						
1 burrito	290	7	48	460	9	5
Amy's Texas Veggie Burger						
1 patty	120	2.5	14	350	12	3
Amy's Thai Stir-Fry						
1 box	310	11	45	420	8	5
Amy's Tofu Scramble						
1 box	320	19	19	580	19	4
Amy's Tofu Scramble in a Pocket Sandwich						
1 piece	180	6	23	520	11	<1
Amy's Tofu Vegetable Lasagna						
1 box	310	11	41	680	13	6
Amy's Tortilla Casserole & Black Beans Bowl						
1 box	390	18	41	780	17	7
Amy's Vegetable Lasagna						
1 box	310	12	35	680	16	5
Amy's Vegetable Pie in a Pocket Sandwich						
1 piece	300	9	45	490	8	3
Amy's Vegetable Pot Pie						
1 pie	420	19	54	590	9	4
Amy's Veggie Loaf Whole Meal						
1 meal	290	8	47	690	9	7
Amy's Veggie Steak & Gravy Whole Meal						
1 meal	380	16	50	680	12	7
Banquet Beef Pot Pie						
1 pie	390	22	36	1010	12	3
Banquet Chicken Pot Pie						
1 pie	370	21	35	1040	10	3
Banquet Turkey Pot Pie						
1 pie	380	21	36	1030	10	3
Kashi Frozen Entrée Black Bean Mango						
1 entrée	340	8	58	430	8	7
Kashi Frozen Entrée Chicken Florentine						
1 entrée	290	9	31	550	22	5
Kashi Frozen Entrée Chicken Pasta Pomodoro						
1 entrée	280	6	38	470	19	6
Kashi Frozen Entrée Lemongrass Coconut Chicken						
1 entrée	300	8	38	680	18	7
Kashi Frozen Entrée Mayan Harvest Bake						
1 entrée	340	9	58	380	9	8

BRAND/FOOD ITEM SERVING SIZE	CALORIES	FAT	CARBS	SODIUM	PROTEIN	FIBER
Kashi Frozen Entrée Pesto Pasta Primavera						
1 entrée	290	11	37	750	11	7
Kashi Frozen Entrée Ranchero Beans						
1 entrée	340	7	56	570	12	11
Kashi Frozen Entrée Red Curry Chicken						
1 entrée	300	9	40	490	18	5
Kashi Frozen Entrée Southwest Style Chicken						
1 entrée	240	5	32	680	16	6
Kashi Frozen Entrée Sweet & Sour Chicken						
1 entrée	320	3.5	55	380	18	6
Kashi Frozen Entrée Tuscan Veggie Bake						
1 entrée	260	9	42	700	7	8
Kashi Frozen Entrée Veggie Chana Masala						
1 entrée	310	9	44	690	11	8
Kashi GoLean Waffles Blueberry						
2 waffles	170	3	33	300	8	6
Kashi GoLean Waffles Original						
2 waffles	170	3	33	330	8	6
Kashi GoLean Waffles Strawberry Flax						
2 waffles	160	3	31	300	8	6
Kashi Heart to Heart Waffles Honey Oat						
2 waffles	160	3	31	370	6	3
Kashi Pizza Caribbean Carnival						
⅓ pizza	280	8	39	590	14	5
Kashi Pizza Mediterranean Original Crust						
⅓ pizza	290	9	37	640	15	5
Kashi Pizza Sicilian Veggie						
⅓ pizza	220	5	37	530	11	5
Kashi Pocket Bread Chicken Rustico						
1 piece	300	8	41	670	18	4
Kashi Pocket Bread Turkey Fiesta						
1 piece	270	6	42	660	15	4
Kashi Pocket Bread Veggie Medley						
1 stuffed bread	280	7	49	570	10	6
Kashi Thin Crust Pizza Margherita						
⅓ pizza	260	9	29	630	14	4
Kashi Thin Crust Pizza Mushroom Trio & Spinach						
⅓ pizza	250	9	28	660	14	4
Kashi Thin Crust Pizza Roasted Vegetable						
⅓ pizza	250	9	28	630	14	4
Lean Cuisine Alfredo Pasta with Chicken & Broccoli						
1 package	300	6	45	660	16	3
Lean Cuisine Angel Hair Pomodoro						
1 package	250	5	42	620	8	4

BRAND/FOOD ITEM SERVING SIZE	CALORIES	FAT	CARBS	SODIUM	PROTEIN	FIBER
Lean Cuisine Asian-Style Pot Stickers						
1 package	260	4	47	530	9	3
Lean Cuisine Baja-Style Chicken Quesadilla						
1 package	280	8	34	690	18	8
Lean Cuisine BBQ Chicken Quesadilla						
1 package	260	7	35	630	16	2
Lean Cuisine Cheddar Potatoes with Broccoli						
1 package	230	5	35	640	12	4
Lean Cuisine Cheese Ravioli						
1 package	220	5	33	620	11	3
Lean Cuisine Chicken Chow Mein with Rice						
1 package	260	4	41	550	14	3
Lean Cuisine Chicken Enchilada Suiza						
1 package	280	5	48	600	10	3
Lean Cuisine Chicken Fettuccini						
1 package	270	6	32	690	22	0
Lean Cuisine Chicken Florentine Lasagna						
1 package	280	6	36	650	20	3
Lean Cuisine Chicken Fried Rice						
1 package	260	5	41	530	12	4
Lean Cuisine Chicken Teriyaki Stir Fry						
1 package	250	2	46	570	12	3
Lean Cuisine Classic Five Cheese Lasagna						
1 package	360	8	51	600	21	4
Lean Cuisine Classic Macaroni & Beef						
1 package	310	9	38	630	20	3
Marie Callender's Beef Pot Pie						
1 cup	510	29	47	780	15	4
Marie Callender's Chicken Pot Pie						
1 pie	640	38	56	1100	16	4
Marie Callender's Turkey Pot Pie						
1 pie	630	35	58	1180	19	4
Morningstar Farms Garden Veggie Patties						
1 pattie	110	3.5	9	350	10	3
Morningstar Farms Grillers Original						
1 burger	130	6	5	260	15	2
Morningstar Farms Maple Flavored Veggie Sausage Patties						
1 pattie	80	3	5	250	10	<1

BRAND/FOOD ITEM SERVING SIZE	CALORIES	FAT	CARBS	SODIUM	PROTEIN	FIBER
Morningstar Farms Sausage Patties						
1 pattie	80	3	3	260	10	1
Morningstar Farms Veggie Bacon Strips						
2 strips	60	4.5	2	230	2	1
Morningstar Farms Veggie Sausage Links						
2 links	80	3	3	300	9	2
Newman's Own Four Cheese Thin & Crispy Pizza						
⅓ pizza	300	13	31	610	16	2
Newman's Own Margherita Thin & Crispy Pizza						
⅓ pizza	280	12	31	650	12	1
Newman's Own Roasted Garlic & Chicken Thin & Crispy Pizza						
⅓ pizza	270	10	31	540	14	2
Newman's Own Supreme Thin & Crispy Pizza						
⅓ pizza	320	15	32	680	14	2
Newman's Own Uncured Pepperoni Thin & Crispy Pizza						
⅓ pizza	320	16	31	680	14	2
Stouffer's Baked Chicken Breast						
1 container	250	10	20	730	20	1
Stouffer's Beef Stroganoff						
1 container	380	17	34	990	22	2
Stouffer's Cheesy Spaghetti Bake						
1 container	460	24	39	950	21	4
Stouffer's Chicken Fettuccini						
1 container	840	38	94	1050	31	5
Stouffer's Fish Filet						
1 container	400	16	36	1050	27	4
Stouffer's Fried Chicken Breast						
1 container	360	18	30	880	20	2
Stouffer's Pork Cutlet						
1 container	370	21	31	1110	13	3
Stouffer's Roasted Chicken						
1 container	460	24	34	990	26	5
Stouffer's Spaghetti with Meat Sauce						
1 container	350	12	44	660	17	5
Stouffer's Veal Parmigiana						
1 container	430	18	46	970	20	5
Stouffer's Vegetable Lasagna						
1 container	390	18	40	730	17	4

BRAND/FOOD ITEM SERVING SIZE	CALORIES	FAT	CARBS	SODIUM	PROTEIN	FIBER

Frozen Fruit

APPLES

Frozen, unsweetened, heated
1 cup sliced

	97	1	25	6	1	4

Frozen, unsweetened, heated, organic
1 cup sliced

	97	1	25	6	1	4

Frozen, unsweetened, unheated
1 cup sliced

	83	1	21	5	0	3

Frozen, unsweetened, unheated, organic
1 cup sliced

	83	1	21	5	0	3

APRICOTS

Frozen, sweetened

1 cup	237	0	61	10	2	5

BLACKBERRIES

Frozen, unsweetened

1 cup	97	1	24	2	2	8

Frozen, unsweetened, organic

1 cup	**97**	**1**	**24**	**2**	**2**	**8**

BLUEBERRIES

Frozen, sweetened
1 cup thawed

	186	0	50	2	1	5

Frozen, unsweetened
1 cup thawed

	79	1	19	2	1	4

Frozen, unsweetened, organic
1 cup thawed

	79	1	19	2	1	4

Wild, frozen

1 cup	71	0	19	4	0	6

Wild, frozen, organic

1 cup	**71**	**0**	**19**	**4**	**0**	**6**

BOYSENBERRIES

Frozen, unsweetened

1 cup	128	1	31	3	3	14

Frozen, unsweetened, organic

1 cup	**128**	**1**	**31**	**3**	**3**	**14**

CHERRIES

Sour, red, frozen, unsweetened

1 cup	71	1	17	2	1	2

Sour, red, frozen, unsweetened, organic

1 cup	**71**	**1**	**17**	**2**	**1**	**2**

Sweet, frozen, sweetened
1 cup thawed

	231	0	58	3	3	5

BRAND/FOOD ITEM SERVING SIZE		CALORIES	FAT	CARBS	SODIUM	PROTEIN	FIBER
LEMONS							
Juice, frozen, unsweetened, single strength							
	1 oz	7	0	2	0	0	0
Juice, frozen, unsweetened, single strength							
	1 cup	54	1	16	2	1	1
Juice, frozen, unsweetened, single strength, organic							
	1 oz	**7**	**0**	**2**	**0**	**0**	**0**
Juice, frozen, unsweetened, single strength, organic							
	1 cup	**54**	**1**	**16**	**2**	**1**	**1**
LOGANBERRIES							
Frozen							
	1 cup	81	0	19	1	2	8
Frozen, organic							
	1 cup	**81**	**0**	**19**	**1**	**2**	**8**
MELONS							
Melon balls, frozen							
	1 cup	57	0	14	54	1	1
Melon balls, frozen, organic							
	1 cup	**57**	**0**	**14**	**54**	**1**	**1**
PEACHES							
Frozen, sliced, sweetened							
	1 cup thawed						
		235	0	60	15	2	4
RASPBERRIES							
Frozen, red, sweetened							
	1 cup	258	0	65	3	2	11
RHUBARB							
Frozen, cooked, with sugar							
	1 cup	278	0	75	2	1	5
Frozen, uncooked							
	1 cup diced						
		29	0	7	3	1	2
Frozen, uncooked, organic							
	1 cup diced						
		29	**0**	**7**	**3**	**1**	**2**
STRAWBERRIES							
Frozen, sweetened, sliced							
	1 cup thawed						
		245	0	66	8	1	5
Frozen, sweetened, whole							
	1 cup thawed						
		199	0	54	3	1	5
Frozen, unsweetened							
	1 cup thawed						
		77	0	20	4	1	5
Frozen, unsweetened							
	1 berry	4	0	1	0	0	0

BRAND/FOOD ITEM SERVING SIZE	CALORIES	FAT	CARBS	SODIUM	PROTEIN	FIBER
Frozen, unsweetened, organic						
1 cup thawed	77	0	20	4	1	5
Frozen, unsweetened, organic						
1 berry	4	0	1	0	0	0
Cascadian Farm Blackberries, Frozen						
1 cup	80	1	22	0	1	7
Cascadian Farm Blueberries, Frozen						
1 cup	70	1	17	0	<1	4
Cascadian Farm Harvest Berries, Frozen						
1 cup	60	1	17	0	1	4
Cascadian Farm Red Raspberries, Frozen						
1 cup	70	0	16	15	1	3
Cascadian Farm Sliced Peaches, Frozen						
1 cup	50	0	14	0	<1	2
Cascadian Farm Strawberries, Frozen						
1 cup	45	0	13	0	<1	3
Cascadian Farm Sweet Cherries, Frozen						
1 cup	90	0	22	0	1	3

Frozen Vegetables

BROCCOLI

Frozen, chopped, boiled, drained, with salt						
1 cup	52	0	10	478	6	6
Frozen, chopped, boiled, drained, with salt, organic						
1 cup	52	0	10	478	6	6
Frozen, chopped, boiled, drained, without salt						
1 cup	52	0	10	20	6	6
Frozen, chopped, boiled, drained, without salt, organic						
1 cup	52	0	10	20	6	6
Frozen, chopped, unprepared						
1 cup	41	0	7	37	4	5
Frozen, chopped, unprepared, organic						
1 cup	41	0	7	37	4	5
Frozen, spears, boiled, drained, with salt						
½ cup	26	0	5	239	3	3
Frozen, spears, boiled, drained, with salt, organic						
½ cup	26	0	5	239	3	3
Frozen, spears, boiled, drained, without salt						
½ cup	26	0	5	22	3	3
Frozen, spears, boiled, drained, without salt, organic						
½ cup	26	0	5	22	3	3
Frozen, spears, unprepared						
1 package (10 oz)	82	1	15	48	9	9
Frozen, spears, unprepared, organic						
1 package (10 oz)	82	1	15	48	9	9

BRAND/FOOD ITEM SERVING SIZE	CALORIES	FAT	CARBS	SODIUM	PROTEIN	FIBER
CARROTS						
Frozen, boiled, drained, with salt						
1 cup sliced	54	1	11	431	1	5
Frozen, boiled, drained, with salt, organic						
1 cup sliced	**54**	**1**	**11**	**431**	**1**	**5**
Frozen, boiled, drained, without salt						
1 cup sliced	54	1	11	86	1	5
Frozen, boiled, drained, without salt, organic						
1 cup sliced	**54**	**1**	**11**	**86**	**1**	**5**
Frozen, unprepared						
½ cup sliced	23	0	5	44	0	2
Frozen, unprepared, organic						
½ cup sliced	**23**	**0**	**5**	**44**	**0**	**2**
CAULIFLOWER						
Frozen, boiled, drained, with salt						
1 cup	31	0	6	457	3	5
Frozen, boiled, drained, with salt, organic						
1 cup	**31**	**0**	**6**	**457**	**3**	**5**
Frozen, boiled, drained, without salt						
1 cup	34	0	7	32	3	5
Frozen, boiled, drained, without salt, organic						
1 cup	**34**	**0**	**7**	**32**	**3**	**5**
Frozen, unprepared						
½ cup	16	0	3	16	1	2
Frozen, unprepared, organic						
½ cup	**16**	**0**	**3**	**16**	**1**	**2**
KALE						
Frozen, boiled, drained, with salt						
1 cup chopped	39	1	7	326	4	3
Frozen, boiled, drained, with salt, organic						
1 cup chopped	**39**	**1**	**7**	**326**	**4**	**3**
Frozen, boiled, drained, without salt						
1 cup chopped	39	1	7	20	4	3
Frozen, boiled, drained, without salt, organic						
1 cup chopped	**39**	**1**	**7**	**20**	**4**	**3**
Frozen, unprepared						
1 package (10 oz)	80	1	14	43	8	6
Frozen, unprepared, organic						
1 package (10 oz)	**80**	**1**	**14**	**43**	**8**	**6**

BRAND/FOOD ITEM SERVING SIZE	CALORIES	FAT	CARBS	SODIUM	PROTEIN	FIBER
MUSTARD GREENS						
Frozen, boiled, drained, with salt						
½ cup chopped or diced	14	0	2	196	2	2
Frozen, boiled, drained, with salt, organic						
½ cup chopped or diced	**14**	**0**	**2**	**196**	**2**	**2**
Frozen, boiled, drained, without salt						
1 cup chopped	29	0	5	38	3	4
Frozen, boiled, drained, without salt, organic						
1 cup chopped	**29**	**0**	**5**	**38**	**3**	**4**
Frozen, unprepared						
1 cup chopped	29	0	5	42	4	5
Frozen, unprepared, organic						
1 cup chopped	**29**	**0**	**5**	**42**	**4**	**5**
ONIONS						
Frozen, chopped, boiled, drained, with salt						
½ cup chopped or diced	27	0	6	260	1	2
Frozen, chopped, boiled, drained, with salt, organic						
½ cup chopped or diced	**27**	**0**	**6**	**260**	**1**	**2**
Frozen, chopped, boiled, drained, without salt						
½ cup chopped or diced	29	0	7	13	1	2
Frozen, chopped, boiled, drained, without salt, organic						
½ cup chopped or diced	**29**	**0**	**7**	**13**	**1**	**2**
Frozen, chopped, unprepared						
1 package (10 oz)	82	0	19	34	2	5
Frozen, chopped, unprepared, organic						
1 package (10 oz)	**82**	**0**	**19**	**34**	**2**	**5**
Frozen, whole, boiled, drained, with salt						
1 cup	55	0	13	512	1	3
Frozen, whole, boiled, drained, with salt, organic						
1 cup	**55**	**0**	**13**	**512**	**1**	**3**
Frozen, whole, boiled, drained, without salt						
1 cup	59	0	14	17	1	3
Frozen, whole, boiled, drained, without salt, organic						
1 cup	**59**	**0**	**14**	**17**	**1**	**3**
Frozen, whole, unprepared						
1 package (10 oz)	99	0	24	28	3	5

BRAND/FOOD ITEM SERVING SIZE	CALORIES	FAT	CARBS	SODIUM	PROTEIN	FIBER
Frozen, whole, unprepared, organic						
1 package (10 oz)	99	0	24	28	3	5

SPINACH

BRAND/FOOD ITEM SERVING SIZE	CALORIES	FAT	CARBS	SODIUM	PROTEIN	FIBER
Frozen, chopped or leaf, boiled, drained, with salt						
½ cup	32	1	5	306	4	4
Frozen, chopped or leaf, boiled, drained, with salt, organic						
½ cup	32	1	5	306	4	4
Frozen, chopped or leaf, boiled, drained, without salt						
½ cup	32	1	5	92	4	4
Frozen, chopped or leaf, boiled, drained, without salt, organic						
½ cup	32	1	5	92	4	4
Frozen, chopped or leaf, unprepared						
1 cup	45	1	7	115	6	5
Frozen, chopped or leaf, unprepared, organic						
1 cup	45	1	7	115	6	5

SQUASH

BRAND/FOOD ITEM SERVING SIZE	CALORIES	FAT	CARBS	SODIUM	PROTEIN	FIBER
Summer, crookneck and straightneck, frozen, boiled, drained						
1 cup sliced	48	0	11	465	2	3
Summer, crookneck and straightneck, frozen, boiled, drained, organic						
1 cup sliced	48	0	11	465	2	3
Summer, crookneck and straightneck, frozen, unprepared						
1 cup sliced	26	0	6	7	1	2
Summer, crookneck and straightneck, frozen, unprepared, organic						
1 cup sliced	26	0	6	7	1	2
Summer, zucchini, includes skin, frozen, boiled, drained, with salt						
1 cup	33	0	7	555	3	1
Summer, zucchini, includes skin, frozen, boiled, drained, with salt, organic						
1 cup	33	0	7	555	3	1
Summer, zucchini, includes skin, frozen, boiled, drained, without salt						
1 cup	38	0	8	4	3	3
Summer, zucchini, includes skin, frozen, boiled, drained, without salt, organic						
1 cup	38	0	8	4	3	3
Summer, zucchini, includes skin, frozen, unprepared						
1 package (10 oz)	48	0	10	6	3	4
Summer, zucchini, includes skin, frozen, unprepared, organic						
1 package (10 oz)	48	0	10	6	3	4
Winter, butternut, frozen, boiled, with salt						
1 cup mashed	94	0	24	571	3	n/a

BRAND/FOOD ITEM SERVING SIZE	CALORIES	FAT	CARBS	SODIUM	PROTEIN	FIBER
Winter, butternut, frozen, boiled, with salt, organic						
1 cup mashed	**94**	**0**	**24**	**571**	**3**	**n/a**
Winter, butternut, frozen, boiled, without salt						
1 cup mashed	94	0	24	5	3	n/a
Winter, butternut, frozen, boiled, without salt, organic						
1 cup mashed	**94**	**0**	**24**	**5**	**3**	**n/a**
Winter, butternut, frozen, unprepared						
1 package (12 oz)	194	0	49	7	6	4
Winter, butternut, frozen, unprepared, organic						
1 package (12 oz)	**194**	**0**	**49**	**7**	**6**	**4**
TURNIP GREENS						
Frozen, boiled, drained, with salt						
½ cup	24	0	4	206	3	3
Frozen, boiled, drained, with salt, organic						
½ cup	**24**	**0**	**4**	**206**	**3**	**3**
Frozen, boiled, drained, without salt						
½ cup	24	0	4	12	3	3
Frozen, boiled, drained, without salt, organic						
½ cup	**24**	**0**	**4**	**12**	**3**	**3**
Cascadian Farm Frozen Bagged Vegetables Broccoli Florets						
⅔ cup	**20**	**0**	**4**	**20**	**2**	**2**
Cascadian Farm Frozen Bagged Vegetables Cut Green Beans						
¾ cup	**30**	**0**	**6**	**0**	**1**	**2**
Cascadian Farm Frozen Bagged Vegetables Edamame Soybeans in the Pod						
⅔ cup	120	5	9	10	10	3
Cascadian Farm Frozen Bagged Vegetables Edamame Soybeans Shelled						
⅔ cup	120	5	9	10	10	3
Cascadian Farm Frozen Bagged Vegetables Peas & Carrots						
⅔ cup	**50**	**0**	**10**	**75**	**2**	**3**
Cascadian Farm Frozen Bagged Vegetables Sweet Corn						
¾ cup	**90**	**1**	**19**	**0**	**3**	**2**
Cascadian Farm Frozen Bagged Vegetables Sweet Peas						
⅔ cup	70	0	12	95	4	4
Cascadian Farm Frozen Boxed Vegetables Asparagus Cuts						
⅔ cup	**20**	**0**	**3**	**85**	**2**	**<1**
Cascadian Farm Frozen Boxed Vegetables Broccoli Florets						
1⅓ cup	20	0	3	120	1	2
Cascadian Farm Frozen Boxed Vegetables Cut Spinach						
⅓ cup	**25**	**0**	**3**	**160**	**2**	**1**
Cascadian Farm Frozen Boxed Vegetables French Green Beans with Almonds						
⅔ cup	60	3	7	190	2	1
Cascadian Farm Frozen Boxed Vegetables Peas & Pearl Onions						
¾ cup	**60**	**0**	**11**	**90**	**3**	**3**

BRAND/FOOD ITEM SERVING SIZE	CALORIES	FAT	CARBS	SODIUM	PROTEIN	FIBER
Cascadian Farm Frozen Boxed Vegetables Petite Whole Green Beans						
1 cup	25	0	5	95	1	2
Cascadian Farm Frozen Boxed Vegetables Sugar Snap Peas						
¾ cup	35	0	6	0	2	2
Cascadian Farm Frozen Boxed Vegetables Super Sweet Corn						
⅔ cup	60	1	11	85	2	2
Cascadian Farm Frozen Boxed Vegetables Winter Squash						
½ cup	50	0	11	0	1	2
Cascadian Farm Frozen Potatoes Country-Style						
¾ cup	50	0	12	10	1	1
Cascadian Farm Frozen Potatoes Crinkle Cut French Fries						
3 oz	130	4	21	15	2	2
Cascadian Farm Frozen Potatoes French Fries Straight Cut						
3 oz	130	4	21	15	2	2
Cascadian Farm Frozen Potatoes Hash Browns						
1 cup	60	0	14	10	2	1
Cascadian Farm Frozen Potatoes Oven Fries Wedge Cut						
3 oz	110	3	21	15	2	2
Cascadian Farm Frozen Potatoes Shoe String Fries						
3 oz	140	5	21	15	2	2
Cascadian Farm Frozen Potatoes Spud Puppies						
3 oz	160	7	23	400	2	2
Cascadian Farm Frozen Purely Steam Broccoli and Carrots						
1½ cups	60	3	8	250	2	3
Cascadian Farm Frozen Purely Steam Garden Vegetable Medley						
1 cup	60	1	12	270	2	1
Cascadian Farm Frozen Purely Steam Petite Sweet Peas						
⅔ cup	50	1	10	90	4	4
Cascadian Farm Frozen Vegetable Blends California-Style Blend						
⅔ cup	25	0	5	25	1	2
Cascadian Farm Frozen Vegetable Blends Chinese Stirfry						
1 cup	25	0	6	15	2	2
Cascadian Farm Frozen Vegetable Blends Gardener's Blend						
¾ cup	50	0	11	35	2	3
Cascadian Farm Frozen Vegetable Blends Mixed Vegetables						
⅔ cup	60	0	12	20	2	2
Cascadian Farm Frozen Vegetable Blends Thai Stirfry						
¾ cup	25	0	5	15	1	2

GRAINS, BREADS, CEREALS, AND PASTA

Grains are a girl's or guy's best friend in these tough economic times. Besides being better for the earth, grain-based vegetarian meals are a hell of a lot cheaper than meat-based meals. Combine grains with legumes, and your protein needs are taken care of—you'll never have to eat another piece of yucky, hormone-riddled meat again.

When it comes to bread, always go for the least refined brands with the fewest ingredients. Choose brands with 100 percent whole wheat and no high-fructose corn syrup or hydrogenated oils. My favorite bread brand is Food for Life's Ezekiel. Check out foodforlife.com to find it in a store near you. If you can't get it in the store, you can have it delivered by online retailers like low-carb.com. It's worth it.

Starting the day with a good high-fiber cereal has been shown to decrease your hunger and calorie intake throughout the day. Luckily, many of the best brands are so minimally processed that they actually qualify for MYM status. Parents, check out the stats on those sugar-bomb cereals you've been giving your kids before school. I know they love their Froot Loops, but that crap will not give them the energy they need; it's essentially like dumping the whole sugar bowl into their mouths. Look for cereals from Health Valley, Arrowhead Mills, Kashi,

Erewhon, Amy's, and Nature's Path—they won't steer you wrong.

And don't forget: A bowl of pasta represents some of the densest concentration of calories and carbs in any foods. I know it's delicious, but please stick to whole grain or legume-based pasta and *watch your portion sizes.*

BRAND/FOOD ITEM SERVING SIZE	CALORIES	FAT	CARBS	SODIUM	PROTEIN	FIBER
Grains						
BARLEY						
Pearled, cooked						
1 cup	193	1	44	5	4	6
Pearled, cooked, organic						
1 cup	**193**	**1**	**44**	**5**	**4**	**6**
BULGUR						
Cooked						
1 cup	151	8	34	9	6	8
Cooked						
1 tbsp	7	0	2	0	0	0
Cooked, organic						
1 cup	**151**	**8**	**34**	**9**	**6**	**8**
COUSCOUS						
Cooked						
1 cup	176	0	36	8	6	2
Cooked, organic						
1 cup	**176**	**0**	**36**	**8**	**6**	**2**
MILLET						
Cooked						
1 cup	207	2	41	3	6	2
Cooked, organic						
1 cup	**207**	**2**	**41**	**3**	**6**	**2**
QUINOA						
Cooked						
1 cup	222	4	39	13	8	5
Cooked, organic						
1 cup	**222**	**4**	**39**	**13**	**8**	**5**
RICE						
Brown, long-grain, cooked						
1 cup	216	2	45	10	5	4

BRAND/FOOD ITEM SERVING SIZE	CALORIES	FAT	CARBS	SODIUM	PROTEIN	FIBER
Brown, long-grain, cooked, organic						
1 cup	216	2	45	10	5	4
Brown, medium-grain, cooked						
1 cup	218	2	46	2	5	4
Brown, medium-grain, cooked, organic						
1 cup	218	2	46	2	5	4
White, long-grain, regular, cooked						
1 cup	205	0	45	2	4	1
White, long-grain, regular, cooked, organic						
1 cup	205	0	45	2	4	1
White, medium-grain, cooked						
1 cup	242	0	53	0	4	1
White, medium-grain, cooked, organic						
1 cup	242	0	53	0	4	1
White, short-grain, cooked						
1 cup	242	0	53	0	4	0
White, short-grain, cooked, organic						
1 cup	242	0	53	0	4	0
Wild rice, cooked						
1 cup	166	1	35	5	7	3
Wild rice, cooked, organic						
1 cup	166	1	35	5	7	3
SPELT						
Cooked						
1 cup	246	2	51	10	11	8
Cooked, organic						
1 cup	246	2	51	10	11	8
WHEAT FLOUR						
Whole grain						
1 cup	407	2	87	6	16	15
Whole grain, organic						
1 cup	407	2	87	6	16	15
Arrowhead Mills Brown Basmati Rice						
¼ cup	140	1.5	31	0	3	2
Arrowhead Mills Long Grain Brown Rice						
¼ cup	160	1	32	0	3	1
Arrowhead Mills Short Grain Brown Rice						
¼ cup	180	1	38	0	4	2
Arrowhead Mills White Basmati Rice						
¼ cup	150	0.5	33	0	3	<1
Eden Foods Organic Buckwheat						
¼ cup uncooked						
	160	1	0	31	5	5
Eden Foods Organic Millet						
¼ cup uncooked						
	160	2	30	5	5	4
Eden Foods Quinoa						
¼ cup	180	3.5	29	10	7	11
Eden Foods Red Quinoa						
¼ cup uncooked						
	170	2	32	5	6	5

BRAND/FOOD ITEM SERVING SIZE	CALORIES	FAT	CARBS	SODIUM	PROTEIN	FIBER
Kashi 7 Whole Grain Pilaf						
½ cup cooked	170	2.5	33	0	6	6
Nature's Path FlaxPlus Flaxseeds						
2 tbsp	110	8	6	5	4	5
RiceSelect Organic Texmati Brown Rice						
¼ cup uncooked	170	1	35	0	4	2
RiceSelect Organic Toasted Almond Pilaf						
¼ cup uncooked	200	2	34	540	4	0
RiceSelect Organic Whole Wheat Couscous						
¼ cup uncooked	210	1	45	0	8	7
RiceSelect Texmati Brown Rice						
¼ cup uncooked	170	1	35	0	4	2

Breads

BRAND/FOOD ITEM SERVING SIZE	CALORIES	FAT	CARBS	SODIUM	PROTEIN	FIBER
French or Vienna (includes sourdough)						
1 slice	185	1	36	416	8	2
Multigrain (includes whole-grain)						
1 slice	69	1	11	109	3	2
Multigrain, toasted (includes whole-grain)						
1 slice	69	1	11	110	3	2
Whole wheat, commercially prepared						
1 slice	69	1	12	132	4	2
Whole wheat, commercially prepared, toasted						
1 slice	76	1	13	146	4	2
Whole wheat, prepared from recipe						
1 slice	128	2	24	159	4	3
Whole wheat, prepared from recipe, toasted						
1 slice	128	2	24	160	4	3
Arnold Country Oat Bran						
1 slice	120	1.5	21	230	4	1
Arnold Flax + Fiber						
1 slice	100	2	21	170	5	5
Arnold Health Nut						
1 slice	120	2	21	220	5	2
Arnold Stone Ground 100% Whole Wheat						
2 slices	130	2	22	260	6	3
Arnold Whole Wheat						
1 slice	110	1	21	220	5	3
English muffins, whole wheat						
1 muffin	134	1	27	312	6	4
Food for Life 7 Sprouted Grains Bread						
1 slice	80	0.5	15	80	4	3
Food for Life Bran for Life Bread						
1 slice	**80**	**1**	**17**	**140**	**4**	**5**

BRAND/FOOD ITEM SERVING SIZE	CALORIES	FAT	CARBS	SODIUM	PROTEIN	FIBER
Food for Life Cinnamon Raisin						
1 slice	80	0	18	65	3	2
Food for Life Ezekiel 4:9 Bread						
1 slice	80	0.5	15	75	4	3
Food for Life Ezekiel 4:9 Bread Sesame						
1 slice	80	0.5	14	80	4	3
Food for Life Ezekiel 4:9 Burger Bun						
1 bun	170	1.5	34	170	9	6
Food for Life Genesis 1:29 English Muffin						
½ muffin	90	2	15	70	4	3
Food for Life Tortilla						
1 slice	150	3.5	24	140	6	5
Oroweat 100% Whole Wheat Bread						
1 slice	90	1	18	190	4	3
Oroweat 100% Whole Wheat English Muffins						
1 muffin	130	1.5	25	240	5	4
Oroweat 100% Whole Wheat Hot Dog Buns						
1 bun	160	2.5	28	320	8	6
Oroweat 100% Whole Wheat Sandwich Rolls						
1 roll	180	3	31	350	8	6
Oroweat Country White Bread						
1 slice	110	1.5	20	240	3	<1
Oroweat Health Nut Bread						
1 slice	100	2	18	190	4	2
Oroweat Jewish Rye Bread						
1 slice	80	1	15	170	3	1
Oroweat Whole Grain & Flax Bread						
1 slice	100	1.5	17	160	4	3
Oroweat Whole Grain & Flax English Muffins						
1 muffin	150	2.5	29	160	5	5
Oroweat Whole Grain & Oat Bread						
1 slice	90	1	17	180	4	3
Oroweat Whole Grain 9 Grain Bread						
1 slice	90	1	17	160	4	3
Pepperidge Farm 100% Natural German Dark Wheat Bread						
1 slice	100	1.5	20	150	4	3
Pepperidge Farm 100% Natural Honey Flax Bread						
1 slice	100	2	19	120	5	3
Pepperidge Farm 100% Natural Nine Grain Bread						
1 slice	100	2	20	130	4	3
Pepperidge Farm Deli Flats 7 Grain Thin Rolls						
1 slice	100	1	19	170	6	5
Pepperidge Farm Deli Flats Soft 100% Whole Wheat Thin Rolls						
1 slice	100	1.5	19	170	6	5
Pepperidge Farm Deli Flats Soft Oatmeal Thin Rolls						
1 slice	100	1.5	20	170	6	5
Pepperidge Farm Whole Grain 100% Whole Wheat Bread						
1 slice	100	1.5	20	105	5	4
Pepperidge Farm Whole Grain 15 Grain Bread						
1 slice	100	2	20	115	5	4
Pepperidge Farm Whole Grain Oatmeal Bread						
1 slice	100	1.5	20	110	4	4

BRAND/FOOD ITEM SERVING SIZE	CALORIES	FAT	CARBS	SODIUM	PROTEIN	FIBER
Pepperidge Farm Whole Grain Soft Honey Oat Bread						
1 slice	100	2	19	115	5	4
Pepperidge Farm Whole Grain Soft Honey Whole Wheat Bread						
1 slice	100	1.5	21	115	4	4
Thomas' English Muffin Cinnamon Raisin						
1 muffin	140	1	29	170	4	1
Thomas' English Muffin Hearty Grain						
1 muffin	150	1	27	160	5	2
Thomas' English Muffin Original						
1 muffin	130	1	26	220	4	2
Thomas' Pita Pocket 100% Whole Wheat						
1 pita	140	1.5	28	320	6	4
Thomas' Pita Pocket White						
1 pita	170	1.5	32	350	5	2
Weight Watchers Pita Pocket						
1 pita	100	1	24	260	7	9
Wonder Whole Grain White						
2 slices	130	2	25	300	6	4

Cereals

BRAND/FOOD ITEM SERVING SIZE	CALORIES	FAT	CARBS	SODIUM	PROTEIN	FIBER
Amy's Cream of Rice Hot Cereal Bowl						
1 bowl	170	1	39	220	2	2
Amy's Multi-Grain Hot Cereal Bowl						
1 bowl	190	1.5	40	300	4	5
Amy's Rolled Oats Hot Cereal Bowl						
1 bowl	220	3.5	42	220	6	5
Amy's Steel-Cut Oats Hot Cereal Bowl						
1 bowl	220	3.5	42	190	6	5
Arrowhead Mills 4 Grain Plus Flax Hot Cereal						
¼ cup	140	1.5	28	0	5	9
Arrowhead Mills Amaranth Flakes Cereal						
1 cup	140	2	26	120	4	3
Arrowhead Mills Ancient Grain Flakes, Granola & Fruit Organic Harvest Apple Cereal						
½ cup	200	4	38	180	4	4
Arrowhead Mills Bear Mush Hot Cereal						
¼ cup	150	1	32	0	5	2
Arrowhead Mills Blueberry 'n Cream Cereal						
½ cup	210	6	36	0	6	4
Arrowhead Mills Bulgur Wheat Cereal						
¼ cup	150	0.5	34	0	5	4
Arrowhead Mills Corn Flakes Cereal						
1 cup	120	0	27	70	2	2
Arrowhead Mills Crunchy Oat Bran with Almonds & Raisins Cereal						
½ cup	210	8	33	0	5	4
Arrowhead Mills Honey Gone Nuts Cereal						
½ cup	240	10	33	0	6	4
Arrowhead Mills Kamut & Cranberries Flakes Cereal						
1 cup	170	1	36	90	5	3

BRAND/FOOD ITEM SERVING SIZE	CALORIES	FAT	CARBS	SODIUM	PROTEIN	FIBER
Arrowhead Mills Kamut Flakes Cereal						
1 cup	120	1	25	70	4	2
Arrowhead Mills Maple Apple Spice Instant Oatmeal Hot Cereal						
1 packet	140	2	26	45	4	3
Arrowhead Mills Maple Buckwheat Flakes Cereal						
1 cup	170	1	35	190	4	1
Arrowhead Mills Mocha Almond Crunch Cereal						
½ cup	210	8	33	40	5	4
Arrowhead Mills Multigrain Flakes Cereal						
1 cup	170	2	33	180	5	3
Arrowhead Mills Oat Bran Flakes Cereal						
1 cup	140	2.5	24	80	5	4
Arrowhead Mills Oat Bran Hot Cereal						
1 packet	130	2.5	21	0	6	4
Arrowhead Mills Oat Flakes Hot Cereal						
1 packet	130	2	23	0	5	4
Arrowhead Mills Old Fashioned Oatmeal Hot Cereal						
1 packet	130	2	23	0	5	4
Arrowhead Mills Organic Cinnamon Raisin Cereal						
½ cup	220	7	39	65	4	4
Arrowhead Mills Organic Instant Oatmeal Hot Cereal with Flax						
1 packet	140	3	24	70	5	4
Arrowhead Mills Organic Vermont Maple Cereal						
½ cup	220	7	34	85	5	4
Arrowhead Mills Original Plain Instant Oatmeal Hot Cereal						
1 packet	110	2	1	0	4	2
Arrowhead Mills Pralines 'n Cream Cereal						
½ cup	210	8	32	45	5	4
Arrowhead Mills Puffed Corn Cereal						
1 cup	60	1	12	5	2	2
Arrowhead Mills Puffed Kamut Cereal						
1 cup	50	0	11	0	3	2
Arrowhead Mills Puffed Millet Cereal						
1 cup	60	0.5	11	0	2	1
Arrowhead Mills Puffed Rice Cereal						
1 cup	60	0	14	50	1	<1
Arrowhead Mills Puffed Wheat Cereal						
1 cup	60	0	12	0	3	2
Arrowhead Mills Raspberry 'n Cream Cereal						
½ cup	220	8	34	0	5	4
Arrowhead Mills Rice and Shine Hot Cereal						
¼ cup	150	1	32	0	3	2
Arrowhead Mills Rice Flakes Sweetened Cereal						
1 cup	180	1	40	190	3	1
Arrowhead Mills Seven Grain Hot Cereal						
⅓ cup	140	1	28	0	8	6
Arrowhead Mills Shredded Wheat Cereal						
½ cup	190	1	38	5	6	6
Arrowhead Mills Spelt & Cranberries Flake Cereal						
1 cup	170	1	35	120	5	4
Arrowhead Mills Spelt Flakes Cereal						
1 cup	120	1	24	100	4	3

BRAND/FOOD ITEM SERVING SIZE	CALORIES	FAT	CARBS	SODIUM	PROTEIN	FIBER
Arrowhead Mills Steel Cut Oats Hot Cereal						
¼ cup	160	3	27	0	6	8
Arrowhead Mills Strawberry 'n Cream Cereal						
½ cup	220	8	34	0	5	4
Arrowhead Mills Supernatural with Almonds & Raisins Cereal						
½ cup	220	8	34	5	5	3
Arrowhead Mills Sweetened Shredded Wheat Cereal						
½ cup	200	1	42	5	5	5
Arrowhead Mills Triple Berry Crunch Cereal						
½ cup	210	8	34	65	5	4
Arrowhead Mills Yellow Corn Grits Hot Cereal						
¼ cup	130	0	30	0	3	1
B&G Cream of Rice						
¼ cup	170	0	36	0	3	0
B&G Cream of Wheat						
3 tbsp	120	0	23	85	4	1
B&G Cream of Wheat Maple Sugar Instant						
1 packet	130	0	28	140	2	1
Barbara's Bakery Puffins Cinnamon Cereal						
⅔ cup	100	1	26	150	2	6
Barbara's Bakery Puffins Multi-Grain Cereal						
¾ cup	110	0	25	80	2	3
Cascadian Farms Cinnamon Crunch						
1 cup	110	2.5	22	105	2	3
Cascadian Farms Cinnamon Raisin Granola						
⅔ cup	210	3	42	200	5	3
Cascadian Farms Clifford Crunch						
1 cup	100	1	25	160	2	5
Cascadian Farms Dark Chocolate Almond Granola						
¾ cup	210	4.5	39	160	4	4
Cascadian Farms Fiber Right Honey Clusters						
1 cup	190	1	44	135	4	9
Cascadian Farms Fruit & Nut Granola						
¾ cup	210	5	38	80	5	3
Cascadian Farms Hearty Morning						
¾ cup	200	2.5	44	360	5	8
Cascadian Farms Honey Nut O's						
1 cup	110	1	25	180	2	3
Cascadian Farms Maple Brown Sugar Granola						
⅔ cup	220	4.5	42	160	5	3
Cascadian Farms Multi Grain Squares						
¾ cup	110	0.5	25	125	3	2
Cascadian Farms Oats & Honey Granola						
⅔ cup	230	6	42	110	5	3
Cascadian Farms Purely O's						
1 cup	110	2	22	250	3	3
Cascadian Farms Raisin Bran						
1 cup	180	1.5	43	310	5	6
Cascadian Farms Vanilla Almond Crunch						
¾ cup	200	2.5	41	200	4	3
Erewhon Apple Cinnamon Instant Oatmeal						
1 packet	130	2	24	100	5	3

BRAND/FOOD ITEM SERVING SIZE	CALORIES	FAT	CARBS	SODIUM	PROTEIN	FIBER
Erewhon Aztec Crunchy Corn & Amaranth Cereal						
1 cup	110	0	26	70	2	1
Erewhon Barley Plus Cereal						
1 packet	170	1	37	0	5	4
Erewhon Brown Rice Cream Cereal						
1 packet	170	1	36	30	5	1
Erewhon Cinnamon, Raisin & Flax Organic Instant Oatmeal						
1 packet	130	2.5	24	100	4	4
Erewhon Cocoa Crispy Brown Rice Cereal						
1 cup	200	1.5	44	190	3	1
Erewhon Corn Flakes						
1 cup	130	0	30	60	3	1
Erewhon Crispy Brown Rice Cereal						
1 cup	110	0	25	180	2	1
Erewhon Crispy Brown Rice Cereal Gluten Free						
1 cup	110	0.5	25	160	2	0
Erewhon Crispy Brown Rice Cereal Salt Free						
1 cup	110	0	25	10	2	1
Erewhon Crispy Brown Rice with Mixed Berries Cereal						
1 cup	120	0.5	27	100	2	1
Erewhon Kamut Flakes						
⅔ cup	110	0	25	75	5	4
Erewhon Maple Spice Instant Oatmeal						
1 packet	130	2	25	100	5	3
Erewhon Organic Instant Oatmeal with Added Oat Bran						
1 packet	130	2.5	25	0	6	4
Erewhon Raisin Bran Cereal						
1 cup	170	1	40	100	5	6
Erewhon Rice Twice Cereal						
¾ cup	120	0	26	60	2	0
Erewhon Strawberry Crisp Cereal						
¾ cup	120	0.5	28	125	2	1
General Mills Apple Cinnamon Cheerios						
¾ cup	120	1.5	25	120	2	1
General Mills Banana Nut Cheerios						
¾ cup	100	1	23	160	1	1
General Mills Basic 4						
1 cup	200	2	43	320	4	3
General Mills Berry Berry Kix						
¾ cup	100	1	22	180	1	1
General Mills Berry Burst Cheerios—Triple Berry						
¾ cup	100	1	22	170	2	2
General Mills Boo Berry						
1 cup	130	1	28	190	1	1
General Mills Cheerios						
1 cup	100	2	20	190	3	3
General Mills Cheerios Oat Cluster Crunch						
¾ cup	100	1	22	135	2	2
General Mills Chex Chocolate						
¾ cup	130	2.5	26	240	2	<1
General Mills Chex Cinnamon						
¾ cup	120	2	25	190	2	7

BRAND/FOOD ITEM SERVING SIZE	CALORIES	FAT	CARBS	SODIUM	PROTEIN	FIBER
General Mills Chex Corn						
1 cup	120	0.5	26	290	2	1
General Mills Chex Honey Nut						
¾ cup	120	0.5	28	230	2	1
General Mills Chex Multi Bran						
¾ cup	160	1.5	39	310	3	6
General Mills Chex Rice						
1 cup	100	0	23	250	2	0
General Mills Chex Strawberry						
¾ cup	130	2	26	200	1	<1
General Mills Chex Wheat						
¾ cup	160	1	38	340	5	7
General Mills Chocolate Lucky Charms						
¾ cup	110	1	24	160	1	1
General Mills Cinnamon Toast Crunch						
¾ cup	130	3	25	220	1	1
General Mills Cocoa Puffs						
¾ cup	110	1.5	23	150	1	1
General Mills Cookie Crisp						
¾ cup	100	1	22	150	1	1
General Mills Cookie Crisp Double Chocolate						
¾ cup	120	1.5	26	140	1	1
General Mills Count Chocula						
¾ cup	110	1	23	160	1	1
General Mills Country Corn Flakes						
1 cup	120	0.5	28	300	2	1
General Mills Dora The Explorer						
¾ cup	100	1.5	23	180	1	3
General Mills Fiber One						
½ cup	60	1	25	105	2	14
General Mills Fiber One Caramel Delight						
1 cup	180	3	41	260	3	9
General Mills Fiber One Frosted Shredded Wheat						
1 cup	200	1	50	0	5	9
General Mills Fiber One Honey Clusters						
1 cup	160	1.5	42	290	5	13
General Mills Fiber One Raisin Bran Clusters						
1 cup	160	1.5	42	290	5	13
General Mills Franken Berry						
1 cup	130	1.5	28	190	1	1
General Mills Frosted Cheerios						
¾ cup	110	1	23	170	2	2
General Mills Fruity Cheerios						
¾ cup	100	1.5	23	135	1	2
General Mills Golden Grahams						
¾ cup	120	1	26	270	2	1
General Mills Honey Kix						
1¼ cup	120	1	28	230	2	3
General Mills Honey Nut Cheerios						
¾ cup	110	1.5	22	190	2	2
General Mills Honey Nut Clusters						
1 cup	210	1	49	290	4	3

BRAND/FOOD ITEM SERVING SIZE	CALORIES	FAT	CARBS	SODIUM	PROTEIN	FIBER
General Mills Kaboom						
1¼ cup	110	1	28	210	1	4
General Mills Kix						
1¼ cup	110	1	26	210	2	3
General Mills Lucky Charms						
¾ cup	110	1	22	190	2	1
General Mills Multi Grain Cheerios						
1 cup	110	1	23	160	2	3
General Mills Oatmeal Crisp Crunchy Almond						
1 cup	240	4.5	47	130	6	4
General Mills Oatmeal Crisp Hearty Raisin						
1 cup	230	2.5	51	135	5	4
General Mills Raisin Nut Bran						
¾ cup	180	3	38	230	4	5
General Mills Reese's Puffs						
¾ cup	120	3	22	180	2	1
General Mills Sprinkles Cookies Crisp						
¾ cup	100	1	23	150	1	1
General Mills Strawberry Yogurt Burst Cheerios						
¾ cup	120	1.5	24	180	2	2
General Mills Total						
¾ cup	100	0.5	23	190	2	3
General Mills Total Blueberry Pomegranate						
1 cup	170	2	38	95	5	4
General Mills Total Cinnamon Crunch						
1 cup	190	2.5	40	200	4	4
General Mills Total Cranberry Crunch						
1¼ cup	190	1.5	44	230	4	4
General Mills Total Honey Clusters						
¾ cup	170	1	38	230	3	3
General Mills Total Raisin Bran						
1 cup	160	1	40	230	3	5
General Mills Trix						
1 cup	120	1	28	190	1	1
General Mills Vanilla Yogurt Burst Cheerios						
¾ cup	120	1.5	24	180	2	2
General Mills Wheaties						
¾ cup	100	0.5	22	190	3	3
Health Valley Corn Crunch-Ems! Cereal						
1 cup	**110**	**0**	**27**	**160**	**4**	**2**
Health Valley Cranberry Crunch Cereal						
¾ cup	190	4	38	100	4	3
Health Valley Heart Wise Cereal						
1 cup	200	3	37	140	11	5
Health Valley Low Fat Date Almond Flavor Granola						
⅔ cup	**180**	**1**	**43**	**90**	**5**	**6**
Health Valley Low Fat Raisin Cinnamon Granola						
⅔ cup	180	1	43	90	5	6
Health Valley Organic Amaranth Flakes						
1 cup	**100**	**1**	**23**	**90**	**3**	**3**
Health Valley Organic Blue Corn Flakes						
¾ cup	**100**	**0**	**24**	**10**	**3**	**3**

BRAND/FOOD ITEM SERVING SIZE	CALORIES	FAT	CARBS	SODIUM	PROTEIN	FIBER
Health Valley Organic Fiber 7 Cereal						
1 cup	**160**	**1**	**37**	**100**	**6**	**7**
Health Valley Organic Golden Flax Cereal						
1 cup	190	3.5	37	65	6	6
Health Valley Organic Multigrain Apple Cinnamon Square-Ems Cereal						
1¼ cups	210	3	44	125	5	8
Health Valley Organic Multigrain Maple Honey Nut Square-Ems Cereal						
1¼ cups	210	3	44	125	5	8
Health Valley Organic Oat Bran Flakes						
1 cup	**190**	**1.5**	**39**	**190**	**5**	**4**
Health Valley Organic Oat Bran Flakes with Raisins						
1 cup	200	1.5	43	160	5	4
Health Valley Real Oat Bran Almond Crunch Cereal						
½ cup	**200**	**3**	**34**	**90**	**6**	**5**
Health Valley Rice Crunch-Ems! Cereal						
1 cup	**110**	**0**	**26**	**150**	**4**	**2**
Kashi 7 Whole Grain Flakes Cereal						
1 cup	180	1	41	150	6	6
Kashi 7 Whole Grain Nuggets Cereal						
½ cup	210	1.5	47	260	7	7
Kashi 7 Whole Grain Puffs						
1 cup	70	0.5	15	0	2	1
Kashi Apple Orchard Granola						
½ cup	220	7	38	130	6	7
Kashi GoLean Cereal						
1 cup	140	1	30	85	13	10
Kashi GoLean Crunch! Cereal						
1 cup	190	3	37	100	9	8
Kashi GoLean Crunch! Honey Almond Flax Cereal						
1 cup	200	4.5	36	140	9	8
Kashi GoLean Instant Hot Cereal Hearty						
1 packet	150	2	26	100	8	5
Kashi GoLean Instant Hot Cereal Truly Vanilla						
1 packet	150	2	25	100	9	7
Kashi Good Friends Cereal						
1 cup	160	1.5	42	110	5	12
Kashi Good Friends Cinna-Raisin Crunch Cereal						
1 cup	170	1.5	41	105	4	8
Kashi Granola Cocoa Beach Cereal						
½ cup	230	9	36	140	6	7
Kashi Granola Mountain Medley Cereal						
½ cup	220	7	38	120	6	7
Kashi Granola Summer Berry Cereal						
½ cup	220	6	39	150	6	7
Kashi Heart to Heart Honey Toasted Oat Cereal						
¾ cup	120	1.5	25	85	4	5
Kashi Heart to Heart Oat Flakes & Wild Blueberry Clusters Cereal						
1 cup	200	2	44	135	6	4
Kashi Heart to Heart Oatmeal Golden Brown Maple Cereal						
1 packet	160	2	33	100	4	5
Kashi Heart to Heart Warm Cinnamon Oat Cereal						
¾ cup	110	1.5	24	80	4	5

BRAND/FOOD ITEM SERVING SIZE	CALORIES	FAT	CARBS	SODIUM	PROTEIN	FIBER
Kashi Honey Sunshine Cereal						
¾ cup	100	1.5	25	135	2	6
Kashi Mighty Bites Honey Crunch Cereal						
1 cup	120	1.5	23	160	5	3
Kashi Organic Promise Autumn Wheat Cereal						
29 biscuits						
	180	1	43	0	6	6
Kashi Organic Promise Cinnamon Harvest						
28 biscuits						
	180	1	43	0	6	5
Kashi Organic Promise Island Vanilla Cereal						
27 biscuits						
	190	1	44	5	6	6
Kashi Organic Promise Strawberry Fields Cereal						
1 cup	120	0	28	200	2	1
Kellogg's All-Bran Original Cereal						
1 cup	80	1	23	80	4	10
Kellogg's Apple Jacks						
1 cup	100	0.5	25	130	1	3
Kellogg's Cocoa Krispies						
¾ cup	120	1	27	150	1	<1
Kellogg's Froot Loops						
¾ cup	110	1	22	190	2	1
Kellogg's Frosted Flakes						
¾ cup	110	0	27	140	1	1
Kellogg's Raisin Bran Cereal						
1 cup	190	1.5	45	350	5	7
Kellogg's Smart Start Cereal						
1 cup	190	0.5	43	280	3	3
Malt-O-Meal Creamy Hot Wheat Cereal						
3 tbsp dry	130	0	27	0	4	1
Malt-O-Meal Maple & Brown Sugar Hot Wheat Cereal						
¼ cup dry	170	0	37	0	4	1
Malt-O-Meal Original Hot Wheat Cereal						
3 tbsp dry						
	130	0.5	27	0	5	1
Nature's Path Açai Apple Granola						
¾ cup	240	8	39	170	5	4
Nature's Path Agave Plus Granola						
¾ cup	250	9	37	95	6	4
Nature's Path Apple Cinnamon Oatmeal						
1 packet	210	2.5	40	100	5	4
Nature's Path Corn Puffs Cereal						
1 cup	60	0	12	0	2	1
Nature's Path Crispy Rice Cereal						
¾ cup	110	1.5	24	160	2	2
Nature's Path Crunchy Maple Sunrise Cereal						
⅔ cup	110	1	25	130	2	3
Nature's Path Crunchy Vanilla Sunrise Cereal						
⅔ cup	110	1	25	130	2	3
Nature's Path Flax Plus Flakes Cereal						
¾ cup	110	1.5	23	135	4	5

BRAND/FOOD ITEM SERVING SIZE	CALORIES	FAT	CARBS	SODIUM	PROTEIN	FIBER
Nature's Path Flax Plus Maple Pecan Crunch Cereal						
⅔ cup	220	7	38	190	6	5
Nature's Path Flax Plus Oatmeal						
1 packet	**210**	**3**	**38**	**140**	**6**	**5**
Nature's Path Flax Plus Pumpkin Raisin Crunch Cereal						
¾ cup	210	4.5	40	150	6	7
Nature's Path Flax Plus Raisin Bran Flakes						
¾ cup	190	2.5	41	190	6	8
Nature's Path Flax Plus Red Berry Crunch Cereal						
¾ cup	220	4.5	41	170	6	7
Nature's Path Fruit Juice Sweetened Corn Flakes						
¾ cup	**110**	**0**	**24**	**150**	**2**	**2**
Nature's Path Gorilla Munch Cereal						
¾ cup	**120**	**0**	**27**	**110**	**2**	**2**
Nature's Path Hemp Plus Granola						
¾ cup	260	10	36	35	6	5
Nature's Path Hemp Plus Oatmeal						
1 packet	**160**	**2.5**	**30**	**105**	**5**	**4**
Nature's Path Heritage Flakes Cereal						
¾ cup	**120**	**1**	**24**	**130**	**4**	**5**
Nature's Path Honey'd Corn Flakes						
¾ cup	**120**	**0**	**26**	**140**	**2**	**2**
Nature's Path Kamut Puffs Cereal						
1 cup	**50**	**0**	**11**	**0**	**2**	**2**
Nature's Path Koala Crisp Cereal						
¾ cup	**110**	**1**	**25**	**100**	**2**	**2**
Nature's Path Maple Nut Oatmeal						
1 packet	**210**	**4**	**38**	**100**	**5**	**4**
Nature's Path Mesa Sunrise Flakes Cereal						
¾ cup	**120**	**1**	**24**	**125**	**3**	**3**
Nature's Path Millet Puffs Cereal						
1 cup	**50**	**0**	**14**	**0**	**2**	**1**
Nature's Path Millet Rice Flakes Cereal						
¾ cup	**120**	**2**	**22**	**115**	**4**	**3**
Nature's Path Multigrain Oatbran Flakes Cereal						
¾ cup	**110**	**1**	**24**	**110**	**4**	**5**
Nature's Path MultiGrain Raisin Spice Oatmeal						
1 packet	180	1	39	100	4	4
Nature's Path Optimum Banana Almond Cereal						
¾ cup	190	6	35	140	10	5
Nature's Path Optimum Blueberry Cinnamon Cereal						
1 cup	200	3	38	230	9	7
Nature's Path Optimum Cinnamon Blueberry Flaxseed Oatmeal						
1 packet	150	2.5	29	115	9	3
Nature's Path Optimum Cranberry Ginger Cereal						
¾ cup	190	2.5	41	95	5	8
Nature's Path Optimum Cranberry Ginger Oatmeal						
1 packet	150	2	30	160	5	3
Nature's Path Optimum Slim Cereal						
1 cup	210	2	40	290	9	9
Nature's Path Optimum Strawberry & Yogurt Cereal						
1 cup	170	3	40	190	5	7

BRAND/FOOD ITEM SERVING SIZE	CALORIES	FAT	CARBS	SODIUM	PROTEIN	FIBER
Nature's Path Original Oatmeal						
1 packet	210	3.5	37	160	7	6
Nature's Path Peanut Butter Granola						
¾ cup	260	11	35	75	7	4
Nature's Path Pomegran Plus Granola						
¾ cup	250	9	38	60	5	4
Nature's Path Pumpkin Flax Plus Granola						
¾ cup	260	10	37	45	6	5
Nature's Path Rice Puffs Cereal						
1 cup	50	0	14	0	1	1
Nature's Path Shredded Heritage Bites Cereal						
¾ cup	110	0.5	24	160	3	5
Nature's Path Shredded Oaty Bites Cereal						
¾ cup	120	1	25	140	2	2
Nature's Path SmartBran Cereal						
⅔ cup	90	1	24	130	3	13
Nature's Path Synergy 8 Grain Flakes Cereal						
¾ cup	100	1	24	0	3	5
Nature's Path Vanilla Almond Flax Plus Granola						
¾ cup	250	9	36	80	6	5
Nature's Path Whole O's Cereal						
⅔ cup	110	1.5	25	115	2	3
Newman's Own Sweet Enough Flakes'N Strawberries Cereal						
¾ cup	100	0.5	25	130	2	2
Newman's Own Sweet Enough Honey Flax Flakes Cereal						
¾ cup	100	0.5	24	80	3	4
Newman's Own Sweet Enough Honey Nut O's Cereal						
¾ cup	100	1.5	22	170	3	<1
Newman's Own Sweet Enough Vanilla Almond Cereal						
¾ cup	110	0.5	25	130	2	2
Post Bran Flakes						
¾ cup	100	0.5	24	220	3	5
Post Cocoa Pebbles						
¾ cup	120	1	26	190	1	0
Post Frosted Shredded Wheat						
1 cup	180	1	43	0	4	5
Post Fruity Pebbles						
¾ cup	120	1	26	190	1	0
Post Grape-Nuts						
½ cup	200	1	48	290	6	7
Post Honey Bunches of Oats						
¾ cup	120	1.5	25	150	2	2
Post Honeycomb						
1½ cups	120	1.5	27	180	2	2
Post Raisin Bran						
1 cup	190	1	46	300	4	8
Post Selects Banana Nut Crunch						
1 cup	240	6	44	230	5	4
Post Shredded Wheat						
1 cup	160	1	40	0	5	6
Quaker Cinnamon Swirl High Fiber Instant Oatmeal						
1 packet	180	2	34	210	7	10

BRAND/FOOD ITEM SERVING SIZE	CALORIES	FAT	CARBS	SODIUM	PROTEIN	FIBER
Quaker Life Cereal						
¾ cup	120	1.5	25	160	3	2
Quaker Maple & Brown Sugar Lower Sugar Instant Oatmeal						
1 packet	120	2	24	290	4	3
Quaker Oatmeal Squares, Brown Sugar, Cereal						
1 cup	210	2.5	44	250	6	5
Quaker Organic Instant Oatmeal						
1 packet	**100**	**2**	**19**	**0**	**4**	**3**
Quaker Quick Oats						
½ cup	150	3	27	0	5	4
Quaker Steel Cut Oats						
¼ cup	150	2.5	27	0	5	4
Quaker Take Heart Instant Oatmeal, Golden Maple						
1 packet	160	2.5	33	110	4	5
Quaker Weight Control Instant Oatmeal, Maple & Brown Sugar						
1 packet	160	3	29	310	7	6
U.S. Mills Farina Cream of Wheat Cereal						
3 tbsp	120	0	22	0	3	<1

Pasta

MACARONI
Cooked, enriched, elbow shaped						
1 cup	221	1	43	1	8	3
Cooked, enriched, elbow shaped, organic						
1 cup	221	1	43	1	8	3
Cooked, enriched, small shells						
1 cup	182	1	35	1	7	2
Cooked, enriched, small shells, organic						
1 cup	182	1	35	1	7	2
Cooked, enriched, spiral shaped						
1 cup	212	1	41	1	8	2
Cooked, enriched, spiral shaped, organic						
1 cup	212	1	41	1	8	2
Whole-wheat, cooked, elbow shaped						
1 cup	174	1	37	4	7	4
Whole-wheat, cooked, elbow shaped, organic						
1 cup	174	1	37	4	7	4

SPAGHETTI
Cooked, enriched, without added salt						
1 cup	221	1	43	1	8	3
Cooked, enriched, without added salt, organic						
1 cup	221	1	43	1	8	3
Whole-wheat, cooked						
1 cup	174	1	37	4	7	6
Whole-wheat, cooked, organic						
1 cup	174	1	37	4	7	6
Barilla Angel Hair						
2 oz	200	1	42	0	7	2
Barilla Plus Penne						
2 oz	210	2	38	25	10	4

BRAND/FOOD ITEM SERVING SIZE	CALORIES	FAT	CARBS	SODIUM	PROTEIN	FIBER
Barilla Plus Rotini						
2 oz	210	2	38	25	10	4
Barilla Plus Spaghetti						
2 oz	210	2	38	25	10	4
Barilla Rotini						
2 oz	200	1	42	0	7	2
Barilla Spaghetti						
2 oz	200	1	42	0	7	2
Barilla Tri-Color Rotini						
2 oz	200	1	42	0	7	2
De Cecco Capellini						
2 oz	200	1	41	0	7	2
De Cecco Elbows						
2 oz	200	1	41	0	7	2
De Cecco Fettuccine						
2 oz	200	1	41	0	7	2
De Cecco Linguine						
2 oz	200	1	41	0	7	2
De Cecco Penne						
2 oz	200	1	41	0	7	2
De Cecco Spaghetti						
2 oz	200	1	41	0	7	2
De Cecco Whole Grain Angel Hair						
2 oz	180	1.5	35	0	8	7
De Cecco Whole Grain Fusilli						
2 oz	180	1.5	35	0	8	7
De Cecco Whole Grain Linguini						
2 oz	180	1.5	35	0	8	7
De Cecco Whole Grain Spaghetti						
2 oz	180	1.5	35	0	8	7
De Cecco Ziti						
2 oz	200	1	41	0	7	2
Eden Foods Brown Rice Udon						
2 oz	190	1	38	510	8	2
Eden Foods Harusame Pasta						
2 oz	190	0	47	5	0	0
Eden Foods Japanese Bifun (Rice) Pasta						
2 oz	200	0.5	44	5	5	0
Eden Foods Kuzu Pasta						
2 oz	200	0	48	0	0	2
Eden Foods Lotus Root Soba						
2 oz	190	1	37	470	9	4
Eden Foods Mugwort Soba						
2 oz	190	0.5	37	550	8	2
Eden Foods Organic Artichoke Ribbons Pasta						
½ cup	210	1.5	40	10	9	2
Eden Foods Organic Kamut & Buckwheat Rigatoni						
½ cup	200	1.5	39	10	9	5
Eden Foods Organic Kamut & Quinoa Twisted Pair						
½ cup	210	2	40	0	8	5
Eden Foods Organic Kamut Ditalini						
½ cup	210	1.5	38	0	10	6

BRAND/FOOD ITEM SERVING SIZE	CALORIES	FAT	CARBS	SODIUM	PROTEIN	FIBER
Eden Foods Organic Kamut Elbows						
½ cup	210	1.5	38	0	10	6
Eden Foods Organic Kamut Soba						
½ cup	200	1	38	120	7	3
Eden Foods Organic Kamut Spaghetti						
½ cup	210	1.5	38	0	10	6
Eden Foods Organic Kamut Udon						
½ cup	200	1.5	37	120	10	3
Eden Foods Organic Kamut Vegetable Spirals						
½ cup	210	2	40	45	8	6
Eden Foods Organic Parsley Garlic Ribbons Pasta						
½ cup	210	1.5	40	0	9	3
Eden Foods Organic Saffron Ribbons Pasta						
½ cup	210	1.5	40	0	9	3
Eden Foods Organic Spelt & Buckwheat Gemelli						
½ cup	210	2	41	15	6	4
Eden Foods Organic Spelt Ribbons						
½ cup	210	2	41	10	7	5
Eden Foods Organic Spelt Spaghetti						
½ cup	210	2	41	10	7	5
Eden Foods Organic Spelt Ziti Rigati						
½ cup	210	2	41	10	7	5
Eden Foods Organic Vegetable Ribbons Pasta						
½ cup	210	1.5	40	0	9	3
Eden Foods Organic Vegetable Shells						
½ cup	200	1	40	0	8	2
Eden Foods Organic Vegetable Spirals						
½ cup	200	1	40	0	8	2
Eden Foods Soba 100% Buckwheat Pasta						
2 oz	200	1	43	5	6	3
Eden Foods Udon						
2 oz	190	1.5	37	660	8	3
Eden Foods Wheat & Rice Udon						
½ cup	200	2	38	120	8	3
Eden Foods Wild Yam Soba						
2 oz	190	0.5	37	510	9	2
RiceSelect Original Orzo ⅓ cup uncooked	210	1	42	0	7	2
Ronzoni Acini Di Pepe						
2 oz	210	1	42	0	7	2
Ronzoni Alphabets						
2 oz	210	1	42	0	7	2
Ronzoni Angel Hair						
2 oz	210	1	42	0	7	2
Ronzoni Bow Ties						
2 oz	210	1	42	0	7	2
Ronzoni Capellini						
2 oz	210	1	42	0	7	2
Ronzoni Healthy Harvest 7 Grain Fusilli						
2 oz	180	2	40	0	8	5

BRAND/FOOD ITEM SERVING SIZE	CALORIES	FAT	CARBS	SODIUM	PROTEIN	FIBER
Ronzoni Healthy Harvest 7 Grain Spaghetti						
2 oz	180	2	40	0	8	5
Ronzoni Healthy Harvest Whole Wheat Lasagna						
2 oz	180	2	41	0	7	6
Ronzoni Healthy Harvest Whole Wheat Linguini						
2 oz	180	2	41	0	7	6
Ronzoni Healthy Harvest Whole Wheat Penne Rigate						
2 oz	180	2	41	0	7	6
Ronzoni Healthy Harvest Whole Wheat Rotini						
2 oz	180	2	41	0	7	6
Ronzoni Healthy Harvest Whole Wheat Wide Noodle						
2 oz	180	1	41	15	8	7
Ronzoni Jumbo Shells						
2 oz	210	1	42	0	7	2
Ronzoni Orzo						
2 oz	210	1	42	0	7	2
Ronzoni Tri Color Rotini						
2 oz	210	1	42	0	7	2
Ronzoni Ziti						
2 oz	210	1	42	0	7	2
San Giorgio Pastina						
2 oz	210	1	42	0	7	2

MEAT, FISH, AND EGGS

In fruits and vegetables, choosing organic is a huge plus. In meat and eggs, it is essential. Seriously, *do not even consider* putting nonorganic meat or eggs into your body—you're basically ingesting every single hormone, antibiotic, and pesticide that that animal has eaten in its entire life and possibly the *other* animals that were ground up and fed to it, too. Ewww. Organic, free-range beef (grass-fed), poultry, and eggs are more nutritious and have higher counts of heart-healthy, inflammation-reducing omega-3 fatty acids. Even their trans fats could have health benefits. While there is no such thing as organic fish—yet—some fish are less toxic with heavy-metal contamination than others. Consult Seafood Safety on page 150 to pick the best ones, and stick with the bolded options.

BRAND/FOOD ITEM SERVING SIZE	CALORIES	FAT	CARBS	SODIUM	PROTEIN	FIBER

Meat, Fish, and Eggs

BEEF

Chuck, Denver cut, steak, trimmed to 0" fat, choice, lean only, grilled

	CALORIES	FAT	CARBS	SODIUM	PROTEIN	FIBER
3 oz	193	11	0	75	22	0

Chuck, Denver Cut, steak, trimmed to 0" fat, choice, lean only, grilled, organic

3 oz	193	11	0	75	22	0

Chuck, shoulder clod, shoulder tender, medallion, trimmed to 0" fat, choice, lean only, grilled

3 oz	56	7	0	51	22	0

SEAFOOD SAFETY

Many fish are excellent sources of omega-3s, but you do have to watch out for heavy metals and other toxicity. Because many environmental toxins are absorbed into the fish's fatty tissues, when we eat them, we become the unhappy recipients of every bad chemical the fish has been exposed to. Toxins in fish include exogenous estrogens, PCBs, dioxins, and other pollutants that affect our hormone levels and raise cancer risk. Keep yourself safe by choosing fish that are raised or harvested safely and sustainably. The folks at Seafood Watch at the Monterey Bay Aquarium have created great regional seafood guides (www.mbayaq.org)—check out the best choices, for both environmental and health reasons, in your area.

Here are my suggestions for the best and worst choices for fish.

Go with These	Stay Away from These
Abalone	Atlantic cod
Alaska wild salmon	Atlantic flounder or sole
(fresh, frozen, or canned)	Blue and king crab
Anchovies	Bluefin tuna
Atlantic char	Bluefish
Atlantic herring	Chilean sea bass
Atlantic mackerel	Croaker
Barramundi	Eel
(U.S. farmed, not imported)	Grouper
Black sea bass	King mackerel
Clams (steamers)	Lingcod
Halibut	Marlin
Oysters (farmed)	Orange roughy
Pacific cod	Pacific roughy
Pacific halibut	Shad
Pacific pollock	Shark
Pacific rockfish	Summer and winter flounder
Rainbow trout (farmed)	Swordfish
Sablefish	Wahoo
Sardines	White sea bass
Snapper	Wild striped bass
Stone, Kona,	
and Dungeness crab	
Tilefish	

BRAND/FOOD ITEM SERVING SIZE	CALORIES	FAT	CARBS	SODIUM	PROTEIN	FIBER
Chuck, shoulder clod, shoulder tender, medallion, trimmed to 0" fat, choice, lean only, grilled, organic						
3 oz	**56**	**7**	**0**	**51**	**22**	**0**
Chuck, shoulder top and center, steak, trimmed to 0" fat, choice, lean only, grilled						
3 oz	157	7	0	50	22	0
Chuck, shoulder top and center, steak, trimmed to 0" fat, choice, lean only, grilled, organic						
3 oz	**157**	**7**	**0**	**50**	**22**	**0**
Flank, steak, trimmed to 0" fat, choice, lean only, broiled						
3 oz	165	7	0	48	24	0
Flank, steak, trimmed to 0" fat, choice, lean only, broiled, organic						
3 oz	**165**	**7**	**0**	**48**	**24**	**0**
Ground, 95% lean meat / 5% fat, crumbled, pan-browned						
3 oz	164	6	0	72	25	0
Ground, 95% lean meat / 5% fat, crumbled, pan-browned, organic						
3 oz	**164**	**6**	**0**	**72**	**25**	**0**
Ground, 95% lean meat / 5% fat, loaf, baked						
3 oz	148	5	0	49	23	0
Ground, 95% lean meat / 5% fat, loaf, baked, organic						
3 oz	**148**	**5**	**0**	**49**	**23**	**0**
Ground, 95% lean meat / 5% fat, patty, broiled						
3 oz	145	6	0	55	22	0
Ground, 95% lean meat / 5% fat, patty, broiled, organic						
3 oz	**145**	**6**	**0**	**55**	**22**	**0**
Ground, 95% lean meat / 5% fat, patty, pan-broiled						
3 oz	139	5	0	60	22	0
Ground, 95% lean meat / 5% fat, patty, pan-broiled, organic						
3 oz	**139**	**5**	**0**	**60**	**22**	**0**
Loin, tenderloin, steak, trimmed to ⅛" fat, choice, lean only, broiled						
3 oz	175	8	0	51	25	0
Loin, tenderloin, steak, trimmed to ⅛" fat, choice, lean only, broiled, organic						
3 oz	**175**	**8**	**0**	**51**	**25**	**0**
Loin, top sirloin, steak, trimmed to ⅛" fat, choice, lean only, broiled						
3 oz	159	6	0	52	25	0
Loin, top sirloin, steak, trimmed to ⅛" fat, choice, lean only, broiled, organic						
3 oz	**159**	**6**	**0**	**52**	**25**	**0**
Loin, tri-tip, roast, trimmed to 0" fat, choice, lean only, roasted						
3 oz	164	8	0	46	22	0
Loin, tri-tip, roast, trimmed to 0" fat, choice, lean only, roasted, organic						
3 oz	**164**	**8**	**0**	**46**	**22**	**0**
Round, outside round, steak, trimmed to 0" fat, choice, lean only, grilled						
3 oz	162	7	0	48	23	0
Round, outside round, steak, trimmed to 0" fat, choice, lean only, grilled, organic						
3 oz	**162**	**7**	**0**	**48**	**23**	**0**
Round, tip round, roast, trimmed to 0" fat, choice, lean only, roasted						
3 oz	150	5	0	31	24	0

BRAND/FOOD ITEM SERVING SIZE	CALORIES	FAT	CARBS	SODIUM	PROTEIN	FIBER
Round, tip round, roast, trimmed to 0" fat, choice, lean only, roasted, organic						
3 oz	**150**	**5**	**0**	**31**	**24**	**0**
CHICKEN						
Broilers or fryers, back, meat only, fried						
½ back, bone and skin removed						
	167	9	3	57	17	0
Broilers or fryers, back, meat only, roasted						
½ back, bone and skin removed						
	96	5	0	38	11	0
Broilers or fryers, back, meat only, roasted, organic						
½ back, bone and skin removed						
	96	**5**	**0**	**38**	**11**	**0**
Broilers or fryers, back, meat only, stewed						
½ back, bone and skin removed						
	88	5	0	28	11	0
Broilers or fryers, back, meat only, stewed, organic						
½ back, bone and skin removed						
	88	**5**	**0**	**28**	**11**	**0**
Broilers or fryers, breast, meat only, fried						
½ breast, bone and skin removed						
	161	4	0	68	29	0
Broilers or fryers, breast, meat only, roasted						
½ breast, bone and skin removed						
	142	3	0	64	27	0
Broilers or fryers, breast, meat only, roasted, organic						
½ breast, bone and skin removed						
	142	**3**	**0**	**64**	**27**	**0**
Broilers or fryers, breast, meat only, rotisserie, original seasoning						
½ breast, bone and skin removed						
	127	3	0	293	25	0
Broilers or fryers, breast, meat only, rotisserie, original seasoning, organic						
½ breast, bone and skin removed						
	127	**3**	**0**	**293**	**25**	**0**
Broilers or fryers, breast, meat only, stewed						
½ breast, bone and skin removed						
	143	3	0	60	28	0
Broilers or fryers, breast, meat only, stewed						
1 cup chopped or diced						
	211	4	0	88	41	0
Broilers or fryers, breast, meat only, stewed, organic						
½ breast, bone and skin removed						
	143	**3**	**0**	**60**	**28**	**0**
Broilers or fryers, breast, meat only, stewed, organic						
1 cup chopped or diced						
	211	**4**	**0**	**88**	**41**	**0**
Broilers or fryers, dark meat, meat only, fried						
1 cup	335	16	4	136	41	0
Broilers or fryers, dark meat, meat only, roasted						
1 cup chopped or diced						
	287	14	0	130	38	0

BRAND/FOOD ITEM SERVING SIZE	CALORIES	FAT	CARBS	SODIUM	PROTEIN	FIBER
Broilers or fryers, dark meat, meat only, roasted, organic						
1 cup chopped or diced						
	287	**14**	**0**	**130**	**38**	**0**
Broilers or fryers, dark meat, meat only, stewed						
1 cup chopped or diced						
	269	13	0	104	36	0
Broilers or fryers, dark meat, meat only, stewed, organic						
1 cup chopped or diced						
	269	**13**	**0**	**104**	**36**	**0**
Broilers or fryers, drumstick, meat only, fried						
1 drumstick						
	82	3	0	40	12	0
Broilers or fryers, drumstick, meat only, roasted						
1 drumstick						
	76	2	0	42	12	0
Broilers or fryers, drumstick, meat only, roasted, organic						
1 drumstick						
	76	**2**	**0**	**42**	**12**	**0**
Broilers or fryers, drumstick, meat only, stewed						
1 drumstick						
	78	3	0	37	13	0
Broilers or fryers, drumstick, meat only, stewed, organic						
1 drumstick						
	78	**3**	**0**	**37**	**13**	**0**
Broilers or fryers, leg, meat only, fried						
1 leg, bone and skin removed						
	196	9	1	90	27	0
Broilers or fryers, leg, meat only, roasted						
1 leg, bone and skin removed						
	181	8	0	86	26	0
Broilers or fryers, leg, meat only, roasted, organic						
1 leg, bone and skin removed						
	181	**8**	**0**	**86**	**26**	**0**
Broilers or fryers, leg, meat only, stewed						
1 leg, bone and skin removed						
	187	8	0	79	27	0
Broilers or fryers, leg, meat only, stewed, organic						
1 leg, bone and skin removed						
	187	**8**	**0**	**79**	**27**	**0**
Broilers or fryers, light meat, meat only, fried						
1 cup	269	8	1	113	46	0
Broilers or fryers, light meat, meat only, roasted						
1 cup chopped or diced						
	242	6	0	108	43	0
Broilers or fryers, light meat, meat only, roasted, organic						
1 cup chopped or diced						
	242	**6**	**0**	**108**	**43**	**0**
Broilers or fryers, light meat, meat only, stewed						
1 cup chopped or diced						
	223	6	0	91	40	0

BRAND/FOOD ITEM SERVING SIZE	CALORIES	FAT	CARBS	SODIUM	PROTEIN	FIBER
Broilers or fryers, light meat, meat only, stewed, organic						
1 cup chopped or diced						
	223	**6**	**0**	**91**	**40**	**0**
Broilers or fryers, meat only, fried						
1 cup, chopped or diced						
	307	13	2	127	43	0
Broilers or fryers, meat only, roasted						
1 cup chopped or diced						
	266	10	0	120	41	0
Broilers or fryers, meat only, roasted, organic						
1 cup chopped or diced						
	266	**10**	**0**	**120**	**41**	**0**
Broilers or fryers, meat only, stewed						
1 cup chopped or diced						
	248	9	0	98	38	0
Broilers or fryers, meat only, stewed, organic						
1 cup chopped or diced						
	248	**9**	**0**	**98**	**38**	**0**
Broilers or fryers, thigh, meat only, fried						
1 thigh, bone and skin removed						
	113	5	1	49	15	0
Broilers or fryers, thigh, meat only, roasted						
1 thigh, bone and skin removed						
	109	6	0	46	13	0
Broilers or fryers, thigh, meat only, roasted, organic						
1 thigh, bone and skin removed						
	109	**6**	**0**	**46**	**13**	**0**
Broilers or fryers, thigh, meat only, stewed						
1 thigh, bone and skin removed						
	107	5	0	41	14	0
Broilers or fryers, thigh, meat only, stewed, organic						
1 thigh, bone and skin removed						
	107	**5**	**0**	**41**	**14**	**0**
Broilers or fryers, wing, meat only, fried						
1 wing, bone and skin removed						
	42	2	0	18	6	0
Broilers or fryers, wing, meat only, roasted						
1 wing, bone and skin removed						
	43	2	0	19	6	0
Broilers or fryers, wing, meat only, roasted, organic						
1 wing, bone and skin removed						
	43	**2**	**0**	**19**	**6**	**0**
Broilers or fryers, wing, meat only, stewed						
1 wing, bone and skin removed						
	43	2	0	18	7	0
Broilers or fryers, wing, meat only, stewed, organic						
1 wing, bone and skin removed						
	43	**2**	**0**	**18**	**7**	**0**
EGGS						
Chicken, white, raw, fresh						
1 cup	117	0	2	403	26	0

BRAND/FOOD ITEM SERVING SIZE	CALORIES	FAT	CARBS	SODIUM	PROTEIN	FIBER
Chicken, white, raw, fresh						
1 large	16	0	0	55	4	0
Chicken, white, raw, fresh, organic						
1 cup	**117**	**0**	**2**	**403**	**26**	**0**
Chicken, white, raw, fresh, organic						
1 large	16	0	0	55	4	0
Chicken, whole, fried						
1 egg	90	7	0	94	6	0
Chicken, whole, hard-boiled						
1 egg	78	5	1	62	6	0
Chicken, whole, hard-boiled						
1 cup chopped						
	211	14	2	169	17	0
Chicken, whole, hard-boiled, organic						
1 egg	**78**	**5**	**1**	**62**	**6**	**0**
Chicken, whole, hard-boiled, organic						
1 cup chopped						
	211	**14**	**2**	**169**	**17**	**0**
Chicken, whole, omelet (plain)						
1 egg	96	7	0	98	6	0
Chicken, whole, omelet, organic (plain)						
1 egg	**96**	**7**	**0**	**98**	**6**	**0**
Chicken, whole, poached						
1 egg	71	5	0	147	6	0
Chicken, whole, poached, organic						
1 egg	**71**	**5**	**0**	**147**	**6**	**0**
Chicken, whole, scrambled						
1 egg	102	7	1	171	7	0
Chicken, whole, scrambled						
1 cup	367	27	5	616	24	0
Chicken, whole, scrambled, organic						
1 egg	**102**	**7**	**1**	**171**	**7**	**0**
Chicken, whole, scrambled, organic						
1 cup	**367**	**27**	**5**	**616**	**24**	**0**
Duck, whole, fresh, raw						
1 egg	130	10	1	102	9	0
Duck, whole, fresh, raw, organic						
1 egg	**130**	**10**	**1**	**102**	**9**	**0**
Goose, whole, fresh, raw						
1 egg	266	19	2	199	20	0
Goose, whole, fresh, raw, organic						
1 egg	**266**	**19**	**2**	**199**	**20**	**0**
Quail, whole, fresh, raw						
1 egg	14	1	0	13	1	0
Quail, whole, fresh, raw, organic						
1 egg	**14**	**1**	**0**	**13**	**1**	**0**
Turkey, whole, fresh, raw						
1 egg	135	9	1	119	11	0
Turkey, whole, fresh, raw, organic						
1 egg	**135**	**9**	**1**	**119**	**11**	**0**

BRAND/FOOD ITEM SERVING SIZE	CALORIES	FAT	CARBS	SODIUM	PROTEIN	FIBER
FISH						
Bass, striped, dry heat						
3 oz	105	3	0	75	19	0
Bluefish, dry heat						
3 oz	135	5	0	65	22	0
Carp, dry heat						
3 oz	138	6	0	54	19	0
Caviar, black and red, granular						
1 tbsp	40	3	1	240	4	0
Cod, Atlantic, dry heat						
3 oz	89	1	0	66	19	0
Cod, Pacific, dry heat						
3 oz	89	1	0	77	20	0
Grouper, mixed species, dry heat						
3 oz	100	1	0	45	21	0
Halibut, Atlantic and Pacific, dry heat						
3 oz	119	3	0	59	23	0
Mackerel, Atlantic, dry heat						
3 oz	223	15	0	71	20	0
Mackerel, Atlantic, dry heat, organic						
3 oz	223	15	0	71	20	0
Mackerel, jack, canned, drained solids						
1 cup	296	12	0	720	44	0
Mackerel, king, dry heat						
3 oz	114	2	0	173	22	0
Mackerel, Pacific and jack, mixed species, dry heat						
1 fillet	354	18	0	194	45	0
Mackerel, Pacific and jack, mixed species, dry heat						
3 oz	171	9	0	94	22	0
Mackerel, salted						
1 cup cooked						
	415	34	0	6052	25	0
Mackerel, Spanish, dry heat						
3 oz	134	5	0	56	20	0
Pike, northern, dry heat						
3 oz	96	1	0	42	21	0
Salmon, Atlantic, farmed, dry heat						
3 oz	175	11	0	52	19	0
Salmon, Atlantic, wild, dry heat						
3 oz	155	7	0	48	22	0
Salmon, chinook, dry heat						
3 oz	196	11	0	51	22	0
Salmon, chinook, smoked (lox), regular						
1 oz	33	1	0	567	5	0
Salmon, coho, farmed, dry heat						
3 oz	151	7	0	44	21	0
Salmon, coho, wild, dry heat						
3 oz	118	4	0	49	20	0
Salmon, sockeye, dry heat						
3 oz	184	9	0	56	23	0

BRAND/FOOD ITEM SERVING SIZE	CALORIES	FAT	CARBS	SODIUM	PROTEIN	FIBER
Sardine, canned in oil, drained solids with bone						
2 sardines	50	3	0	121	6	0
Sea bass, mixed species, dry heat						
3 oz	105	2	0	74	20	0
Snapper, mixed species, dry heat						
3 oz	109	1	0	48	22	0
Trout, mixed species, dry heat						
3 oz	162	7	0	57	23	0
Tuna, fresh, bluefin, dry heat						
3 oz	156	5	0	42	25	0
Tuna, light, canned in oil, drained solids						
1 cup solid or chunks						
	289	12	9	517	43	0
Tuna, light, canned in water, drained solids						
1 cup solid or chunks						
	179	1	0	521	39	0
Tuna, white, canned in oil, drained solids						
3 oz	158	7	0	337	23	0
Tuna, white, canned in water, drained solids						
3 oz	109	3	0	320	20	0
Tuna, yellowfin, fresh, dry heat						
3 oz	118	1	0	40	25	0
Whitefish, mixed species, dry heat						
3 oz	146	6	0	55	21	0
Yellowtail, mixed species, dry heat						
3 oz	159	6	0	42	25	0
*PORK**						
Cured, bacon, baked						
1 slice	44	4	0	178	3	0
Cured, bacon, baked, organic						
1 slice	44	4	0	178	3	0
Cured, bacon, broiled, pan-fried, or roasted						
1 slice	43	3	0	185	3	0
Cured, bacon, broiled, pan-fried, or roasted, reduced sodium						
1 slice	43	3	0	82	3	0
Cured, bacon, microwaved						
1 slice	25	2	0	104	2	0
Cured, bacon, microwaved, organic						
1 slice	25	2	0	104	2	0
Cured, bacon, pan-fried						
1 slice	42	3	0	192	3	0
Cured, breakfast strips, cooked						
3 slices	156	12	0	714	10	0
Cured, breakfast strips, organic						
3 slices	156	12	0	714	10	0
Cured, Canadian-style bacon, grilled						
2 slices	87	4	1	727	11	0
Cured, Canadian-style bacon, grilled, organic						
2 slices	87	4	1	727	11	0

*To improve taste, texture, and color, many pork products are enhanced with solutions of water, salts, and other flavorings.

BRAND/FOOD ITEM SERVING SIZE	CALORIES	FAT	CARBS	SODIUM	PROTEIN	FIBER
Composite of trimmed retail cuts (leg, loin, and shoulder), separable lean only, cooked						
3 oz	180	8	0	50	25	0
Composite of trimmed retail cuts (leg, loin, and shoulder), separable lean only, cooked, organic						
3 oz	**180**	**8**	**0**	**50**	**25**	**0**
Composite of trimmed retail cuts (leg, loin, shoulder, and spareribs), separable lean and fat, cooked						
3 oz	232	15	0	53	23	0
Composite of trimmed retail cuts (leg, loin, shoulder, and spareribs), separable lean and fat, cooked, organic						
3 oz	**232**	**15**	**0**	**53**	**23**	**0**
Composite of trimmed retail cuts (loin and shoulder blade), separable lean and fat, cooked						
3 oz	200	12	0	47	22	0
Composite of trimmed retail cuts (loin and shoulder blade), separable lean and fat, cooked, organic						
3 oz	**200**	**12**	**0**	**47**	**22**	**0**
Composite of trimmed retail cuts (loin and shoulder blade), separable lean only, cooked						
3 oz	179	8	0	48	25	0
Composite of trimmed retail cuts (loin and shoulder blade), separable lean only, cooked, organic						
3 oz	**179**	**8**	**0**	**48**	**25**	**0**
Enhanced, loin, tenderloin, separable lean and fat, roasted						
1 roast	615	19	2	1168	109	0
Enhanced, loin, tenderloin, separable lean and fat, roasted, organic						
1 roast	**615**	**19**	**2**	**1168**	**109**	**0**
Enhanced, loin, tenderloin, separable lean only, roasted						
1 roast	589	16	2	1173	110	0
Enhanced, loin, tenderloin, separable lean only, roasted, organic						
1 roast	**589**	**16**	**2**	**1173**	**110**	**0**
Enhanced, loin, top loin (chops), boneless, separable lean and fat, broiled						
1 chop	176	5	0	318	33	0
Enhanced, loin, top loin (chops), boneless, separable lean and fat, broiled, organic						
1 chop	**176**	**5**	**0**	**318**	**33**	**0**
Enhanced, loin, top loin (chops), boneless, separable lean only, broiled						
1 chop	190	7	0	314	33	0
Enhanced, loin, top loin (chops), boneless, separable lean only, broiled, organic						
1 chop	**190**	**7**	**0**	**314**	**33**	**0**
Enhanced, shoulder (Boston butt), blade (steaks), separable lean and fat, braised						
1 steak	676	45	0	399	68	0
Enhanced, shoulder (Boston butt), blade (steaks), separable lean and fat, braised, organic						
1 steak	**676**	**45**	**0**	**399**	**68**	**0**

*To improve taste, texture, and color, many pork products are enhanced with solutions of water, salts, and other flavorings.

BRAND/FOOD ITEM SERVING SIZE	CALORIES	FAT	CARBS	SODIUM	PROTEIN	FIBER
Enhanced, shoulder (Boston butt), blade (steaks), separable lean only, braised						
1 steak	599	32	0	407	73	0
Enhanced, shoulder (Boston butt), blade (steaks), separable lean only, braised, organic						
1 steak	**599**	**32**	**0**	**407**	**73**	**0**
Leg (ham), rump half, separable lean and fat, roasted						
3 oz	214	12	0	53	25	0
Leg (ham), rump half, separable lean and fat, roasted, organic						
3 oz	**214**	**12**	**0**	**53**	**25**	**0**
Leg (ham), rump half, separable lean only, roasted						
3 oz	175	7	0	55	26	0
Leg (ham), rump half, separable lean only, roasted, organic						
3 oz	**175**	**7**	**0**	**55**	**26**	**0**
Leg (ham), shank half, separable lean and fat, roasted						
3 oz	246	17	0	50	22	0
Leg (ham), shank half, separable lean and fat, roasted, organic						
3 oz	**246**	**17**	**0**	**50**	**22**	**0**
Leg (ham), shank half, separable lean only, roasted						
3 oz	183	9	0	54	24	0
Leg (ham), shank half, separable lean only, roasted, organic						
3 oz	**183**	**9**	**0**	**54**	**24**	**0**
Leg (ham), whole, separable lean and fat, roasted						
3 oz	232	15	0	51	23	0
Leg (ham), whole, separable lean and fat, roasted, organic						
3 oz	**232**	**15**	**0**	**51**	**23**	**0**
Leg (ham), whole, separable lean only, roasted						
3 oz	179	8	0	54	25	0
Leg (ham), whole, separable lean only, roasted, organic						
3 oz	**179**	**8**	**0**	**54**	**25**	**0**
Loin, blade (chops), bone-in, separable lean and fat, braised						
3 oz	275	22	0	47	19	0
Loin, blade (chops), bone-in, separable lean and fat, braised, organic						
3 oz	**275**	**22**	**0**	**47**	**19**	**0**
Loin, blade (chops), bone-in, separable lean and fat, broiled						
3 oz	272	21	0	60	19	0
Loin, blade (chops), bone-in, separable lean and fat, broiled, organic						
3 oz	**272**	**21**	**0**	**60**	**19**	**0**
Loin, blade (chops), bone-in, separable lean and fat, pan-fried						
3 oz	291	24	0	57	18	0
Loin, blade (chops), bone-in, separable lean only, braised						
3 oz	191	11	0	53	21	0
Loin, blade (chops), bone-in, separable lean only, braised, organic						
3 oz	**191**	**11**	**0**	**53**	**21**	**0**
Loin, blade (chops), bone-in, separable lean only, broiled						
3 oz	199	12	0	68	22	0
Loin, blade (chops), bone-in, separable lean only, broiled, organic						
3 oz	**199**	**12**	**0**	**68**	**22**	**0**
Loin, blade (chops), bone-in, separable lean only, pan-fried						
3 oz	205	13	0	66	21	0

*To improve taste, texture, and color, many pork products are enhanced with solutions of water, salts, and other flavorings.

BRAND/FOOD ITEM SERVING SIZE	CALORIES	FAT	CARBS	SODIUM	PROTEIN	FIBER
Loin, blade (roasts), bone-in, separable lean and fat, roasted						
3 oz	275	21	0	26	20	0
Loin, blade (roasts), bone-in, separable lean and fat, roasted, organic						
3 oz	**275**	**21**	**0**	**26**	**20**	**0**
Loin, blade (roasts), bone-in, separable lean only, roasted						
3 oz	210	13	0	25	23	0
Loin, blade (roasts), bone-in, separable lean only, roasted, organic						
3 oz	**210**	**13**	**0**	**25**	**23**	**0**
Loin, center loin (chops), bone-in, separable lean and fat, braised						
3 oz	210	12	0	50	24	0
Loin, center loin (chops), bone-in, separable lean and fat, braised, organic						
3 oz	**210**	**12**	**0**	**50**	**24**	**0**
Loin, center loin (chops), bone-in, separable lean and fat, broiled						
3 oz	178	9	0	47	22	0
Loin, center loin (chops), bone-in, separable lean and fat, broiled, organic						
3 oz	**178**	**9**	**0**	**47**	**22**	**0**
Loin, center loin (chops), bone-in, separable lean and fat, pan-fried						
3 oz	235	14	0	68	25	0
Loin, center loin (chops), bone-in, separable lean only, braised						
3 oz	172	7	0	53	25	0
Loin, center loin (chops), bone-in, separable lean only, braised, organic						
3 oz	**172**	**7**	**0**	**53**	**25**	**0**
Loin, center loin (chops), bone-in, separable lean only, broiled						
3 oz	153	6	0	48	23	0
Loin, center loin (chops), bone-in, separable lean only, broiled, organic						
3 oz	**153**	**6**	**0**	**48**	**23**	**0**
Loin, center loin (chops), bone-in, separable lean only, pan-fried						
3 oz	197	9	0	73	27	0
Loin, center loin (roasts), bone-in, separable lean and fat, roasted						
3 oz	199	11	0	54	22	0
Loin, center loin (roasts), bone-in, separable lean and fat, roasted, organic						
3 oz	**199**	**11**	**0**	**54**	**22**	**0**
Loin, center loin (roasts), bone-in, separable lean only, roasted						
3 oz	169	8	0	56	23	0
Loin, center loin (roasts), bone-in, separable lean only, roasted, organic						
3 oz	**169**	**8**	**0**	**56**	**23**	**0**
Loin, center rib (chops), bone-in, lean only, broiled						
3 oz	158	7	0	48	22	0
Loin, center rib (chops), bone-in, lean only, broiled, organic						
3 oz	**158**	**7**	**0**	**48**	**22**	**0**
Loin, center rib (chops), boneless, separable lean only, braised						
3 oz	211	10	0	41	28	0

*To improve taste, texture, and color, many pork products are enhanced with solutions of water, salts, and other flavorings.

BRAND/FOOD ITEM SERVING SIZE	CALORIES	FAT	CARBS	SODIUM	PROTEIN	FIBER
Loin, center rib (chops), boneless, separable lean only, braised, organic						
3 oz	**211**	**10**	**0**	**41**	**28**	**0**
Loin, center rib (chops), boneless, separable lean only, broiled						
3 oz	216	10	0	65	29	0
Loin, center rib (chops), boneless, separable lean only, broiled, organic						
3 oz	**216**	**10**	**0**	**65**	**29**	**0**
Loin, center rib (chops), boneless, separable lean only, broiled, pan-fried						
3 oz	224	12	0	52	28	0
TURKEY						
All classes, dark meat, roasted						
1 cup chopped or diced						
	262	10	0	111	40	0
All classes, dark meat, roasted, organic						
1 cup chopped or diced						
	262	**10**	**0**	**111**	**40**	**0**
All classes, light meat, roasted						
1 cup chopped or diced						
	220	5	0	90	42	0
All classes, light meat, roasted, organic						
1 cup chopped or diced						
	220	**5**	**0**	**90**	**42**	**0**
All classes, meat only, roasted						
1 cup chopped or diced						
	238	7	0	98	41	0
All classes, meat only, roasted, organic						
1 cup chopped or diced						
	238	**7**	**0**	**98**	**41**	**0**
Diced, light and dark meat, seasoned						
1 oz	39	2	0	241	5	0
Diced, light and dark meat, seasoned, organic						
1 oz	**39**	**2**	**0**	**241**	**5**	**0**
Fryer-roasters, breast, meat only, roasted						
½ breast	413	2	0	159	92	0
Fryer-roasters, breast, meat only, roasted, organic						
½ breast	**413**	**2**	**0**	**159**	**92**	**0**
Fryer-roasters, leg, meat only, roasted						
1 leg, bone and skin removed						
	356	8	0	181	65	0
Fryer-roasters, leg, meat only, roasted, organic						
1 leg, bone and skin removed						
	356	**8**	**0**	**181**	**65**	**0**
Fryer-roasters, wing, meat only, roasted						
1 wing, bone and skin removed						
	98	2	0	47	19	0
Fryer-roasters, wing, meat only, roasted, organic						
1 wing, bone and skin removed						
	98	**2**	**0**	**47**	**19**	**0**

*To improve taste, texture, and color, many pork products are enhanced with solutions of water, salts, and other flavorings.

NUTS AND SEEDS

Nuts and seeds can definitely hit the spot when you're trying to wean off of salty chips or crackers. But keep in mind, despite their numerous health benefits, nuts and seeds are ridiculously high in calories. (Extra salt and oil roasting make things even worse.) Just a small handful can completely blow your calorie allotment for the day. So pay close attention to the portion sizes and get ready to do some nut counting.

BRAND/FOOD ITEM SERVING SIZE	CALORIES	FAT	CARBS	SODIUM	PROTEIN	FIBER
Nuts						
ALMONDS						
Blanched						
1 tbsp	53	5	2	3	2	1
Blanched						
1 oz	165	14	6	8	6	3
Blanched, organic						
1 tbsp	53	5	2	3	2	1
Blanched, organic						
1 oz	165	14	6	8	6	3
Dry roasted, with salt added						
1 oz (22 nuts)	169	15	5	96	6	3
Dry roasted, with salt added, organic						
1 oz (22 nuts)	169	15	5	96	6	3
Dry roasted, without salt added						
1 oz (22 nuts)	169	15	5	0	6	3
Dry roasted, without salt added, organic						
1 oz (22 nuts)	169	15	5	0	6	3
Honey roasted, unblanched						
1 oz	168	14	8	37	5	4

BRAND/FOOD ITEM SERVING SIZE	CALORIES	FAT	CARBS	SODIUM	PROTEIN	FIBER
Honey roasted, unblanched, organic						
1 oz	**168**	**14**	**8**	**37**	**5**	**4**
Oil roasted, with salt added						
1 oz (22 nuts)						
	172	16	5	96	6	3
Oil roasted, with salt added, organic						
1 oz (22 nuts)						
	172	16	5	96	6	3
Oil roasted, without salt added						
1 oz (22 nuts)						
	172	16	5	0	6	3
Oil roasted, without salt added, organic						
1 oz (22 nuts)						
	172	16	5	0	6	3
BRAZIL NUTS						
Dried, unblanched						
1 kernel	**33**	**3**	**1**	**0**	**1**	**0**
Dried, unblanched						
1 oz (6 nuts)						
	186	**19**	**3**	**1**	**4**	**2**
Dried, unblanched, organic						
1 kernel	**33**	**3**	**1**	**0**	**1**	**0**
Dried, unblanched, organic						
1 oz (6 nuts)						
	186	**19**	**3**	**1**	**4**	**2**
CASHEWS						
Cashew butter, plain, with salt added						
1 tbsp	94	8	4	98	3	0
Cashew butter, plain, with salt added, organic						
1 tbsp	94	8	4	98	3	0
Cashew butter, plain, without salt added						
1 tbsp	**94**	**8**	**4**	**2**	**3**	**0**
Cashew butter, plain, without salt added, organic						
1 tbsp	**94**	**8**	**4**	**2**	**3**	**0**
Cashew dry roasted, with salt added						
1 oz	163	13	9	181	4	1
Cashew dry roasted, with salt added, organic						
1 oz	163	13	9	181	4	1
Cashew dry roasted, without salt added						
1 oz	**163**	**13**	**9**	**5**	**4**	**1**
Cashew dry roasted, without salt added, organic						
1 oz	**163**	**13**	**9**	**5**	**4**	**1**
Cashew oil roasted, with salt added						
1 oz (18 nuts)						
	165	14	9	87	5	1
Cashew oil roasted, with salt added, organic						
1 oz (18 nuts)						
	165	14	9	87	5	1
Cashew oil roasted, without salt added						
1 oz (18 nuts)						
	164	14	8	4	5	1

BRAND/FOOD ITEM SERVING SIZE	CALORIES	FAT	CARBS	SODIUM	PROTEIN	FIBER
Cashew oil roasted, without salt added, organic						
1 oz (18 nuts)	164	14	8	4	5	1
Cashew raw						
1 oz	157	12	9	3	5	1
Cashew raw, organic						
1 oz	157	12	9	3	5	1
HAZELNUTS OR FILBERTS						
Blanched						
1 oz	178	17	5	0	4	3
Blanched, organic						
1 oz	178	17	5	0	4	3
Dry roasted, without salt added						
1 oz	183	18	5	0	4	3
Dry roasted, without salt added, organic						
1 oz	183	18	5	0	4	3
MACADAMIA NUTS						
Dry roasted, with salt added						
1 oz (10–12 nuts)	203	22	4	75	2	2
Dry roasted, with salt added, organic						
1 oz (10–12 nuts)	203	22	4	75	2	2
Dry roasted, without salt added						
1 oz (10–12 nuts)	203	22	4	1	2	2
Dry roasted, without salt added, organic						
1 oz (10–12 nuts)	203	22	4	1	2	2
Raw						
1 oz (10–12 nuts)	204	21	4	1	2	2
Raw, organic						
1 oz (10–12 nuts)	204	21	4	1	2	2
PEANUTS						
Boiled, with salt						
1 oz shelled	90	6	6	213	4	3
Boiled, with salt						
33 nuts	89	6	6	210	4	3
Boiled, with salt, organic						
1 oz shelled	90	6	6	213	4	3
Boiled, with salt, organic						
33 nuts	89	6	6	210	4	3
Dry roasted, with salt						
1 oz	166	14	6	230	7	2
Dry roasted, with salt						
1 peanut	6	1	0	8	0	0
Dry roasted, with salt, organic						
1 oz	166	14	6	230	7	2

BRAND/FOOD ITEM SERVING SIZE	CALORIES	FAT	CARBS	SODIUM	PROTEIN	FIBER
Dry roasted, with salt, organic						
1 peanut	6	1	0	8	0	0
Dry roasted, without salt						
1 oz	166	14	6	2	7	2
Dry roasted, without salt						
1 peanut	6	1	0	0	0	0
Dry roasted, without salt, organic						
1 oz	166	14	6	2	7	2
Dry roasted, without salt, organic						
1 peanut	6	1	0	0	0	0
Oil roasted, with salt						
½ cup halves/wholes						
	431	38	11	230	20	7
Oil roasted, with salt						
1 peanut	5	0	0	3	0	0
Oil roasted, with salt, organic						
½ cup halves/wholes						
	431	38	11	230	20	7
Oil roasted, with salt, organic						
1 peanut	5	0	0	3	0	0
Raw						
1 cup	828	72	24	26	38	12
Raw						
1 oz	161	14	5	5	7	2
Raw, organic						
1 cup	828	72	24	26	38	12
Raw, organic						
1 oz	161	14	5	5	7	2
PECANS						
Dry roasted, with salt added						
1 oz	201	21	4	109	3	3
Dry roasted, with salt added, organic						
1 oz	201	21	4	109	3	3
Dry roasted, without salt added						
1 oz	**201**	**21**	**4**	**0**	**3**	**3**
Dry roasted, without salt added, organic						
1 oz	**201**	**21**	**4**	**0**	**3**	**3**
Oil roasted, with salt added						
1 oz (15 halves)						
	203	21	4	111	3	3
Oil roasted, with salt added, organic						
1 oz (15 halves)						
	203	21	4	111	3	3
Oil roasted, without salt added						
1 oz (15 halves)						
	203	21	4	0	3	3
Oil roasted, without salt added, organic						
1 oz (15 halves)						
	203	21	4	0	3	3

BRAND/FOOD ITEM SERVING SIZE	CALORIES	FAT	CARBS	SODIUM	PROTEIN	FIBER
PINE NUTS						
Dried						
1 oz (167 nuts)	191	19	4	1	4	1
Dried						
10 nuts	11	1	0	0	0	0
Dried, organic						
1 oz (167 nuts)	191	19	4	1	4	1
Dried, organic						
10 nuts	11	1	0	0	0	0
PISTACHIOS						
Dry roasted, with salt added						
1 oz (49 nuts)	161	13	8	115	6	3
Dry roasted, with salt added, organic						
1 oz (49 nuts)	161	13	8	115	6	3
Dry roasted, without salt added						
1 oz (49 nuts)	161	13	8	3	6	3
Dry roasted, without salt added, organic						
1 oz (49 nuts)	161	13	8	3	6	3
Raw						
1 oz (49 nuts)	159	13	8	0	6	3
Raw, organic						
1 oz (49 nuts)	159	13	8	0	6	3
WALNUTS						
Black, dried						
1 tbsp	48	5	1	0	2	1
Black, dried						
1 oz	175	17	3	1	7	2
Black, dried, organic						
1 tbsp	48	5	1	0	2	1
Black, dried, organic						
1 oz	175	17	3	1	7	2
English						
1 cup, in shell, edible yield (7 nuts)	183	18	4	1	4	2
English						
1 oz (14 halves)	185	18	4	1	4	2
English, organic						
1 cup, in shell, edible yield (7 nuts)	183	18	4	1	4	2
English, organic						
1 oz (14 halves)	185	18	4	1	4	2

BRAND/FOOD ITEM SERVING SIZE	CALORIES	FAT	CARBS	SODIUM	PROTEIN	FIBER
MIXED NUTS						
Eden Foods All Mixed Up Nut Mix						
3 tbsp	160	12	7	70	8	4
Eden Foods Organic Pistachios, Shelled & Dry Roasted						
3 tbsp	**160**	**12**	**7**	**60**	**6**	**3**
Eden Foods Organic Tamari Almonds, Dry Roasted						
3 tbsp	**160**	**11**	**8**	**65**	**8**	**4**
Eden Foods Organic Wild Berry Trail Mix						
3 tbsp	150	8	13	10	5	4

Seeds

BRAND/FOOD ITEM SERVING SIZE	CALORIES	FAT	CARBS	SODIUM	PROTEIN	FIBER
PUMPKIN OR SQUASH SEEDS						
Dried						
1 oz	158	14	3	2	9	2
Dried, organic						
1 oz	158	14	3	2	9	2
Roasted, with salt added						
1 oz	163	14	4	73	8	2
Roasted, with salt added, organic						
1 oz	163	14	4	73	8	2
Roasted, without salt						
1 oz	163	14	4	5	8	2
Roasted, without salt, organic						
1 oz	163	14	4	5	8	2
Roasted, with salt added						
1 oz (85 seeds)	126	6	15	720	5	5
Roasted, with salt added, organic						
1 oz (85 seeds)	126	6	15	720	5	5
Roasted, without salt						
1 oz (85 seeds)	126	6	15	5	5	5
Roasted, without salt, organic						
1 oz (85 seeds)	126	6	15	5	5	5
SESAME SEEDS						
Whole, dried						
1 tbsp	52	4	2	1	2	1
Whole, dried, organic						
1 tbsp	52	4	2	1	2	1
Whole, roasted and toasted						
1 oz	160	14	7	3	5	4
Whole, roasted and toasted, organic						
1 oz	160	14	7	3	5	4
SUNFLOWER SEEDS						
Dried						
1 cup, with hulls	269	24	9	4	10	4

BRAND/FOOD ITEM SERVING SIZE	CALORIES	FAT	CARBS	SODIUM	PROTEIN	FIBER
Dried, organic						
1 cup, with hulls	**269**	**24**	**9**	**4**	**10**	**4**
Dry roasted, with salt added						
1 oz	165	14	7	116	5	3
Dry roasted, with salt added, organic						
1 oz	165	14	7	116	5	3
Dry roasted, without salt						
1 oz	**165**	**14**	**7**	**1**	**5**	**3**
Dry roasted, without salt, organic						
1 oz	**165**	**14**	**7**	**1**	**5**	**3**
Oil roasted, with salt added						
1 oz	168	15	6	116	6	3
Oil roasted, with salt added, organic						
1 oz	168	15	6	116	6	3
Oil roasted, without salt						
1 oz	168	15	6	1	6	3
Oil roasted, without salt, organic						
1 oz	168	15	6	1	6	3
Toasted, with salt added						
1 oz	175	16	6	174	5	3
Toasted, with salt added, organic						
1 oz	175	16	6	174	5	3
Toasted, without salt						
1 oz	**175**	**16**	**6**	**1**	**5**	**3**
Toasted, without salt, organic						
1 oz	**175**	**16**	**6**	**1**	**5**	**3**
Eden Foods Organic Pumpkin Seeds, Dry Roasted & Salted						
¼ cup	200	16	5	100	10	5
Eden Foods Organic Spicy Pumpkin Seeds, Dry Roasted with Tamari						
¼ cup	200	16	5	75	10	5

SAUCES AND DRESSINGS

Herein lie some of the biggest offenders for mystery calories. Sauces and salad dressings can turn an MYM-approved food into a Master Disaster in a flash. If you order a salad at a fast-food restaurant, check out the contents of the dressing packet (especially the sodium, thickeners, glutamates, sugar, and other garbage) as well as the calories. McDonald's offers Newman's Own dressings—and their Low-Fat Balsamic Vinaigrette can be a lifeline in an otherwise vast wasteland of yuck. To make it easier for you to get your allotment of tomatoes in the off-season, I've designated a few jarred marinara sauces as MYM-approved. (Keep an eye out for sodium, added sugar, and total calories.)

BRAND/FOOD ITEM SERVING SIZE	CALORIES	FAT	CARBS	SODIUM	PROTEIN	FIBER
Condiments and Spreads						
Arrowhead Mills Almond Butter, Creamy						
2 tbsp	200	17	6	0	7	4
Arrowhead Mills Almond Butter, Crunchy						
2 tbsp	200	17	6	0	7	4
Arrowhead Mills Cashew Butter, Creamy						
2 tbsp	160	13	9	0	4	<1
Arrowhead Mills Cashew Butter, Crunchy						
2 tbsp	160	13	9	0	4	<1
Arrowhead Mills Honey Sweetened Peanut Butter, Creamy						
2 tbsp	190	16	7	100	7	2
Arrowhead Mills Honey Sweetened Peanut Butter, Crunchy						
2 tbsp	190	16	7	100	7	2

BRAND/FOOD ITEM SERVING SIZE	CALORIES	FAT	CARBS	SODIUM	PROTEIN	FIBER
Arrowhead Mills Organic Valencia Peanut Butter, Creamy						
2 tbsp	190	17	6	0	8	2
Arrowhead Mills Organic Valencia Peanut Butter, Crunchy						
2 tbsp	190	17	6	0	8	2
Arrowhead Mills Sesame Tahini, Organic						
2 tbsp	190	18	3	10	8	<1
Arrowhead Mills Valencia Peanut Butter, Creamy						
2 tbsp	190	17	6	0	8	2
Arrowhead Mills Valencia Peanut Butter, Crunchy						
2 tbsp	190	17	6	0	8	2
Cascadian Farm Apricot Fruit Spread						
1 tbsp	40	0	10	0	0	0
Cascadian Farm Fruit Spread Blackberry						
1 tbsp	45	0	11	0	0	0
Cascadian Farm Fruit Spread Blueberry						
1 tbsp	45	0	11	0	0	0
Cascadian Farm Fruit Spread Concord Grape						
1 tbsp	40	0	10	0	0	0
Cascadian Farm Fruit Spread Raspberry						
1 tbsp	45	0	11	0	0	0
Cascadian Farm Fruit Spread Strawberry						
1 tbsp	40	0	10	0	0	0
Cascadian Farm Sweet Relish						
1 tbsp	15	0	4	65	0	0
Eden Foods Organic Apple Butter						
1 tbsp	20	0	4	0	0	1
Eden Foods Organic Apple Cherry Butter						
1 tbsp	25	0	6	0	0	<1
Eden Foods Organic Apple Cherry Sauce						
½ cup	70	0	17	10	0	3
Eden Foods Organic Apple Cinnamon Sauce						
½ cup	60	0	14	10	0	2
Eden Foods Organic Apple Sauce						
½ cup	60	0	13	10	0	2
Eden Foods Organic Apple Strawberry Sauce						
½ cup	60	0	13	10	0	2
Eden Foods Organic Barley Malt Syrup						
1 tbsp	60	0	14	0	1	0
Eden Foods Organic Brown Mustard Squeeze Bottle						
1 tsp	0	0	1	80	0	0
Eden Foods Organic Cherry Butter						
1 tbsp	35	0	9	0	0	1
Eden Foods Organic Yellow Mustard Squeeze Bottle						
1 tsp	0	0	0	80	0	0
Muir Glen Tomato Ketchup						
1 tbsp	40	0	4	230	0	0
Newman's Own All-Natural Steak Sauce						
2 tbsp	20	0.5	4	85	0	0
Newman's Own Organic Balsamic Vinegar						
1 tbsp	20	0	5	0	0	0

BRAND/FOOD ITEM SERVING SIZE	CALORIES	FAT	CARBS	SODIUM	PROTEIN	FIBER

Pasta Sauces

Amy's Organic Family Marinara Pasta Sauce
½ cup	80	4.5	10	590	1	3

Amy's Organic Light in Sodium Tomato Basil Pasta Sauce
½ cup	90	4.5	11	290	2	2

Amy's Organic Low Sodium Marinara Sauce
½ cup	40	1	7	100	1	1

Amy's Organic Tomato Basil Pasta Sauce
½ cup	110	6	11	580	2	3

Classico Creamy Alfredo Sauce
¼ cup	100	9	3	410	2	0

Classico Organic Spinach & Garlic Sauce
½ cup	70	0	11	330	2	2

Classico Organic Tomato, Herbs & Spices Sauce
½ cup	70	1	12	400	2	2

Classico Roasted Garlic Alfredo Sauce
¼ cup	70	6	3	430	1	1

Classico Roasted Garlic Sauce
½ cup	50	1	9	350	2	2

Classico Tomato & Basil Sauce
½ cup	50	1	11	310	2	2

Eden Foods Organic Spaghetti Sauce
½ cup	70	2.5	9	10	2	5

Muir Glen Cabernet Marinara Pasta Sauce
½ cup	60	1	11	360	2	2

Muir Glen Chef Inspirations Beef Bolognese Pasta Sauce
½ cup	70	2	10	410	3	2

Muir Glen Chef Inspirations Italian Sausage with Peppers Pasta Sauce
½ cup	80	3	10	420	3	2

Muir Glen Chef Inspirations Vodka Pasta Sauce
½ cup	90	4.5	10	360	3	2

Muir Glen Chunky Tomato & Herb Pasta Sauce
½ cup	60	0.5	11	350	2	2

Muir Glen Chunky Tomato Sauce
¼ cup	15	0	4	230	2	<1

Muir Glen Fire Roasted Tomato Pasta Sauce
½ cup	70	2	11	340	2	2

Muir Glen Four Cheese Pasta Sauce
½ cup	80	2.5	11	380	4	2

Muir Glen Garden Vegetable Pasta Sauce
½ cup	60	1	10	350	2	2

Muir Glen Italian Herb Pasta Sauce
½ cup	60	0.5	11	350	2	2

Muir Glen Pizza Sauce
¼ cup	40	2	6	290	1	1

Muir Glen Portobello Mushroom Pasta Sauce
½ cup	50	0	10	350	2	2

Muir Glen Roasted Garlic Pasta Sauce
½ cup	60	0.5	12	380	2	2

Muir Glen Salsa Black Bean & Corn Medium
2 tbsp	20	0	4	135	<1	<1

BRAND/FOOD ITEM SERVING SIZE	CALORIES	FAT	CARBS	SODIUM	PROTEIN	FIBER
Muir Glen Tomato Basil Pasta Sauce						
½ cup	60	1	12	370	2	2
Muir Glen Tomato Paste						
2 tbsp	30	0	6	20	1	1
Muir Glen Tomato Puree						
¼ cup	25	0	6	30	1	1
Muir Glen Tomato Sauce						
¼ cup	25	0	5	310	1	1
Muir Glen Tomato Sauce No Salt Added						
¼ cup	25	0	5	10	1	1
Newman's Own Alfredo Pasta Sauce						
½ cup	90	8	3	460	1	0
Newman's Own Bombolina Sauce						
½ cup	90	4.5	13	620	2	<1
Newman's Own Cabernet Marinara Sauce						
½ cup	70	3	10	590	2	<1
Newman's Own Fire Roasted Tomato & Garlic Pasta Sauce						
½ cup	70	3.5	9	500	2	2
Newman's Own Five Cheese Sauce						
½ cup	80	3	10	610	3	<1
Newman's Own Fra Diavolo Sauce						
½ cup	70	3	10	510	0	3
Newman's Own Italian Sausage & Peppers Sauce						
½ cup	90	4	11	630	4	<1
Newman's Own Marinara Sauce						
½ cup	70	2	12	510	2	<1
Newman's Own Marinara with Mushrooms Sauce						
½ cup	70	2	12	520	2	<1
Newman's Own Pesto & Tomato Sauce						
½ cup	80	4	10	640	2	<1
Newman's Own Roasted Garlic & Peppers Sauce						
½ cup	70	2.5	11	460	2	4
Newman's Own Roasted Garlic Sauce						
½ cup	70	2.5	11	580	2	<1
Newman's Own Sockarooni Sauce						
½ cup	70	2	12	520	2	<1
Newman's Own Sweet Onion and Roasted Garlic Pasta Sauce						
½ cup	60	1.5	12	530	2	<1
Newman's Own Vodka Sauce						
½ cup	110	5	11	440	5	0
Prego Organic Mushroom Italian Sauce						
½ cup	90	3	13	470	2	4
Prego Organic Tomato & Basil Sauce						
½ cup	90	3	13	470	2	4
Prego Traditional Italian Sauce						
½ cup	70	1.5	13	480	2	3
Prego Traditional Marinara Sauce						
½ cup	80	3	10	480	2	3
Ragu Cheesy Double Cheddar Sauce						
¼ cup	100	9	3	450	2	0
Ragu Cheesy Roasted Garlic Parmesan Sauce						
¼ cup	110	10	3	350	2	0

BRAND/FOOD ITEM SERVING SIZE	CALORIES	FAT	CARBS	SODIUM	PROTEIN	FIBER
Ragu Chunky Mama's Special Garden Sauce						
½ cup	90	3	14	510	2	2
Ragu Light Tomato Basil Sauce						
½ cup	50	0	11	360	2	2
Ragu Old World Style Mushroom Sauce						
½ cup	70	2.5	10	460	2	2
Ragu Old World Style Traditional Sauce						
½ cup	70	2.5	10	480	2	2
Ragu Organic Traditional Sauce						
½ cup	80	3	11	510	2	2
Ragu Robusto Chopped Tomato Olive Oil & Garlic Sauce						
½ cup	90	4	12	680	2	2

Dressings and Marinades

	CALORIES	FAT	CARBS	SODIUM	PROTEIN	FIBER
Bolthouse Farms Caesar Parmigiano Dressing						
2 tbsp	80	6.5	3	220	1	0
Bolthouse Farms Chunky Blue Cheese Dressing						
2 tbsp	70	6.5	2	150	2	0
Bolthouse Farms Classic Ranch Dressing						
2 tbsp	80	7.5	3	290	1	0
Bolthouse Farms Creamy Italian Dressing						
2 tbsp	70	7	2	105	1	0
Bolthouse Farms Honey Mustard Dressing						
2 tbsp	45	2	7	80	1	0
Bolthouse Farms Original Coleslaw Dressing						
2 tbsp	70	4	10	170	1	0
Bolthouse Farms Poppy Seed Dressing						
2 tbsp	70	4.5	8	120	1	0
Bolthouse Farms Thousand Island Dressing						
2 tbsp	70	5.5	4	180	1	<1
Kraft Catalina Dressing						
2 tbsp	130	11	7	380	0	0
Kraft Creamy French Dressing						
2 tbsp	150	14	5	260	1	0
Kraft Creamy Italian Dressing						
2 tbsp	100	11	2	250	0	0
Kraft Peppercorn Dressing						
2 tbsp	120	12	2	320	0	0
Kraft Ranch Dressing						
2 tbsp	120	12	3	370	0	0
Kraft Thousand Island Dressing						
2 tbsp	110	10	5	330	0	0
Newman's Own Balsamic Vinaigrette Dressing						
2 tbsp	90	9	3	350	0	0
Newman's Own Caesar Dressing						
2 tbsp	150	16	1	420	1	0
Newman's Own Creamy Caesar Dressing						
2 tbsp	150	16	1	450	1	0
Newman's Own Creamy Italian Dressing						
2 tbsp	140	14	2	270	1	0

BRAND/FOOD ITEM SERVING SIZE	CALORIES	FAT	CARBS	SODIUM	PROTEIN	FIBER
Newman's Own Family Recipe Italian Dressing						
2 tbsp	120	13	1	400	1	0
Newman's Own Greek Vinaigrette Dressing						
2 tbsp	100	10	1	270	0	0
Newman's Own Herb & Roasted Garlic Marinade						
1 tbsp	20	1	3	370	0	0
Newman's Own Lemon Pepper Marinade						
1 tbsp	15	0	3	300	0	0
Newman's Own Lighten Up Balsamic Vinaigrette Dressing						
2 tbsp	45	4	2	470	0	0
Newman's Own Lighten Up Caesar Dressing						
2 tbsp	70	6	3	520	1	0
Newman's Own Lighten Up Honey Mustard Dressing						
2 tbsp	70	4	7	290	0	0
Newman's Own Lighten Up Italian Dressing						
2 tbsp	60	6	0	260	0	0
Newman's Own Lighten Up Light Cranberry Walnut Dressing						
2 tbsp	70	4	8	230	1	0
Newman's Own Lighten Up Light Lime Vinaigrette						
2 tbsp	60	5	4	280	0	0
Newman's Own Lighten Up Low Fat Sesame Ginger Dressing						
2 tbsp	35	1.5	5	390	0	0
Newman's Own Lighten Up Raspberry & Walnut Dressing						
2 tbsp	70	5	7	120	0	0
Newman's Own Lighten Up Red Wine Vinegar & Olive Oil Dressing						
2 tbsp	50	4.5	2	390	0	0
Newman's Own Lighten Up Roast Garlic Balsamic Dressing						
2 tbsp	50	4	3	420	0	0
Newman's Own Lighten Up Sun Dried Tomato Dressing						
2 tbsp	60	4	5	380	0	0
Newman's Own Mesquite with Lime Marinade						
1 tbsp	20	1	3	190	0	0
Newman's Own Olive Oil & Vinegar Dressing						
2 tbsp	150	16	1	150	0	0
Newman's Own Orange Ginger Dressing						
2 tbsp	80	4.5	9	340	0	0
Newman's Own Organic Extra Virgin Olive Oil						
1 tbsp	130	14	0	0	0	0
Newman's Own Organic Light Balsamic Dressing						
2 tbsp	45	4	3	450	0	0
Newman's Own Organic Low Fat Asian Dressing						
2 tbsp	35	2	5	440	0	0
Newman's Own Organic Tuscan Italian Dressing						
2 tbsp	100	11	1	380	0	0
Newman's Own Parmesan & Roasted Garlic Dressing						
2 tbsp	110	11	2	250	0	0
Newman's Own Ranch Dressing						
2 tbsp	140	15	2	250	0	0
Newman's Own Sesame Ginger Marinade						
1 tbsp	25	1	4	300	0	0
Newman's Own Southwest Dressing						
2 tbsp	90	8	4	280	1	0

BRAND/FOOD ITEM SERVING SIZE	CALORIES	FAT	CARBS	SODIUM	PROTEIN	FIBER
Newman's Own Teriyaki Marinade						
1 tbsp	25	0	6	330	0	0
Newman's Own Three Cheese Balsamic Vinaigrette Dressing						
2 tbsp	100	11	2	380	0	0
Newman's Own Two Thousand Island Dressing						
2 tbsp	140	14	4	260	0	0
South Beach Living Balsamic Dressing						
2 tbsp	50	4	4	350	0	0
South Beach Living Italian Dressing						
2 tbsp	30	4.5	3	300	0	0
South Beach Living Ranch Dressing						
2 tbsp	70	7	2	300	1	0

Salsa

BRAND/FOOD ITEM SERVING SIZE	CALORIES	FAT	CARBS	SODIUM	PROTEIN	FIBER
Amy's Organic Black Bean & Corn Salsa						
2 tbsp	15	0	3	170	1	0
Amy's Organic Medium Salsa						
2 tbsp	10	0	2	190	0	0
Amy's Organic Mild Salsa						
2 tbsp	10	0	2	190	0	0
Amy's Organic Spicy Chipotle Salsa						
2 tbsp	10	0	2	160	0	0
Muir Glen Chipotle Medium Salsa						
2 tbsp	10	0	2	140	0	0
Muir Glen Garlic Cilantro Medium Salsa						
2 tbsp	10	0	2	130	0	0
Muir Glen Medium Salsa						
2 tbsp	10	0	3	130	0	0
Muir Glen Mild Salsa						
2 tbsp	10	0	3	130	0	0
Newman's Own All-Natural Bandito Chunky Peach Salsa						
2 tbsp	25	0	6	90	0	<1
Newman's Own All-Natural Bandito Chunky Roasted Garlic Salsa						
2 tbsp	10	0	2	150	1	1
Newman's Own All-Natural Bandito Hot Salsa						
2 tbsp	10	0	2	105	0	1
Newman's Own All-Natural Bandito Medium Salsa						
2 tbsp	10	0	2	105	0	1
Newman's Own All-Natural Bandito Mild Salsa						
2 tbsp	10	0	2	105	0	1
Newman's Own All-Natural Bandito Pineapple Salsa						
2 tbsp	15	0	3	90	0	1
Newman's Own All-Natural Bandito Tequila Lime Salsa						
2 tbsp	15	0	3	170	0	0
Newman's Own Black Bean & Corn Salsa						
2 tbsp	14	0	5	140	1	2
Newman's Own Farmer's Garden Salsa						
2 tbsp	15	0	4	220	1	0
Newman's Own Mango Salsa						
2 tbsp	20	0	5	140	1	2

SNACKS AND SWEETS

Okay, here are some of the biggest offenders to avoid. This is where you'll find the calories you can absolutely live without. Before you go for an Oreo, check out the list and realize that each cookie is 50 calories—and who eats just one of those? This is your fast-carb, high-blood-sugar, bad-mood, crash-and-burn list. Some foods will be better than others. Choose Kashi and Newman's Own before Fritos and Chips Ahoy. But if you ask me? Be smart, don't start. (That doesn't mean you never get to have dessert again, just stay away from the fake crap. There are delicious, healthy desserts to be found, and you can even make your own chemical-free ones with my Master cookbook.)

Your best options here are the energy bars. Bars are sometimes sold as "meal replacements." That's a pretty accurate description, because I would never say they are food. They can help out in emergencies, period. For my thyroid people, keep in mind that most of these bars have soy. And definitely keep an eye on the calories here.

BRAND/FOOD ITEM SERVING SIZE	CALORIES	FAT	CARBS	SODIUM	PROTEIN	FIBER

Salty Snacks

BRAND/FOOD ITEM SERVING SIZE	CALORIES	FAT	CARBS	SODIUM	PROTEIN	FIBER
Cape Cod Classic Potato Chips						
1 oz (19 chips)	150	8	17	110	2	1
Cape Cod Potato Chips, Reduced Fat						
1 oz (23 chips)	130	6	18	110	2	1
Cape Cod Sea Salt & Cracked Pepper Potato Chips						
1 oz (18 chips)	150	8	17	130	2	1
Cape Cod Sweet & Salty Popcorn						
1 oz (1½ cups)	110	1	25	160	1	2
Cape Cod Sweet Cream Butter Popcorn						
1 oz (2¼ cups)	170	12	14	210	2	3
Cape Cod Sweet Mesquite Barbeque						
1 oz (18 chips)	140	6	18	150	2	2
Cape Cod White Cheddar Popcorn						
1 oz (2¼ cups)	160	11	12	250	4	2
Cheetos Baked! Crunchy Cheese Flavored Snacks						
1 oz	130	5	19	240	2	0
Cheetos Crunchy Cheese Flavored Snacks						
1 oz	160	10	15	290	2	<1
Chips Ahoy! Original						
3 cookies	160	8	22	110	2	<1
Doritos Cool Ranch Flavored Tortilla Chips						
1 oz	150	8	18	180	2	2
Doritos Nacho Cheese Flavored Tortilla Chips						
1 oz	150	8	17	180	2	1
Eden Foods 5 Flavor Arare Rice Puffs Snack						
30 puffs	110	0	24	160	3	2
Eden Foods Brown Rice Chips						
50 chips	150	7	19	100	2	0
Eden Foods Brown Rice Crackers						
8 crackers	120	2	22	230	3	2
Eden Foods Nori Maki Rice Crackers						
15 crackers	110	0	24	160	3	2
Eden Foods Organic Yellow Popcorn						
2 tbsp	80	1	20	0	2	5
Eden Foods Sea Vegetable Chips						
25 chips	140	5	23	220	<1	0
Eden Foods Vegetable Chips						
25 chips	140	5	23	260	<1	0

BRAND/FOOD ITEM SERVING SIZE	CALORIES	FAT	CARBS	SODIUM	PROTEIN	FIBER
Eden Foods Wasabi Chips—Hot 'n Spicy						
25 chips	130	4	24	260	<1	0
Fritos BBQ Flavored Corn Chips						
1 oz	150	10	16	280	2	1
Fritos Original Corn Chips						
1 oz	160	10	15	170	2	1
Genisoy Apple Cinnamon Crunch Soy Crisps						
1 oz	120	3	17	270	7	2
Genisoy Potato Bake BBQ Chips						
17 crisps	110	2.5	16	190	5	2
Genisoy Potato Bake Parmesan & Roasted Garlic Chips						
17 crisps	110	2.5	16	270	5	2
Genisoy Potato Bake Ranch Chips						
17 crisps	110	2.5	16	270	5	2
Genisoy Potato Bake Sea Salt & Black Pepper Chips						
17 crisps	110	2.5	16	270	5	2
Genisoy Rich Cheddar Cheese Soy Crisps						
1 oz	110	3	14	270	7	2
Genisoy Tangy Salt 'N Vinegar Soy Crisps						
1 oz	110	3	14	270	7	2
Genisoy Tortilla Nacho Chips						
17 crisps	110	3	13	260	8	2
Genisoy Zesty BBQ Soy Chips						
1 oz	120	3	17	270	7	2
Guiltless Gourmet Blue Corn Tortilla Chips						
1 oz (about 18 chips)						
	120	3	23	250	3	2
Guiltless Gourmet Chili Lime Tortilla Chips						
1 oz (about 18 chips)						
	120	3	19	250	2	2
Guiltless Gourmet Chipotle Tortilla Chips						
1 oz (about 18 chips)						
	123	3	22	250	2	2
Guiltless Gourmet Mucho Nacho Tortilla Chips						
1 oz (about 18 chips)						
	120	3	22	250	2	2
Guiltless Gourmet Spicy Black Bean Tortilla Chips						
1 oz (about 18 chips)						
	120	3	19	250	2	2
Guiltless Gourmet Spinach Artichoke Parmesan Tortilla Chips						
1 oz (about 18 chips)						
	110	3	19	200	2	2
Guiltless Gourmet Unsalted Tortilla Chips						
1 oz (about 18 chips)						
	120	2	22	26	3	2
Guiltless Gourmet Yellow Corn Tortilla Chips						
1 oz (about 18 chips)						
	120	3	19	250	2	2
Health Valley Organic Bruschetta Vegetable Crackers						
4 crackers						
	70	3	10	210	1	0

BRAND/FOOD ITEM SERVING SIZE	CALORIES	FAT	CARBS	SODIUM	PROTEIN	FIBER
Health Valley Organic Cracked Pepper Crackers						
4 crackers	70	3	10	190	1	0
Health Valley Organic Garden Herb Crackers						
4 crackers	70	3	10	170	1	0
Health Valley Organic Sesame Crackers						
4 crackers	70	3	10	200	1	<1
Health Valley Organic Stoned Wheat Crackers						
4 crackers	70	3	10	170	1	<1
Health Valley Organic Whole Wheat Crackers						
4 crackers	70	3	9	170	2	1
Health Valley Original Amaranth Bran Graham Crackers						
6 crackers	120	3	22	80	3	3
Health Valley Original Oat Bran Graham Crackers						
6 crackers	120	3	22	80	3	3
Health Valley Original Rice Bran Graham Crackers						
6 crackers	110	3	19	70	3	3
Kashi Heart to Heart Whole Grain Crackers						
7 crackers	120	3.5	22	85	3	4
Kashi Heart to Heart Whole Grain Crackers Roasted Garlic						
7 crackers	120	3.5	22	75	3	4
Kashi TLC Country Cheddar Crackers						
18 crackers	130	4.5	20	220	3	<1
Kashi TLC Fire Roasted Vegetable Crackers						
15 crackers	130	3.5	21	210	3	2
Kashi TLC Honey Sesame Crackers						
15 crackers	120	3	22	140	3	2
Kashi TLC Mediterranean Bruschetta Party Crackers						
4 crackers	120	4	18	140	3	3
Kashi TLC Original 7 Grain Crackers						
15 crackers	130	3	22	160	3	2
Kashi TLC Roasted Garlic & Thyme Party Crackers						
4 crackers	130	4.5	18	140	3	3
Kashi TLC Stoneground 7 Grain Party Crackers						
4 crackers	130	5	17	140	3	3

BRAND/FOOD ITEM SERVING SIZE	CALORIES	FAT	CARBS	SODIUM	PROTEIN	FIBER
Kashi TLC Toasted Asiago Crackers						
15 crackers	130	4	21	200	3	2
Kettle Baked Potato Chips, Lightly Salted						
1 oz (20 chips)	120	3	21	135	2	2
Kettle Baked Sea Salt & Vinegar Potato Chips						
1 oz (20 chips)	120	3	21	170	2	2
Kettle Blue Corn Tortilla Chips						
1 oz	140	7	18	100	3	2
Kettle Krinkle Cut Classic Barbeque Potato Chips						
1 oz (9 chips)	150	9	15	170	2	2
Kettle Krinkle Cut Lightly Salted Potato Chips						
1 oz (9 chips)	150	9	16	115	2	1
Kettle Lightly Salted Organic Potato Chips						
1 oz	150	9	16	105	2	1
Kettle Multi Grain Tortilla Chips						
1 oz	140	7	18	100	3	2
Kettle Potato Chips, Lightly Salted						
1 oz (13 chips)	150	9	16	115	2	1
Kettle Roaster Fresh Nut Butters Organic Unsalted Peanut Butter						
1 oz (2 tbsp)	160	14	5	0	7	2
Kettle Sea Salt & Black Pepper Organic Potato Chips						
1 oz (13 chips)	150	9	16	200	2	2
Kettle Yellow Corn Tortilla Chips						
1 oz	140	7	18	100	3	2
Lay's Baked! Barbecue Flavored Potato Crisps						
1 oz	120	3	22	210	2	2
Lay's Baked! Original Potato Crisps						
1 oz	120	2	23	180	2	2
Lay's Baked! Sour Cream & Onion Flavored Potato Crisps						
1 oz	120	3	21	210	2	2
Lay's Barbecue Flavored Potato Chips						
1 oz	150	10	15	200	2	1
Lay's Cheddar & Sour Cream Flavored Potato Chips						
1 oz	160	10	15	230	2	<1
Lay's Classic Potato Chips						
1 oz	150	10	15	180	2	1
Lay's Kettle Cooked Original Potato Chips						
1 oz	150	8	18	110	2	1
Lay's Kettle Cooked Reduced Fat Original Flavored Potato Chips						
1 oz	140	6	19	160	2	2
Lay's Light Original Potato Chips						
1 oz	75	0	17	200	2	1
Lay's Salt & Vinegar Flavored Potato Chips						
1 oz	150	10	15	380	2	1

BRAND/FOOD ITEM SERVING SIZE	CALORIES	FAT	CARBS	SODIUM	PROTEIN	FIBER
Lay's Sour Cream & Onion Flavored Potato Chips						
1 oz	160	10	15	210	2	1
Lay's Wavy Original Potato Chips						
1 oz	150	10	15	180	2	1
Newman's Own 94% Fat Free Microwave Popcorn						
3½ cups	110	1.5	20	250	3	4
Newman's Own Butter Boom Microwave Popcorn						
3½ cups	130	5	18	290	2	3
Newman's Own Butter Microwave Popcorn						
3½ cups	130	5	18	180	2	3
Newman's Own Light Butter Microwave Popcorn						
3½ cups	120	4	19	170	3	4
Newman's Own Low Sodium Butter Microwave Popcorn						
3½ cups	130	5	18	100	2	3
Newman's Own Natural 100 Calorie Mini Bags Popcorn						
1 bag	100	2.5	18	210	2	4
Newman's Own Natural Flavor Microwave Popcorn						
3½ cups	130	5	18	200	2	3
Newman's Own Organic Bavarian Sour Dough Pretzels						
1 pretzel	90	0	19	400	2	1
Newman's Own Organic Cinnamon Sugar Soy Crisps						
1 oz	120	4	15	170	7	3
Newman's Own Organic Honey Wheat Pretzels						
20 pretzels						
	110	1	22	180	2	3
Newman's Own Organic Mighty Mini Pretzels						
20 pretzels						
	110	1	22	180	3	4
Newman's Own Organic Pop's Corn Butter Flavored Popcorn						
3½ cups	130	9	17	190	3	1
Newman's Own Organic Pop's Corn Light Butter Flavored Popcorn						
3½ cups	140	4.5	22	20	3	1
Newman's Own Organic Pop's Corn No Butter Popcorn						
3½ cups	110	1.5	21	20	3	5
Newman's Own Organic Salt & Pepper Rounds Pretzels						
8 pretzels						
	100	1	24	400	2	<1
Newman's Own Organic Salt & Pepper Thins Pretzels						
10 pretzels						
	120	1	24	400	2	<1
Newman's Own Organic Salted Nuggets Pretzels						
20 nuggets						
	120	1.5	25	330	3	2
Newman's Own Organic Salted Rods Pretzels						
4 rods	120	1.5	25	330	3	2
Newman's Own Organic Salted Rounds Pretzels						
8 rounds						
	110	1	24	400	2	<1
Newman's Own Organic Salted Sticks Pretzels						
12 sticks	110	1	24	350	2	1
Newman's Own Organic Salted Thins Pretzels						
10 pretzels						
	110	1	24	400	2	<1

BRAND/FOOD ITEM SERVING SIZE	CALORIES	FAT	CARBS	SODIUM	PROTEIN	FIBER
Newman's Own Organic Soy Crisps, Barbeque						
1 oz	110	3.5	14	390	7	3
Newman's Own Organic Soy Crisps, Lightly Salted						
1 oz	110	2.5	14	650	9	3
Newman's Own Organic Soy Crisps, White Cheddar						
1 oz	120	4	13	290	8	3
Newman's Own Organic Spelt Pretzels						
20 pretzels						
	120	1	23	240	4	4
Newman's Own Organic Thin Sticks Pretzels						
22 pretzels						
	110	1.5	22	180	3	4
Newman's Own Organic Unsalted Rounds Pretzels						
8 pretzels						
	110	1	24	105	2	<1
Newman's Own White Kernel Popcorn						
3½ cups	130	5	18	200	2	3
Popchips Barbeque Potato						
1 oz (about 19 chips)						
	120	4	20	250	1	1
Popchips Cheddar Potato						
1 oz (about 20 chips)						
	120	4	20	250	2	1
Popchips Original Potato						
1 oz (about 22 chips)						
	120	4	20	250	1	1
Popchips Parmesan Garlic Potato						
1 oz (about 20 chips)						
	120	4	20	310	2	1
Popchips Salt & Pepper Potato						
1 oz (about 20 chips)						
	120	4	20	250	1	1
Popchips Sea Salt & Vinegar Potato						
1 oz (about 20 chips)						
	120	4	20	250	1	1
Popchips Sour Cream & Onion Potato						
1 oz (about 20 chips)						
	120	4	20	250	2	1
Sun Chips Garden Salsa Flavored Multigrain Snacks						
1 oz	140	6	19	160	2	2
Sun Chips Original Flavored Multigrain Snacks						
1 oz	140	6	18	120	2	2
Tostitos Bite Size Rounds Tortilla Chips						
1 oz	140	7	18	110	2	2
Tostitos Crispy Rounds Tortilla Chips						
1 oz	140	7	18	120	2	2
Tostitos Multigrain Tortilla Chips						
1 oz	150	8	18	135	2	2
Tostitos Natural Blue Corn Restaurant Style Tortilla Chips						
1 oz	140	6	19	80	2	1

BRAND/FOOD ITEM SERVING SIZE	CALORIES	FAT	CARBS	SODIUM	PROTEIN	FIBER
Tostitos Scoops! Tortilla Chips						
1 oz	140	7	19	120	2	2

Energy Bars

Balance Almond Brownie Bar						
1 bar	200	6	22	75	14	2
Balance Chocolate Bar						
1 bar	200	6	23	180	14	1
Balance Chocolate Raspberry Fudge Bar						
1 bar	200	6	22	95	14	2
Balance Cookie Dough Bar						
1 bar	200	7	22	190	15	<1
Balance Honey Peanut Bar						
1 bar	200	7	21	180	15	<1
Balance Mocha Chip Bar						
1 bar	200	6	21	95	15	<1
Balance Peanut Butter Bar						
1 bar	200	7	21	160	15	1
Balance Yogurt Honey Peanut Bar						
1 bar	200	7	21	170	15	<1
Cascadian Farm Chocolate Chip Chewy Granola Bar						
1 bar	140	3.5	25	100	2	1
Cascadian Farm Fiber Right Dark Chocolate Almond Chewy Granola Bar						
1 bar	130	3.5	25	100	2	5
Cascadian Farm Fruit & Nut Chewy Granola Bar						
1 bar	140	4	24	100	2	1
Cascadian Farm Harvest Berries Chewy Granola Bar						
1 bar	130	2	26	115	2	1
Cascadian Farm Multi Grain Chewy Granola Bar						
1 bar	130	2	27	130	2	1
Cascadian Farm Peanut Butter Chip Chewy Granola Bar						
1 bar	140	4	25	130	2	1
Cascadian Farm Sweet & Salty Mixed Nut Chewy Granola Bar						
1 bar	160	8	20	125	3	1
Cascadian Farm Sweet & Salty Peanut Pretzel Chewy Granola Bar						
1 bar	160	7	22	180	3	1
Cascadian Farm Vanilla Chip Chewy Granola Bar						
1 bar	140	3	26	95	2	1
Clif Bar Apricot Bar						
1 bar	230	3	45	125	10	5
Clif Bar Banana Nut Bread Bar						
1 bar	240	6	42	120	9	4
Clif Bar Black Cherry Almond Bar						
1 bar	250	5	44	110	10	5
Clif Bar Blueberry Crisp Bar						
1 bar	240	5	43	150	9	5
Clif Bar Carrot Cake Bar						
1 bar	240	4	46	150	10	5
Clif Bar Chocolate Almond Fudge Bar						
1 bar	250	5	44	140	10	5

BRAND/FOOD ITEM SERVING SIZE	CALORIES	FAT	CARBS	SODIUM	PROTEIN	FIBER
Clif Bar Chocolate Brownie Bar						
1 bar	240	5	44	150	10	5
Clif Bar Chocolate Chip Bar						
1 bar	240	5	44	140	10	5
Clif Bar Chocolate Chip Peanut Crunch Bar						
1 bar	260	6	42	200	11	5
Clif Bar Cool Mint Chocolate Bar						
1 bar	250	5	43	140	10	5
Clif Bar Cranberry Apple Cherry Bar						
1 bar	230	2.5	45	100	10	5
Clif Bar Cranberry Orange Nut Bread Bar						
1 bar	240	6	42	70	9	4
Clif Bar Crunchy Peanut Butter Bar						
1 bar	250	6	42	230	11	5
Clif Bar Iced Gingerbread Bar						
1 bar	250	6	43	160	10	4
Clif Bar Maple Nut Bar						
1 bar	240	5	42	220	10	5
Clif Bar Oatmeal Raisin Walnut Bar						
1 bar	240	5	43	130	10	5
Clif Bar Peanut Toffee Buzz Bar						
1 bar	250	6	42	200	11	5
Clif Bar Spiced Pumpkin Pie Bar						
1 bar	240	5	45	140	10	5
Clif Bar White Chocolate Macadamia Bar						
1 bar	240	7	41	160	9	4
General Mills Cinnamon Toast Crunch Milk 'n Cereal Bar						
1 bar	180	4	32	140	3	1
General Mills Cocoa Puffs Milk 'n Cereal Bar						
1 bar	160	4	29	100	3	1
General Mills Honey Nut Cheerios Milk 'n Cereal Bar						
1 bar	160	4	28	120	3	1
Health Valley Café Creations Cinnamon Danish						
1 bar	130	2.5	27	80	2	2
Health Valley Café Creations Vanilla Crème Sandwich Bar						
1 bar	130	2	28	80	2	1
Health Valley Organic Apple Cobbler Cereal Bar						
1 bar	140	2.5	27	95	2	1
Health Valley Organic Berry Parfait Yogurt Cereal Bar						
1 bar	130	3	24	95	3	2
Health Valley Organic Blueberry Chewy Granola Bar						
1 bar	110	1.5	23	20	1	1
Health Valley Organic Blueberry Cobbler Cereal Bar						
1 bar	140	2.5	27	90	2	1
Health Valley Organic Chocolate Chip Chewy Granola Bar						
1 bar	110	2	22	10	1	<1
Health Valley Organic Double Chocolate Chip Chewy Granola Bar						
1 bar	160	2.5	32	20	2	1
Health Valley Organic Dutch Apple Chewy Granola Bar						
1 bar	100	1.5	20	10	1	<1
Health Valley Organic Fig Cobbler Cereal Bar						
1 bar	130	2.5	26	80	2	2

BRAND/FOOD ITEM SERVING SIZE	CALORIES	FAT	CARBS	SODIUM	PROTEIN	FIBER
Health Valley Organic French Vanilla Yogurt Cereal Bar						
1 bar	130	3	24	95	2	2
Health Valley Organic Peanut Crunch Chewy Granola Bar						
1 bar	110	2.5	21	85	2	<1
Health Valley Organic Raspberry Chewy Granola Bar						
1 bar	110	1.5	23	20	1	<1
Health Valley Organic Strawberry Cobbler Cereal Bar						
1 bar	130	2.5	26	85	2	1
Health Valley Organic Wildberry Chewy Granola Bar						
1 bar	110	1.5	22	10	1	<1
Kashi Baked Apple Spice TLC Tasty Little Cereal Bar						
1 bar	110	3	21	105	2	3
Kashi Blackberry Graham TLC Tasty Little Cereal Bar						
1 bar	110	3	21	125	2	3
Kashi Cherry Dark Chocolate TLC Chewy Granola Bar						
1 bar	120	2	24	65	5	4
Kashi Dark Chocolate Coconut TLC Fruit & Grain Bar						
1 bar	120	3.5	21	50	4	4
Kashi Dark Mocha Almond TLC Chewy Granola Bar						
1 bar	130	3.5	21	90	6	4
Kashi GoLean Chocolate Almond Crunchy! Protein & Fiber Bar						
1 bar	170	5	27	210	8	5
Kashi GoLean Chocolate Almond Toffee Chewy Protein & Fiber Bar						
1 bar	290	6	45	250	13	6
Kashi GoLean Chocolate Caramel Crunchy! Protein & Fiber Bar						
1 bar	150	3	28	220	8	6
Kashi GoLean Chocolate Peanut Crunchy! Protein & Fiber Bar						
1 bar	180	5	30	250	9	6
Kashi GoLean Cinnamon Coffee Cake Crunchy! Protein & Fiber Bar						
1 bar	160	4.5	26	240	8	5
Kashi GoLean Cookies 'n Cream Chewy Protein & Fiber Bar						
1 bar	290	6	50	200	13	6
Kashi GoLean Malted Chocolate Crisp Chewy Protein & Fiber Bar						
1 bar	290	6	49	200	13	6
Kashi GoLean Oatmeal Raisin Cookie Chewy Protein & Fiber Bar						
1 bar	280	5	49	140	13	6
Kashi GoLean Peanut Butter & Chocolate Chewy Protein & Fiber Bar						
1 bar	290	6	48	280	13	6
Kashi Honey Almond Flax TLC Chewy Granola Bar						
1 bar	140	5	19	115	7	4
Kashi Honey Toasted 7 Grain TLC Crunchy Granola Bar						
1 bar	180	6	25	160	6	4
Kashi Peanut Peanut Butter TLC Chewy Granola Bar						
1 bar	140	5	19	90	7	4
Kashi Pumpkin Pie TLC Fruit & Grain Bar						
1 bar	120	3	22	50	4	4
Kashi Pumpkin Spice Flax TLC Crunchy Granola Bar						
1 bar	180	6	26	150	6	4
Kashi Raspberry Chocolate TLC Fruit & Grain Bar						
1 bar	120	3	21	50	4	4
Kashi Ripe Strawberry TLC Tasty Little Cereal Bar						
1 bar	110	3	21	105	2	3

BRAND/FOOD ITEM SERVING SIZE	CALORIES	FAT	CARBS	SODIUM	PROTEIN	FIBER
Kashi Roasted Almond Crunch TLC Crunchy Granola Bar						
1 bar	180	6	25	160	6	4
Kashi Trail Mix TLC Chewy Granola Bar						
1 bar	140	5	20	105	6	4
Lärabar Apple Pie Bar						
1 bar	190	10	24	10	4	5
Lärabar Banana Bread Bar						
1 bar	230	11	30	0	6	5
Lärabar Cashew Cookie Bar						
1 bar	230	13	23	0	6	4
Lärabar Cherry Pie Bar						
1 bar	200	8	30	0	5	5
Lärabar Chocolate Coconut Bar						
1 bar	240	13	29	0	5	5
Lärabar Cinnamon Roll Bar						
1 bar	240	12	30	0	5	4
Lärabar Cocoa Mole Bar						
1 bar	220	9	33	0	4	6
Lärabar Coconut Cream Pie Bar						
1 bar	220	11	31	5	3	6
Lärabar Ginger Snap Bar						
1 bar	240	14	27	0	5	6
Lärabar Jocalat Chocolate Bar						
1 bar	200	10	27	0	4	5
Lärabar Jocalat Chocolate Cherry Bar						
1 bar	200	9	28	0	4	5
Lärabar Jocalat Chocolate Coffee Bar						
1 bar	210	11	27	0	4	5
Lärabar Jocalat Chocolate Hazelnut Bar						
1 bar	200	10	27	0	4	5
Lärabar Jocalat German Chocolate Cake Bar						
1 bar	210	13	25	0	3	4
Lärabar Key Lime Pie Bar						
1 bar	220	10	31	0	4	4
Lärabar Lemon Bar						
1 bar	220	11	28	0	5	4
Lärabar Peanut Butter and Jelly Bar						
1 bar	210	10	27	60	6	4
Lärabar Peanut Butter Cookie Bar						
1 bar	220	12	23	45	7	4
Lärabar Pecan Pie Bar						
1 bar	220	14	24	0	3	4
Lärabar Pistachio Bar						
1 bar	220	10	32	0	5	5
Lärabar Tropical Fruit Tart Bar						
1 bar	210	12	25	0	3	5
LUNA Berry Almond Bar						
1 bar	170	3.5	29	115	9	3
LUNA Caramel Nut Brownie Bar						
1 bar	180	6	27	115	8	4
LUNA Chai Tea Bar						
1 bar	190	5	26	95	9	3

BRAND/FOOD ITEM SERVING SIZE	CALORIES	FAT	CARBS	SODIUM	PROTEIN	FIBER
LUNA Chocolate Peppermint Stick Bar						
1 bar	180	5	28	120	8	3
LUNA Chocolate Raspberry Bar						
1 bar	170	5	27	135	8	5
LUNA Cookies 'n Cream Delight Bar						
1 bar	180	5	27	140	8	3
LUNA Dulce de Leche Bar						
1 bar	170	4	28	135	9	3
LUNA Iced Oatmeal Raisin Bar						
1 bar	180	5	27	150	9	3
LUNA LemonZest Bar						
1 bar	180	5	27	115	9	3
LUNA Nutz Over Chocolate Bar						
1 bar	180	6	25	190	9	3
LUNA Peanut Butter Cookie Bar						
1 bar	180	6	25	140	9	3
LUNA S'Mores Bar						
1 bar	180	5	27	140	9	3
LUNA Sunrise Apple Cinnamon Bar						
1 bar	180	4.5	27	100	8	5
LUNA Sunrise Blueberry Bliss Bar						
1 bar	170	4.5	25	105	8	5
LUNA Sunrise Strawberry Crumble Bar						
1 bar	170	4.5	26	105	8	5
LUNA Sunrise Vanilla Almond Bar						
1 bar	180	4.5	29	95	8	5
LUNA Toasted Nuts 'n Cranberry Bar						
1 bar	170	4.5	26	180	9	3
LUNA White Chocolate Macadamia Bar						
1 bar	190	7	25	210	9	3
Nature Valley Almond Crunch Roasted Nut Bar						
1 bar	190	13	13	180	6	2
Nature Valley Almond Sweet & Salty Nut Granola Bar						
1 bar	160	7	22	170	3	2
Nature Valley Apple Cinnamon Chewy Trail Mix Bar						
1 bar	140	4	25	115	3	1
Nature Valley Apple Crisp Granola Bar						
1 bar	80	3	13	70	2	1
Nature Valley Blueberry Yogurt Chewy Granola Bar						
1 bar	140	3.5	26	110	2	1
Nature Valley Cashew Sweet & Salty Nut Granola Bar						
1 bar	160	7	22	150	2	1
Nature Valley Cinnamon Granola Bar						
1 bar	90	3	15	85	2	1
Nature Valley Cranberry & Pomegranate Chewy Trail Mix Bar						
1 bar	120	3	24	90	2	1
Nature Valley Dark Chocolate & Nut Chewy Trail Mix Bar						
1 bar	140	4	25	100	2	1
Nature Valley Fruit & Nut Chewy Trail Mix Bar						
1 bar	140	4	25	100	3	1
Nature Valley Maple Brown Sugar Granola Bar						
1 bar	90	3.5	15	80	2	1

BRAND/FOOD ITEM SERVING SIZE	CALORIES	FAT	CARBS	SODIUM	PROTEIN	FIBER
Nature Valley Mixed Berry Chewy Trail Mix Bar						
1 bar	140	3.5	26	90	2	1
Nature Valley Oats 'n Honey Granola Bar						
1 bar	90	3	15	80	2	1
Nature Valley Peanut Butter Granola Bar						
1 bar	90	3.5	14	90	2	1
Nature Valley Peanut Crunch Roasted Nut Bar						
1 bar	190	13	13	180	6	2
Nature Valley Peanut Sweet & Salty Nut Granola Bar						
1 bar	170	9	19	150	4	2
Nature Valley Pecan Crunch Granola Bar						
1 bar	90	3.5	14	80	2	1
Nature Valley Roasted Almond Granola Bar						
1 bar	90	4	14	85	2	1
Nature Valley Roasted Mixed Nut Sweet & Salty Nut Granola Bar						
1 bar	160	8	21	150	3	1
Nature Valley Strawberry Yogurt Chewy Granola Bar						
1 bar	140	3.5	26	110	2	1
Nature Valley Vanilla Nut Granola Bar						
1 bar	90	3.5	14	80	2	1
Nature Valley Vanilla Yogurt Chewy Granola Bar						
1 bar	140	3.5	26	110	2	1
Nature's Path Apricot & Nut Granola Bar						
1 bar	160	5	26	85	3	2
Nature's Path Blueberry Flax & Soy Optimum Energy Bar						
1 bar	200	3	38	100	6	5
Nature's Path Chocolate Chip Granola Bar						
1 bar	140	4.5	24	35	2	2
Nature's Path Cranberry Ginger Granola Bar						
1 bar	160	4	27	75	3	3
Nature's Path Hemp Plus Granola Bar						
1 bar	130	3	28	100	3	2
Nature's Path Orange Chocolate Optimum Energy Bar						
1 bar	220	6	37	120	5	4
Nature's Path Peanut Butter Granola Bar						
1 bar	160	5	25	100	4	2
Nature's Path Peanut Butter Optimum Energy Bar						
1 bar	230	8	33	200	7	4
Nature's Path Peanut Choco' Granola Bar						
1 bar	150	6	22	125	3	2
Nature's Path Pomegran Cherry Optimum Energy Bar						
1 bar	230	5	39	140	4	4
Nature's Path Pumpkin Flax Plus Granola Bar						
1 bar	160	4.5	27	90	3	3
Nature's Path ReBound Banana, Nut, Matcha & Flax Bar						
1 bar	190	4	33	140	10	4
PowerBar Fruit Smoothie Energy Berry Blast Bar						
1 bar	220	3.5	43	180	6	<1
PowerBar Fruit Smoothie Energy Creamy Citrus Bar						
1 bar	220	3.5	43	180	6	<1
PowerBar Harvest Apple Cinnamon Crisp Bar						
1 bar	240	4	42	140	10	5

BRAND/FOOD ITEM SERVING SIZE	CALORIES	FAT	CARBS	SODIUM	PROTEIN	FIBER
PowerBar Harvest Double Chocolate Crisp Bar						
1 bar	250	5	42	150	10	5
PowerBar Harvest Oatmeal Raisin Cookie Bar						
1 bar	250	5	43	140	10	5
PowerBar Nut Naturals Fruit & Nut Bar						
1 bar	210	10	20	180	10	3
PowerBar Nut Naturals Trail Mix Bar						
1 bar	210	10	21	220	10	2
PowerBar Performance Chocolate Bar						
1 bar	240	3	45	200	8	3
PowerBar Performance Oatmeal Raisin Bar						
1 bar	230	3.5	45	200	8	2
PowerBar Pria Chocolate Peanut Crunch Bar						
1 bar	110	3.5	16	85	5	1
PowerBar PROTEINplus Chocolate Chip Bar						
1 bar	290	6	37	190	23	2
PowerBar PROTEINplus Chocolate Peanut Butter Bar						
1 bar	300	6	39	210	23	1
PowerBar PROTEINplus Reduced Sugar Chocolate Peanut Butter Bar						
1 bar	270	9	30	290	22	2
PowerBar PROTEINplus Vanilla Yogurt Bar						
1 bar	300	6	38	150	23	1
PowerBar Recovery Peanut Butter Caramel Crisp Bar						
1 bar	260	10	30	180	12	0
PowerBar Triple Threat Chocolate Peanut Butter Crisp Bar						
1 bar	220	6	32	170	11	4
ThinkThin Brownie Crunch Protein Bar						
1 bar	230	8	25	150	20	2
ThinkThin Chocolate Fudge Bar						
1 bar	230	8	24	135	20	1
ThinkThin Chocolate Mudslide Bar						
1 bar	230	7	25	115	20	1
ThinkThin Chunky Peanut Butter Bar						
1 bar	240	8	24	200	20	1
ThinkThin Creamy Peanut Butter Bar						
1 bar	230	9	22	210	20	1
ThinkThin Dark Chocolate Flavor Bar						
1 bar	230	7	26	110	20	2
ThinkThin White Chocolate Chip Bar						
1 bar	230	8	28	15	20	1

Sweets

Cake, chocolate, prepared from recipe without frosting						
1 piece	352	14	51	299	5	2
Cake, pound, commercially prepared, butter						
1 piece	116	6	15	119	2	0
Cake, sponge, prepared from recipe						
1 piece	187	3	36	144	5	0
Cake, white, prepared from recipe without frosting						
1 piece	264	9	42	242	4	1

BRAND/FOOD ITEM SERVING SIZE	CALORIES	FAT	CARBS	SODIUM	PROTEIN	FIBER
Cake, yellow, prepared from recipe without frosting						
1 piece	245	10	36	233	4	1
Health Valley Cookie Cremes Chocolate Sandwich Cookies						
2 cookies	120	5	19	100	1	0
Health Valley Cookie Cremes Vanilla Flavored Sandwich Cookies						
2 cookies	130	5	20	110	1	0
Health Valley Mini Chocolate Chip Cookies						
4 cookies	120	6	16	125	1	1
Health Valley Mini Chocolate Chocolate Chip Cookies						
4 cookies	130	7	16	110	1	1
Health Valley Oatmeal Raisin Cookies						
1 cookie	90	3.5	14	50	2	1
Health Valley Organic Baked Apple Toaster Tarts						
1 bar	150	3	29	110	2	<1
Health Valley Organic Blueberry Toaster Tarts						
1 bar	150	3	29	105	2	1
Health Valley Organic Chocolate Toaster Tarts						
1 bar	150	3	29	85	2	1
Health Valley Organic Raspberry Toaster Tarts						
1 bar	150	3	29	105	2	<1
Health Valley Organic Red Cherry Toaster Tarts						
1 bar	150	3	29	105	2	1
Health Valley Organic Strawberry Toaster Tarts						
1 bar	150	3	28	100	2	<1
Hershey's Kit Kat						
4 sticks (1 package)	210	11	28	30	3	<1
Hershey's Milk Chocolate						
1 bar	210	13	26	35	3	1
Hershey's Milk Chocolate Kisses						
9 pieces	230	13	24	35	3	1
Hershey's Reese's Peanut Butter Cups						
1 package	210	13	24	150	5	1
Hershey's Reese's Pieces						
1 package	210	10	27	80	5	1
Kashi TLC Happy Trail Mix Cookies						
1 cookie	140	5	21	75	2	4
Kashi TLC Oatmeal Dark Chocolate Cookies						
1 cookie	130	5	20	65	2	4
Kashi TLC Oatmeal Raisin Flax Cookies						
1 cookie	130	4.5	20	70	2	4
Kellogg's Pop-Tarts Apple Strudel Pastries						
1 pastry	200	5	35	160	2	<1
Kellogg's Pop-Tarts Blueberry Pastries						
1 pastry	210	5	37	180	2	<1

BRAND/FOOD ITEM SERVING SIZE	CALORIES	FAT	CARBS	SODIUM	PROTEIN	FIBER
Kellogg's Pop-Tarts Frosted Blueberry Pastries						
1 pastry	200	5	38	170	2	<1
Kellogg's Pop-Tarts Low-Fat Frosted Strawberry Pastries						
1 pastry	190	2.5	39	210	2	<1
Kellogg's Pop-Tarts Whole Grain with Fiber Strawberry Toaster Pastries						
1 pastry	190	5	35	150	2	5
LUNA Cookie Berry Pomegranate Cookie						
1 cookie	140	5	27	100	3	4
LUNA Cookie Chocolate Mint Cookie						
1 cookie	130	2.5	26	140	3	4
LUNA Cookie Peanut Butter Chocolate Cookie						
1 cookie	150	6	23	170	4	3
Mars 3 Musketeers						
1 bar	260	8	46	110	2	1
Mars M&Ms						
1 bag (1.69 oz)						
	240	10	34	30	2	1
Mars Snickers						
1 bar (2 oz)						
	280	14	35	140	4	1
Nature Valley Honey Roasted Peanut Nut Cluster						
1 oz	140	7	15	160	5	1
Nature Valley Nut Lovers Nut Clusters						
1 oz	160	10	14	130	4	1
Nature Valley Roasted Almond Nut Clusters						
1 oz	140	7	15	160	4	2
Nature Valley Roasted Cashew Nut Clusters						
1 oz	150	7	18	200	4	1
Nature's Path Apple Cinnamon Frosted Toaster Pastry						
1 pastry	210	4.5	39	130	2	1
Nature's Path Apple Cinnamon Toaster Pastry						
1 pastry	210	4.5	40	150	3	1
Nature's Path Blueberry Frosted Toaster Pastry						
1 pastry	200	4	38	125	2	1
Nature's Path Blueberry Toaster Pastry						
1 pastry	210	4.5	40	150	3	1
Nature's Path Brown Sugar Maple Cinnamon Frosted Toaster Pastry						
1 pastry	210	4.5	39	125	3	1
Nature's Path Brown Sugar Maple Cinnamon Toaster Pastry						
1 pastry	210	5	37	135	3	1
Nature's Path Buckwheat Wildberry Frozen Waffles						
2 waffles						
	180	6	29	350	2	1
Nature's Path Cherry Chocolate Stripes Frosted Toaster Pastries						
1 pastry	200	4.5	38	125	3	1
Nature's Path Cherry Pomegran Frosted Toaster Pastry						
1 pastry	200	4.5	37	150	3	1
Nature's Path Chocolate Frosted Toaster Pastry						
1 pastry	210	5	38	130	3	1
Nature's Path Flax Plus Frozen Waffles						
2 waffles						
	180	7	26	380	5	5

BRAND/FOOD ITEM SERVING SIZE	CALORIES	FAT	CARBS	SODIUM	PROTEIN	FIBER
Nature's Path Flax Plus Red Berry Frozen Waffles						
2 waffles	180	8	26	350	4	4
Nature's Path Flax Plus with Figs Frozen Waffles						
2 waffles	190	9	25	340	4	4
Nature's Path Hemp Plus Frozen Waffles						
2 waffles	190	7	26	360	5	5
Nature's Path Homestyle Frozen Waffles						
2 waffles	270	10	44	420	2	2
Nature's Path Maple Cinn Frozen Waffles						
2 waffles	180	6	28	380	4	4
Nature's Path Mesa Sunrise Frozen Waffles						
2 waffles	200	7	34	450	2	1
Nature's Path Pomegran Plus Frozen Waffles						
2 waffles	160	4.5	27	360	4	4
Nature's Path Raspberry Frosted Toaster Pastries						
1 pastry	210	5	39	150	3	1
Nature's Path Strawberry Frosted Toaster Pastry						
1 pastry	210	4	40	140	3	1
Nature's Path Strawberry Toaster Pastry						
1 pastry	210	4.5	40	150	3	1
Nature's Path Wildberry Acai Frosted Toaster Pastries						
1 pastry	210	5	39	130	3	1
Nestlé Crunch Bar						
1 bar (1.55 oz)	220	12	29	15	2	1
Newman's Own Organic Arrowroot Alphabet Cookies						
10 cookies	120	3	22	135	2	0
Newman's Own Organic Chocolate Alphabet Cookies						
10 cookies	120	3	22	120	2	1
Newman's Own Organic Chocolate Chip Cookies						
4 cookies	160	7	21	100	2	1
Newman's Own Organic Chocolate Chocolate Chip Cookies						
4 cookies	160	8	20	70	2	1
Newman's Own Organic Cinnamon Graham Alphabet Cookies						
10 cookies	120	3	22	90	2	0
Newman's Own Organic Cinnamon Hermits Cookies						
1 cookie	80	1.5	17	60	1	<1
Newman's Own Organic Dark Chocolate						
1 bar (2.25 oz)	330	22	37	5	3	4

BRAND/FOOD ITEM SERVING SIZE	CALORIES	FAT	CARBS	SODIUM	PROTEIN	FIBER
Newman's Own Organic Dark Chocolate Caramel Cups						
1 package	160	9	20	30	1	2
Newman's Own Organic Dark Chocolate Peppermint Cups						
1 package	180	10	20	15	1	1
Newman's Own Organic Double Chocolate Mint Chip Cookies						
4 cookies	160	8	21	70	2	1
Newman's Own Organic Espresso Chocolate Chip Cookies						
4 cookies	150	7	21	100	2	1
Newman's Own Organic Espresso Dark Chocolate						
1 bar (2.25 oz)	320	22	37	5	3	4
Newman's Own Organic Fig Newmans, Fat-Free						
2 bars	120	0	28	140	2	1
Newman's Own Organic Fig Newmans, Low Fat						
2 bars	140	2	28	170	2	1
Newman's Own Organic Fig Newmans, Wheat-Free & Dairy-Free						
2 bars	120	1.5	26	170	2	1
Newman's Own Organic Ginger Hermits Cookies						
1 cookie	80	1.5	16	65	1	<1
Newman's Own Organic Ginger-Os Cookies						
2 cookies	120	4.5	19	160	1	0
Newman's Own Organic Hermits Cookies						
1 cookie	80	1.5	16	65	1	<1
Newman's Own Organic Milk Chocolate						
1 bar (2.5 oz)	340	21	38	35	3	1
Newman's Own Organic Milk Chocolate Caramel Cups						
1 package	160	8	21	40	2	0
Newman's Own Organic Mocha Milk Chocolate						
1 bar (2.25 oz)	340	23	37	30	3	1
Newman's Own Organic Newman-Os Chocolate Crème Cookies						
2 cookies	130	4.5	20	85	2	1
Newman's Own Organic Newman-Os Cookies						
2 cookies	130	4.5	20	85	2	1
Newman's Own Organic Newman-Os Mint Crème Cookies						
2 cookies	130	4.5	20	85	2	1
Newman's Own Organic Orange Chocolate Chip Cookies						
4 cookies	160	7	21	105	2	1

BRAND/FOOD ITEM SERVING SIZE	CALORIES	FAT	CARBS	SODIUM	PROTEIN	FIBER
Newman's Own Organic Peanut Butter Dark Chocolate Cups						
1 package	180	12	17	100	3	2
Newman's Own Organic Peanut Butter Milk Chocolate Cups						
1 package	190	12	17	110	3	1
Newman's Own Organic Super Dark Chocolate						
1 bar (2.25 oz)	330	28	30	0	5	6
Newman's Own Organic Wheat-Free Alphabet Cookies						
10 cookies	110	3	21	115	1	1
Newman's Own Organic Wheat-Free & Dairy-Free Chocolate Chip Cookies						
4 cookies	160	8	21	70	<1	0
Newman's Own Organic Wheat-Free Dairy-Free Cookies						
2 cookies	130	4.5	21	80	1	0
Nutter Butter Cookies						
2 cookies	130	5	20	110	2	1
Oreo Double Stuff						
2 cookies	140	7	21	105	1	<1
Oreo Original						
3 cookies	160	7	25	160	1	1
Pepperidge Farm Milano Cookies						
3 cookies	180	10	21	80	2	
Pepperidge Farm Soft Baked Chocolate Chunk Cookies						
1 cookie	150	7	21	70	1	<1

RESTAURANTS

Obviously, I don't want you to have this stuff. Let's face it—food from restaurant chains is predominantly garbage. It's not organic; it's all processed. Even at Starbucks, that yogurt and fruit might look healthy—but it's not organic. I know, though, that there are many times this food is all that's available to you, and that's the reason it's in this book—so you can choose the best option possible, wherever you are. Because this is basically all bad food, at least keep the calories in mind. Yeah, the grilled chicken sandwich is probably not great, because of antibiotics in the meat, mayo, nonorganic veggies, and the white bread bun, but it's a hell of a lot better than the double bacon cheeseburger at 1,000 calories. And even that salad may have more calories, once you dump the full packet of Caesar on there. Definitely, before you order, *double check the calories.*

RESTAURANT/ FOOD ITEM SERVING SIZE	CALORIES	FAT	CARBS	SODIUM	PROTEIN	FIBER
Arby's All American Roastburger						
241 g	412	18	45	1305	19	2
Arby's Apple Turnover with Icing						
128 g	380	14	58	287	4	3
Arby's Arby-Q						
168 g	340	11	48	1089	17	2

RESTAURANT/ FOOD ITEM SERVING SIZE	CALORIES	FAT	CARBS	SODIUM	PROTEIN	FIBER
Arby's Bacon (Extra)						
4 pieces/17 g	77	6	1	301	5	0
Arby's Bacon & Bleu Roastburger						
231 g	466	23	44	1397	21	2
Arby's Bacon & Egg Croissant						
120 g	337	22	23	651	11	1
Arby's Bacon Biscuit						
95 g	340	21	29	1028	9	1
Arby's Bacon Cheddar Roastburger						
231 g	443	18	44	1448	23	2
Arby's Bacon, Egg & Cheese Biscuit						
158 g	461	30	30	1446	17	1
Arby's Bacon, Egg & Cheese Croissant						
133 g	378	25	23	850	14	1
Arby's Bacon, Egg & Cheese Sourdough						
173 g	437	21	40	1220	20	2
Arby's Bacon, Egg, & Cheese Wrap						
193 g	515	29	50	1367	16	2
Arby's Balsamic Vinaigrette Dressing						
43 g	130	12	5	460	0	0
Arby's BBQ Bacon Cheddar Roastburger						
283 g	581	25	61	2128	25	3
Arby's BBQ Dipping Sauce						
28 g	44	0	11	343	0	0
Arby's Beef 'n Cheddar Sandwich						
Large/329 g	657	36	46	2309	42	3
Arby's Beef 'n Cheddar Sandwich						
Medium/251 g	536	27	44	1701	32	2
Arby's Beef 'n Cheddar Sandwich						
Regular/195 g	440	21	43	1275	22	2
Arby's Biscuit, Plain						
82 g	273	15	28	786	5	1
Arby's Blueberry Muffin						
85 g	320	12	49	490	4	1
Arby's Breakfast Syrup						
28 g	78	0	20	25	0	0
Arby's Bronco Berry Dipping Sauce						
43 g	92	0	23	27	0	0
Arby's Buffalo Dipping Sauce						
28 g	11	1	2	782	0	0
Arby's Buttermilk Ranch Dressing						
43 g	230	24	2	390	1	0
Arby's Cheddar Cheese Sauce, Side						
21 g	25	2	2	182	0	0
Arby's Cheddar Fries						
Medium/198 g	546	33	62	1525	7	6

RESTAURANT/ FOOD ITEM SERVING SIZE	CALORIES	FAT	CARBS	SODIUM	PROTEIN	FIBER
Arby's Cherry Turnover with Icing						
128 g	364	13	58	269	4	1
Arby's Chicken Bacon & Swiss, Crispy						
207 g	544	25	50	1632	32	2
Arby's Chicken Bacon & Swiss, Roast						
194 g	439	18	40	1343	30	2
Arby's Chicken Biscuit						
132 g	417	23	39	1240	15	1
Arby's Chicken Cordon Bleu Sandwich, Crispy						
244 g	577	28	47	1936	37	2
Arby's Chicken Cordon Bleu Sandwich, Roast						
230 g	472	20	37	1646	34	2
Arby's Chicken Fillet Sandwich, Crispy						
203 g	488	23	47	1210	26	2
Arby's Chicken Fillet Sandwich, Roast						
189 g	383	16	37	921	23	2
Arby's Chocolate Malt Swirl Shake						
468 g	620	17	101	454	16	1
Arby's Chocolate Swirl Shake						
468 g	620	17	101	449	16	1
Arby's Chocolate Twist						
71 g	250	12	34	110	4	2
Arby's Chopped Farmhouse Chicken Salad, Crispy						
301 g	395	19	25	857	25	4
Arby's Chopped Farmhouse Chicken Salad, Grilled						
279 g	229	11	9	579	20	3
Arby's Chopped Italian Salad						
303 g	386	28	11	1420	21	3
Arby's Chopped Turkey Club Salad						
279 g	230	11	9	801	22	3
Arby's Cinnamon Twist						
71 g	260	13	32	210	4	2
Arby's Classic Italian Toasted Sub						
290 g	596	27	65	1831	25	3
Arby's Coffee						
12 oz	5	0	0	0	2	0
Arby's Corned Beef Reuben Sandwich						
295 g	590	32	55	1685	32	3
Arby's Croissant						
57 g	190	10	21	190	3	1
Arby's Curly Fries Large/190 g						
	604	36	70	1413	8	7
Arby's Curly Fries Medium/156 g						
	496	29	58	1160	7	6
Arby's Curly Fries Small/106 g						
	338	20	39	791	4	4
Arby's Diet Blackberry Iced FruiTea						
548 g	0	0	4	0	0	0

RESTAURANT/ FOOD ITEM SERVING SIZE	CALORIES	FAT	CARBS	SODIUM	PROTEIN	FIBER
Arby's Diet Peach Iced FruiTea						
548 g	0	0	4	0	0	0
Arby's Dijon Honey Mustard Dressing						
43 g	180	17	8	240	1	0
Arby's Double Meat Roastburger Option, Additional Calories						
71 g	119	9	0	532	13	0
Arby's Egg & Cheese Sourdough						
164 g	392	17	40	1058	17	2
Arby's Fajita Flatbread Melt, Roast Beef						
222 g	514	35	28	1716	26	2
Arby's Fajita Flatbread Melt, Roast Chicken						
222 g	470	26	30	1608	28	2
Arby's French Dip & Swiss Toasted Sub						
296 g	533	19	67	2169	29	3
Arby's French Toastix						
124 g	312	13	44	492	6	1
Arby's Gourmet Chocolate Chunk Cookies						
45 g	209	10	27	163	2	0
Arby's Ham & Cheese Croissant						
120 g	281	15	22	918	14	1
Arby's Ham & Swiss Melt Sandwich						
131 g	268	8	35	1042	17	1
Arby's Ham Biscuit						
132 g	323	17	29	1315	14	1
Arby's Ham, Egg & Cheese Biscuit						
195 g	444	26	31	1734	21	1
Arby's Ham, Egg & Cheese Croissant						
170 g	361	21	23	1138	19	1
Arby's Ham, Egg & Cheese Sourdough						
214 g	442	19	41	1586	26	2
Arby's Ham, Egg, & Cheese Wrap						
249 g	575	31	51	2005	25	2
Arby's Honey Mustard Dipping Sauce						
28 g	129	12	6	151	0	0
Arby's Horsey Sauce						
14 g	62	5	3	173	0	0
Arby's Jalapeno Bites						
Large, 8 pieces/176 g						
	489	34	47	841	9	3
Arby's Jalapeno Bites						
Regular/5 pieces/110 g						
	305	21	29	526	5	2
Arby's Jamocha Swirl Shake						
468 g	611	17	99	485	16	1
Arby's Ketchup Packet						
14 g	13	0	3	158	0	0
Arby's Loaded Potato Bites						
Large/8 pieces/179 g						
	565	35	43	1281	18	4
Arby's Loaded Potato Bites						
Regular/5 pieces/112 g						
	353	22	27	800	11	2

RESTAURANT/ FOOD ITEM SERVING SIZE	CALORIES	FAT	CARBS	SODIUM	PROTEIN	FIBER
Arby's Mandarin Peach Iced FruiTea						
551 g	90	0	23	0	0	0
Arby's Marinara Sauce						
43 g	30	2	4	0	1	1
Arby's Mayonnaise Packet						
14 g	105	11	0	74	0	0
Arby's Melt						
146 g	298	12	36	922	16	2
Arby's Mozzarella Sticks Large/6 pieces/205 g						
	637	42	56	2047	27	3
Arby's Mozzarella Sticks Regular/4 pieces/137 g						
	426	28	38	1370	18	2
Arby's Onion Petals Large/164 g						
	480	33	51	482	6	3
Arby's Onion Petals Regular/85 g						
	248	17	26	249	3	2
Arby's Orange Cream Swirl Shake						
482 g	646	16	113	413	15	1
Arby's Original Gourmet Cinnamon Roll						
100 g	330	15	42	540	6	2
Arby's Passion Fruit Iced FruiTea						
565 g	100	0	25	0	0	0
Arby's Pecan Chicken Salad Sandwich						
322 g	769	39	79	1240	30	9
Arby's Pecan Sticky Bun						
135 g	511	27	60	587	7	3
Arby's Pecan Sticky Bun 4 Pack						
542 g	2044	108	238	2348	29	12
Arby's Philly Beef Toasted Sub						
254 g	610	30	62	1549	29	3
Arby's Popcorn Chicken Large/184 g						
	529	24	39	1354	35	3
Arby's Popcorn Chicken Regular/126 g						
	363	16	27	930	24	2
Arby's Potato Cakes 2 pieces/100 g						
	246	18	26	391	2	2
Arby's Potato Cakes 3 pieces/150 g						
	369	28	39	587	3	3
Arby's Potato Cakes 4 pieces/200 g						
	492	37	52	782	3	5
Arby's Ranch Dipping Sauce						
43 g	158	16	2	277	1	0

RESTAURANT/ FOOD ITEM SERVING SIZE	CALORIES	FAT	CARBS	SODIUM	PROTEIN	FIBER
Arby's Roast Beef Sandwich Large/281 g	547	28	41	1869	42	3
Arby's Roast Beef Sandwich Medium/210 g	415	21	34	1379	31	2
Arby's Roast Beef Sandwich Regular/154 g	320	14	34	953	21	2
Arby's Roast Beef Sandwich, Junior 125 g	272	10	34	740	16	2
Arby's Roast Chicken Club Sandwich 257 g	498	20	46	1540	30	2
Arby's Roast Ham & Swiss Sandwich 345 g	691	31	75	1952	33	5
Arby's Roast Turkey & Swiss Sandwich 345 g	708	30	74	1677	41	5
Arby's Roast Turkey Ranch & Bacon Sandwich 367 g	818	38	75	2146	46	5
Arby's Sauce 14 g	15	0	4	177	0	0
Arby's Sausage & Egg Croissant 147 g	433	32	23	784	12	1
Arby's Sausage Biscuit 122 g	436	31	28	1160	10	1
Arby's Sausage, Egg & Cheese Biscuit 185 g	557	40	30	1579	18	1
Arby's Sausage, Egg & Cheese Croissant 160 g	475	35	23	982	15	1
Arby's Sausage, Egg & Cheese Sourdough 204 g	556	33	40	1431	22	2
Arby's Sausage, Egg & Cheese Wrap 239 g	689	45	50	1849	21	2
Arby's Sausage Gravy Biscuit 238 g	1040	60	107	4700	7	1
Arby's Sausage Patty 51 g	210	20	0	480	6	0
Arby's Spicy Three Pepper Sauce 14 g	22	1	3	140	0	0
Arby's Super Roast Beef 209 g	399	19	40	1061	21	2
Arby's Sweet Tea 16 oz	120	0	32	15	0	0
Arby's Tangy Southwest Sauce 43 g	249	26	3	278	0	0
Arby's TJ Cinnamons Mocha Chill 354 g	306	7	48	214	11	1
Arby's TJ Icing 28 g	119	5	18	58	0	0

RESTAURANT/ FOOD ITEM	SERVING SIZE	CALORIES	FAT	CARBS	SODIUM	PROTEIN	FIBER
Arby's Turkey Bacon Club Toasted Sub							
	290 g	605	24	65	1701	35	3
Arby's Ultimate BLT Sandwich							
	294 g	779	45	75	1571	23	6
Arby's Vanilla Shake							
	482 g	572	18	86	458	17	0
Au Bon Pain Almond Croissant							
	1 serving	600	38	55	300	13	4
Au Bon Pain Angus Steak Teriyaki Hot Wrap							
	1 serving	630	16	99	1650	24	5
Au Bon Pain Apple Croissant							
	1 serving	280	11	44	160	5	3
Au Bon Pain Apple Gingerbread Tulip							
	1 serving	340	13	52	320	4	2
Au Bon Pain Arizona Chicken Sandwich							
	1 serving	690	28	60	1600	47	4
Au Bon Pain Asiago Cheese Bagel							
	1 serving	340	6	56	620	15	2
Au Bon Pain Bacon and Bagel							
	1 serving	340	6	58	650	16	2
Au Bon Pain Bacon and Egg Melt on Ciabatta							
	1 serving	510	26	41	1270	26	2
Au Bon Pain Baja Turkey Sandwich							
	1 serving	700	27	71	1680	46	5
Au Bon Pain Baked BBQ Chicken Sandwich							
	1 serving	680	19	80	1620	44	3
Au Bon Pain Baked Egg and Cheddar Sandwich							
	1 serving	300	9	39	800	16	2
Au Bon Pain Banana Nut Pound Cake							
	1 serving	480	26	56	430	7	1
Au Bon Pain BBQ Brisket Sandwich							
	1 serving	660	21	81	1660	36	5
Au Bon Pain BBQ Chicken Sandwich							
	1 serving	560	13	83	1500	29	6
Au Bon Pain Blondie							
	1 serving	460	33	59	580	5	2
Au Bon Pain Blueberry Muffin							
	1 serving	490	17	74	510	9	2
Au Bon Pain Caffe Americano Large/20 oz							
		15	0	2	30	0	0
Au Bon Pain Caffe Americano Medium/16 oz							
		10	0	2	25	0	0
Au Bon Pain Caffe Americano Small/12 oz							
		5	0	1	15	0	0
Au Bon Pain Caffe Latte Large/20 oz							
		310	16	26	270	16	0

RESTAURANT/ FOOD ITEM SERVING SIZE	CALORIES	FAT	CARBS	SODIUM	PROTEIN	FIBER
Au Bon Pain Caffe Latte Medium/16 oz	260	14	21	220	14	0
Au Bon Pain Caffe Latte Small/12 oz	200	11	17	170	11	0
Au Bon Pain Cappuccino Large/20 oz	200	11	18	150	11	0
Au Bon Pain Cappuccino Medium/16 oz	150	8	13	110	8	0
Au Bon Pain Cappuccino Small/12 oz	120	7	10	85	6	0
Au Bon Pain Caprese Sandwich 1 serving	680	32	65	1200	30	4
Au Bon Pain Caramel Macchiato Large/20 oz	540	15	84	230	15	0
Au Bon Pain Caramel Macchiato Medium/16 oz	430	12	68	190	12	0
Au Bon Pain Caramel Macchiato Small/12 oz	350	10	53	160	10	0
Au Bon Pain Carrot Walnut Muffin	560	27	72	820	9	4
Au Bon Pain Chai Latte Large/20 oz	460	16	62	200	16	0
Au Bon Pain Chai Latte Medium/16 oz	380	14	51	170	14	0
Au Bon Pain Chai Latte Small/12 oz	290	11	38	130	11	0
Au Bon Pain Cherry Danish 1 serving	420	20	54	340	7	1
Au Bon Pain Chicken Artichoke Sandwich 1 serving	500	10	63	1460	39	4
Au Bon Pain Chicken Pesto Sandwich 1 serving	660	24	66	1560	43	4
Au Bon Pain Chocolate Cheesecake Brownie 1 serving	460	19	74	400	5	1
Au Bon Pain Chocolate Cherry Tulip 1 serving	410	21	54	370	5	2
Au Bon Pain Chocolate Chip Brownie 1 serving	510	19	74	380	6	1

RESTAURANT/ FOOD ITEM SERVING SIZE	CALORIES	FAT	CARBS	SODIUM	PROTEIN	FIBER
Au Bon Pain Chocolate Chip Cookie						
1 serving	280	13	40	210	3	2
Au Bon Pain Chocolate Chip Muffin						
1	580	23	83	480	9	3
Au Bon Pain Chocolate Croissant						
1	440	22	58	210	7	3
Au Bon Pain Chocolate Dipped Cranberry Almond Macaroon						
1	300	15	36	190	4	4
Au Bon Pain Chocolate Dipped Shortbread						
1	380	22	42	310	4	1
Au Bon Pain Chocolate Orange Pecan Scone						
1	580	28	74	360	10	3
Au Bon Pain Cinnamon Crisp Bagel						
1	410	7	77	400	11	4
Au Bon Pain Cinnamon Raisin Bagel						
1	320	1	68	450	11	3
Au Bon Pain Cinnamon Scone						
1	530	27	60	400	9	2
Au Bon Pain Confetti Cookie with M&Ms						
1	280	13	39	210	3	0
Au Bon Pain Corn Muffin						
1	490	17	75	600	10	3
Au Bon Pain Cranberry Walnut Muffin						
1	540	25	66	500	10	4
Au Bon Pain Crème de Fleur						
1	500	25	57	410	11	2
Au Bon Pain Crumb Cake						
1	750	40	97	980	8	1
Au Bon Pain Demi Cheese on Baguette						
1	440	15	50	980	27	3
Au Bon Pain Demi Chicken Sandwich on Baguette						
1	370	9	49	850	22	3
Au Bon Pain Demi Ham Sandwich on Baguette						
1	330	5	56	1190	17	3
Au Bon Pain Demi Ham Sandwich with Swiss Cheese						
1	400	10	56	1230	23	3
Au Bon Pain Demi Roast Beef Sandwich on Baguette						
1	360	8	49	830	19	3
Au Bon Pain Demi Roast Beef Sandwich with Brie Cheese on Baguette						
1	460	18	49	1040	24	3
Au Bon Pain Demi Tuna Sandwich on Baguette						
1	320	7	49	770	17	3
Au Bon Pain Demi Tuna Sandwich with Cheddar Cheese on Baguette						
1	400	14	50	900	22	3
Au Bon Pain Demi Turkey Sandwich on Baguette						
1	320	6	49	1000	18	2
Au Bon Pain Demi Turkey Sandwich with Swiss Cheese						
1	400	12	49	1040	24	2

RESTAURANT/ FOOD ITEM	SERVING SIZE	CALORIES	FAT	CARBS	SODIUM	PROTEIN	FIBER
Au Bon Pain Double Chocolate Chunk Muffin							
	1	620	25	86	540	11	4
Au Bon Pain Egg and Broccoli Baked Sandwich							
	1	350	10	42	910	23	3
Au Bon Pain Egg on a Bagel							
	1	360	4	60	790	21	3
Au Bon Pain Egg on a Bagel with Bacon							
	1	420	8	60	1000	25	3
Au Bon Pain Egg on a Bagel with Bacon and Cheese							
	1	510	15	61	1140	31	3
Au Bon Pain Egg on a Bagel with Cheese							
	1	450	10	61	930	26	3
Au Bon Pain Eggplant and Mozzarella Sandwich							
	1	670	30	73	1550	27	6
Au Bon Pain English Toffee Cookie							
	1	250	14	27	170	2	1
Au Bon Pain Everything Bagel							
	1	340	5	61	990	13	3
Au Bon Pain Ginger Squares							
	2 squares	140	5	22	70	2	0
Au Bon Pain Gingerbread Man Cookie							
	1	320	10	53	150	4	1
Au Bon Pain Ham and Cheese Croissant							
	1	400	20	38	660	15	2
Au Bon Pain Hazelnut Fudge Cookie							
	1	310	17	38	160	5	3
Au Bon Pain Hazelnut Mocha Brownie							
	1	490	22	74	350	6	3
Au Bon Pain Holiday Mini Shortbread Cookie							
	2 cookies	190	11	21	160	2	0
Au Bon Pain Honey 9 Grain Bagel							
	1	350	4	69	490	12	6
Au Bon Pain Iced Caffe Latte Large/20 oz							
		190	10	17	140	10	0
Au Bon Pain Iced Caffe Latte Medium/16 oz							
		150	8	13	110	8	0
Au Bon Pain Iced Caffe Latte Small/12 oz							
		110	6	19	80	6	0
Au Bon Pain Iced Caramel Macchiato Large/20 oz							
		490	13	81	200	13	0
Au Bon Pain Iced Caramel Macchiato Medium/16 oz							
		390	10	65	160	10	0
Au Bon Pain Iced Caramel Macchiato Small/12 oz							
		290	7	49	125	7	0

RESTAURANT/ FOOD ITEM SERVING SIZE	CALORIES	FAT	CARBS	SODIUM	PROTEIN	FIBER
Au Bon Pain Iced Chai Latte Large/20 oz						
	340	10	54	125	10	0
Au Bon Pain Iced Chai Latte Medium/16 oz						
	260	7	42	90	7	0
Au Bon Pain Iced Chai Latte Small/12 oz						
	190	5	31	65	5	0
Au Bon Pain Iced Cinnamon Roll						
1	410	15	60	270	8	2
Au Bon Pain Jalapeno Double Cheddar Bagel						
1	340	10	53	640	17	2
Au Bon Pain Lemon Danish						
1	440	20	57	360	7	1
Au Bon Pain Lemon Drop Tulip						
1	410	19	55	330	5	1
Au Bon Pain Lemon Pound Cake						
1	520	25	67	490	6	1
Au Bon Pain Low-fat Triple Berry Muffin						
1	300	3	65	720	4	2
Au Bon Pain Marble Pound Cake						
1	490	26	59	520	6	1
Au Bon Pain Mayan Chicken Hot Wrap						
1	580	13	93	1300	24	6
Au Bon Pain Mini Chocolate Chip Cookie						
1	70	3	10	55	1	0
Au Bon Pain Mini Oatmeal Raisin Cookie						
1	60	3	10	50	1	1
Au Bon Pain Mint Chocolate Pound Cake						
1	530	29	64	580	7	3
Au Bon Pain Mozzarella Chicken Sandwich						
1	680	24	67	1460	48	4
Au Bon Pain Oatmeal Raisin Cookie						
1	230	8	36	190	3	2
Au Bon Pain Onion Dill Bagel						
1	280	1	57	430	11	3
Au Bon Pain Orange Scone						
1	470	23	57	420	10	1
Au Bon Pain Palmier						
1	440	23	53	330	1	1
Au Bon Pain Pecan Roll						
1	810	41	99	430	12	3
Au Bon Pain Plain Bagel						
1	280	1	56	430	11	2
Au Bon Pain Plain Croissant						
1	310	17	31	220	7	1
Au Bon Pain Poppy Bagel						
1	320	4	58	430	12	4

RESTAURANT/ FOOD ITEM SERVING SIZE	CALORIES	FAT	CARBS	SODIUM	PROTEIN	FIBER
Au Bon Pain Portobello and Goat Cheese Sandwich						
1	550	25	62	1340	19	6
Au Bon Pain Portobello, Egg and Cheddar						
1	500	26	42	1160	22	3
Au Bon Pain Prosciutto and Egg on Asiago Bagel						
1	520	16	60	1690	34	1
Au Bon Pain Prosciutto Mozzarella Sandwich						
1	810	41	71	2290	41	4
Au Bon Pain Pumpkin Muffin						
1	530	19	81	560	10	3
Au Bon Pain Raisin Bran Muffin						
1	480	11	85	600	12	10
Au Bon Pain Raspberry Croissant						
1	370	17	46	280	8	2
Au Bon Pain Roast Beef Caesar Sandwich						
1	680	27	68	1560	40	3
Au Bon Pain Rocky Road Brownie						
1	490	22	74	370	6	2
Au Bon Pain Sausage, Egg and Cheddar on Asiago Bagel						
1	810	47	58	1540	38	1
Au Bon Pain Sesame Seed Bagel						
1	330	5	59	440	12	3
Au Bon Pain Shortbread Cookie						
1	340	20	37	300	4	1
Au Bon Pain Smoked Salmon and Wasabi on Onion Dill Bagel						
1	430	11	64	1090	23	1
Au Bon Pain Southwest Jalapeno Muffin						
1	560	30	64	720	8	2
Au Bon Pain Spicy Tuna Sandwich						
1	470	16	60	1180	29	11
Au Bon Pain Spinach and Cheese Croissant						
1	290	16	28	300	10	2
Au Bon Pain Steakhouse on Ciabatta						
1	710	29	73	2400	43	4
Au Bon Pain Sweet Cheese Croissant						
1	400	19	49	320	9	1
Au Bon Pain Sweet Cheese Danish						
1	470	24	54	390	9	1
Au Bon Pain Tuna Melt						
1	690	30	71	1160	42	5
Au Bon Pain Turkey Club Sandwich						
1	700	31	59	1970	45	2
Au Bon Pain Turkey Melt						
1	810	32	79	2040	47	3
Au Bon Pain White Chocolate Chunk Macadamia Nut Cookie						
1	300	16	36	240	3	1
Au Bon Pain White Chocolate Toffee Bagel Braid						
1	350	6	63	500	11	2
Baskin Robbins Cherries Jubilee						
1 scoop (2.5 oz)	150	8	19	50	3	1

RESTAURANT/ FOOD ITEM	SERVING SIZE	CALORIES	FAT	CARBS	SODIUM	PROTEIN	FIBER
Baskin Robbins Chocolate	1 scoop (2.5 oz)	160	9	21	80	3	0
Baskin Robbins Chocolate Chip Cookie Dough	1 scoop (2.5 oz)	190	9	23	85	3	0
Baskin Robbins Chocolate Chip Ice Cream	1 scoop (2.5 oz)	170	10	17	60	3	0
Baskin Robbins Chocolate Fudge	1 scoop (2.5 oz)	170	10	22	90	3	0
Baskin Robbins Cone, Cake	1 cone	25	0	5	15	0	0
Baskin Robbins Cone, Double Header	1 cone	25	0	5	20	1	0
Baskin Robbins Cone, Sugar	1 cone	45	0.5	9	35	1	0
Baskin Robbins Cone, Waffle	1 cone	160	4	28	5	2	0
Baskin Robbins Fat-Free Vanilla Frozen Yogurt	1 scoop (2.5 oz)	90	0	20	65	4	0
Baskin Robbins Gold Medal Ribbon	1 scoop (2.5 oz)	160	8	21	95	3	0
Baskin Robbins Jamoca	1 scoop (2.5 oz)	150	8	16	55	3	0
Baskin Robbins Jamoca Almond Fudge	1 scoop (2.5 oz)	170	9	19	50	3	1
Baskin Robbins Lemon Sorbet	1 scoop (2.5 oz)	80	0	21	10	0	0
Baskin Robbins Mango Sorbet	1 scoop (2.5 oz)	80	0	20	5	0	0
Baskin Robbins Mint Chocolate Chip	1 scoop (2.5 oz)	170	10	17	60	3	0
Baskin Robbins Old Fashioned Butter Pecan	1 scoop (2.5 oz)	170	11	15	60	3	1
Baskin Robbins Oreo Cookies 'n Cream	1 scoop (2.5 oz)	170	9	20	95	3	0
Baskin Robbins Peanut Butter 'n Chocolate	1 scoop (2.5 oz)	200	13	19	115	4	1

RESTAURANT/ FOOD ITEM SERVING SIZE	CALORIES	FAT	CARBS	SODIUM	PROTEIN	FIBER
Baskin Robbins Pistachio Almond						
1 scoop (2.5 oz)	180	12	15	55	4	1
Baskin Robbins Pralines 'n Cream						
1 scoop (2.5 oz)	180	9	22	105	3	0
Baskin Robbins Premium Churned Light Aloha Brownie Ice Cream						
1 scoop (2.5 oz)	150	5	26	95	3	1
Baskin Robbins Premium Churned Light Cappuccino Chip Ice Cream						
1 scoop (2.5 oz)	140	5	20	70	3	1
Baskin Robbins Premium Churned Light Milk Chocolate Ice Cream						
1 scoop (2.5 oz)	130	4.5	20	75	4	1
Baskin Robbins Premium Churned Light Mint Oreo Ice Cream						
1 scoop (2.5 oz)	150	4.5	25	90	3	1
Baskin Robbins Premium Churned Light Raspberry Chip Ice Cream						
1 scoop (2.5 oz)	140	4	24	60	3	1
Baskin Robbins Premium Churned Light Vanilla Ice Cream						
1 scoop (2.5 oz)	130	4.5	19	70	4	1
Baskin Robbins Premium Churned Reduced Fat, No Sugar Added Cabana Berry Banana Ice Cream						
1 scoop (2.5 oz)	90	3.5	17	45	3	2
Baskin Robbins Premium Churned Reduced-Fat, No Sugar Added Caramel Turtle Truffle Ice Cream						
1 scoop (2.5 oz)	120	5	24	75	3	2
Baskin Robbins Premium Churned Reduced-Fat, No Sugar Added Chocolate Overload Ice Cream						
1 scoop (2.5 oz)	120	5	23	70	4	3
Baskin Robbins Premium Churned Reduced-Fat, No Sugar Added Pineapple Coconut Ice Cream						
1 scoop (2.5 oz)	100	4	18	50	3	2
Baskin Robbins Rainbow Sherbet						
1 scoop (2.5 oz)	100	1.5	21	25	1	0
Baskin Robbins Reese's Peanut Butter Cup						
1 scoop (2.5 oz)	190	11	19	80	4	0
Baskin Robbins Rocky Road						
1 scoop (2.5 oz)	180	10	22	75	3	0

RESTAURANT/ FOOD ITEM SERVING SIZE	CALORIES	FAT	CARBS	SODIUM	PROTEIN	FIBER
Baskin Robbins Strawberry Sorbet						
1 scoop (2.5 oz)						
	80	0	21	5	0	0
Baskin Robbins Vanilla						
1 scoop (2.5 oz)						
	170	10	17	45	3	0
Baskin Robbins Very Berry Strawberry						
1 scoop (2.5 oz)						
	140	7	18	45	2	0
Baskin Robbins World Class Chocolate						
1 scoop (2.5 oz)						
	180	10	19	60	3	0
Ben & Jerry's Berry Berry Extraordinary Sorbet						
1 scoop (4 oz)						
	100	0	27	5	0	1
Ben & Jerry's Black Raspberry Swirl Low Fat Frozen Yogurt						
1 scoop (4 oz)						
	140	1.5	28	55	3	1
Ben & Jerry's Butter Pecan						
1 scoop (4 oz)						
	260	20	17	105	4	0
Ben & Jerry's Cake Batter						
1 scoop (4 oz)						
	242	14	24	69	3	0.5
Ben & Jerry's Cherry Garcia						
1 scoop (4 oz)						
	200	11	23	50	3	0
Ben & Jerry's Chocolate						
1 scoop (4 oz)						
	200	12	21	40	3	1
Ben & Jerry's Chocolate Chip Cookie Dough						
1 scoop (4 oz)						
	220	12	26	70	4	0
Ben & Jerry's Chocolate Fudge Brownie						
1 scoop (4 oz)						
	220	11	27	70	3	1
Ben & Jerry's Chocolate Fudge Brownie Low Fat Frozen Yogurt						
1 scoop (4 oz)						
	160	2.5	32	90	4	1
Ben & Jerry's Chocolate Macadamia						
1 scoop (4 oz)						
	253	17	23	62	3	1
Ben & Jerry's Chocolate Peanut Butter Swirl						
1 scoop (4 oz)						
	250	17	22	100	6	2
Ben & Jerry's Chocolate Therapy						
1 scoop (4 oz)						
	210	12	25	65	4	2
Ben & Jerry's Chunky Monkey						
1 scoop (4 oz)						
	240	14	24	35	4	0

RESTAURANT/ FOOD ITEM SERVING SIZE	CALORIES	FAT	CARBS	SODIUM	PROTEIN	FIBER
Ben & Jerry's Cinnamon Buns						
1 scoop (4 oz)	240	12	30	105	3	0
Ben & Jerry's Coconut Seven Layer Bar						
1 scoop (4 oz)	276	17	25	46	3	1
Ben & Jerry's Coffee						
1 scoop (4 oz)	190	11	18	50	3	0
Ben & Jerry's Coffee Coffee Buzz Buzz						
1 scoop (4 oz)	230	14	23	40	4	1
Ben & Jerry's Half Baked						
1 scoop (4 oz)	230	11	28	70	4	1
Ben & Jerry's Half Baked Low Fat Frozen Yogurt						
1 scoop (4 oz)	160	2.5	31	85	4	1
Ben & Jerry's Imagine Whirled Peace						
1 scoop (4 oz)	252	15	26	99	3	0.3
Ben & Jerry's Lemonade Sorbet						
1 scoop (4 oz)	100	0	26	5	0	1
Ben & Jerry's Mango Mango Sorbet						
1 scoop (4 oz)	100	0	27	10	0	1
Ben & Jerry's Mint Chocolate Chunk						
1 scoop (4 oz)	230	14	23	45	3	1
Ben & Jerry's New York Super Fudge Chunk						
1 scoop (4 oz)	250	17	24	45	4	2
Ben & Jerry's Oatmeal Cookie Chunk						
1 scoop (4 oz)	240	13	28	110	4	1
Ben & Jerry's ONE Cheesecake Brownie						
1 scoop (4 oz)	234	14	23	77	3	0.3
Ben & Jerry's Orange and Cream						
1 scoop (4 oz)	152	6	23	30	2	1
Ben & Jerry's Peanut Butter Cookie Dough						
1 scoop (4 oz)	268	17	25	138	6	1
Ben & Jerry's Phish Food						
1 scoop (4 oz)	230	11	32	65	3	1
Ben & Jerry's Strawberry						
1 scoop (4 oz)	170	9	18	35	3	0

RESTAURANT/ FOOD ITEM SERVING SIZE	CALORIES	FAT	CARBS	SODIUM	PROTEIN	FIBER
Ben & Jerry's Strawberry Cheesecake						
1 scoop (4 oz)	210	11	24	35	3	0
Ben & Jerry's Strawberry Kiwi Sorbet						
1 scoop (4 oz)	100	0	27	10	0	1
Ben & Jerry's Sweet Cream & Cookies						
1 scoop (4 oz)	240	13	24	95	4	0
Ben & Jerry's Triple Caramel Chunk						
1 scoop (4 oz)	230	12	28	95	3	0
Ben & Jerry's Vanilla						
1 scoop (4 oz)	190	12	18	50	3	0
Ben & Jerry's Vanilla Fudge Chip No Sugar Added						
1 scoop (4 oz)	180	13	20	40	3	3
Ben & Jerry's Vanilla Heath Bar Crunch						
1 scoop (4 oz)	240	14	24	100	3	0
Ben & Jerry's Vanilla Low Fat Frozen Yogurt						
1 scoop (4 oz)	130	1.5	25	70	4	0
Bob Evans American Cheese						
1 slice	53	4	1	235	n/a	0
Bob Evans Apple Dumpling Pie						
8.7 oz	568	28	77	295	n/a	4
Bob Evans Apple Dumpling Pie a la Mode						
11.5 oz	679	33	90	331	n/a	4
Bob Evans Apple Juice						
Kids	107	0	26	17	n/a	0
Bob Evans Apple Juice						
Large	143	0	35	22	n/a	0
Bob Evans Apple Juice						
Regular	72	0	17	11	n/a	0
Bob Evans Applesauce						
3.3 oz	69	0	18	11	n/a	2
Bob Evans Arnold Palmer						
9.5 oz	47	0	11	7	n/a	0
Bob Evans Bacon (a la Carte)						
1 slice	36	4	0	54	n/a	0
Bob Evans Bacon Cheeseburger						
10.8 oz	719	38	35	1355	n/a	2
Bob Evans Baked Potato						
10.3 oz	220	3	51	525	n/a	6
Bob Evans Banana Nut Bread						
1 piece	215	8	34	125	n/a	2
Bob Evans Biscuit						
1 biscuit	274	14	32	885	n/a	0

RESTAURANT/ FOOD ITEM	SERVING SIZE	CALORIES	FAT	CARBS	SODIUM	PROTEIN	FIBER
Bob Evans Blackberry Cobbler							
	8 oz	566	26	79	517	n/a	1
Bob Evans Blackberry Cobbler a la Mode							
	10.9 oz	682	32	93	554	n/a	1
Bob Evans Blue Cheese							
	1 oz	97	8	0	381	n/a	0
Bob Evans Blue Cheese Dressing (Dinner)							
	2.8 oz	411	44	5	630	n/a	0
Bob Evans Blue Cheese Dressing (Side)							
	1.6 oz	235	25	3	360	n/a	0
Bob Evans Blue Ribbon Apple Pie							
	7.5 oz	503	12	96	712	n/a	4
Bob Evans Blueberry & Banana Yogurt Parfait							
	6.7 oz	177	1	39	61	n/a	3
Bob Evans Blueberry Banana & Yogurt Crepe							
	1 crepe	417	17	59	291	n/a	5
Bob Evans Blueberry Crepe							
	1 crepe	404	25	39	304	n/a	2
Bob Evans Blueberry Hotcake, No Topping (a la Carte)							
	1 cake	343	10	58	792	n/a	2
Bob Evans Blueberry Stuffed French Toast							
	15.3 oz	730	19	90	990	n/a	5
Bob Evans Bob-B-Q Pulled Pork Sandwich							
	7.9 oz	599	25	67	741	n/a	4
Bob Evans Bob's BLT & E							
	9.9 oz	639	41	26	1021	n/a	3
Bob Evans Border Scramble Burrito with Bob Evans Egg Lites							
	19 oz	760	41	56	1775	n/a	9
Bob Evans Border Scramble Burrito with Egg							
	19 oz	873	53	56	1679	n/a	9
Bob Evans Border Scramble Burrito with Egg Whites							
	19 oz	753	41	56	1716	n/a	9
Bob Evans Border Scramble Omelet							
	15.1 oz	660	47	16	1605	n/a	3
Bob Evans Border Scramble Omelet with Bob Evans Egg Lites							
	15 oz	467	28	15	1248	n/a	3
Bob Evans Border Scramble Omelet with Egg Whites							
	15.1 oz	482	31	15	1159	n/a	3
Bob Evans Bowl of Bean Soup							
	10 oz	204	4	28	1016	n/a	8
Bob Evans Bowl of Cheddar Baked Potato Soup							
	8.8 oz	242	13	22	1046	n/a	1
Bob Evans Bowl of Grits							
	10.4 oz	265	10	40	257	n/a	2
Bob Evans Bowl of Oatmeal							
	10.7 oz	167	3	31	259	n/a	4
Bob Evans Bowl of Sausage Gravy							
	11.7 oz	377	26	23	1586	n/a	0
Bob Evans Bowl of Vegetable Beef Soup							
	9.5 oz	135	3	20	759	n/a	3

RESTAURANT/FOOD ITEM SERVING SIZE	CALORIES	FAT	CARBS	SODIUM	PROTEIN	FIBER
Bob Evans Bowl Sausage Chili						
9.8 oz	351	22	24	898	n/a	9
Bob Evans Bread and Celery Dressing						
3.1 oz	148	8	16	427	n/a	1
Bob Evans Broccoli Florets						
5.6 oz	44	1	8	41	n/a	5
Bob Evans Buttermilk Hotcake, No Topping (a la Carte)						
1 cake	337	10	56	792	n/a	2
Bob Evans Buttermilk Ranch Dressing (Dinner)						
2.8 oz	291	29	3	582	n/a	0
Bob Evans Buttermilk Ranch Dressing (Side)						
1.6 oz	166	17	2	333	n/a	0
Bob Evans Caesar Dressing (Dinner)						
2.8 oz	432	47	2	655	n/a	0
Bob Evans Caesar Dressing (Side)						
1.6 oz	247	27	1	375	n/a	0
Bob Evans Caramel Iced Coffee						
10.6 oz	104	4	18	134	n/a	0
Bob Evans Caramel Mocha						
10 oz	268	9	45	149	n/a	1
Bob Evans Chamomile Hot Tea						
9.3 oz	1	0	1	8	n/a	0
Bob Evans Cheeseburger						
10.3 oz	648	31	35	1247	n/a	2
Bob Evans Chicken & Broccoli Alfredo						
27.4 oz	1206	59	108	2432	n/a	8
Bob Evans Chicken & Broccoli Alfredo, Savor Size						
16.6 oz	638	30	58	1282	n/a	7
Bob Evans Chicken-N-Noodles Deep-Dish Dinner						
19.9 oz	785	38	66	2312	n/a	2
Bob Evans Chicken Parmesan with Meat Sauce						
28.3 oz	1520	65	156	3406	n/a	9
Bob Evans Chicken Parmesan with Meat Sauce, Savor Size						
19.1 oz	1016	47	87	2619	n/a	6
Bob Evans Chicken Salad Plate						
21.3 oz	712	43	70	974	n/a	12
Bob Evans Chicken Salad Sandwich						
9.6 oz	637	37	54	1293	n/a	6
Bob Evans Chicken Salad Sandwich, Half						
4.8 oz	319	19	27	646	n/a	3
Bob Evans Chocolate Milk 1%						
Kids	212	3	37	225	n/a	0
Bob Evans Chocolate Milk 1%						
Large	280	4	49	296	n/a	0
Bob Evans Chocolate Milk 1%						
Regular	145	2	25	153	n/a	0
Bob Evans Cinnamon Hotcake, No Topping (a la Carte)						
1 cake	382	12	62	792	n/a	2
Bob Evans Cinnamon Swirl (Frosted)						
5.6 oz	616	30	82	623	n/a	0

RESTAURANT/ FOOD ITEM	SERVING SIZE	CALORIES	FAT	CARBS	SODIUM	PROTEIN	FIBER
Bob Evans Cinnamon Swirl (Unfrosted)							
	4.9 oz	532	28	67	602	n/a	0
Bob Evans Cobb Salad							
	14.6 oz	568	37	10	1673	n/a	3
Bob Evans Cobb Salad, Savor Size							
	10 oz	413	28	7	1146	n/a	2
Bob Evans Coconut Cream Pie							
	7 oz	514	29	59	451	n/a	3
Bob Evans Coleslaw							
	3.6 oz	208	14	19	243	n/a	1
Bob Evans Colonial Dressing (Dinner)							
	2.8 oz	433	38	22	361	n/a	0
Bob Evans Colonial Dressing (Side)							
	1.6 oz	247	22	12	206	n/a	0
Bob Evans Corn							
	3.6 oz	166	11	17	258	n/a	2
Bob Evans Cottage Cheese							
	3.8 oz	92	4	4	310	n/a	1
Bob Evans Country Biscuit Breakfast							
	10.1 oz	666	46	39	1697	n/a	0
Bob Evans Country Caesar Salad							
	16.7 oz	746	53	20	1712	n/a	1
Bob Evans Country Caesar Salad, Savor Size							
	10.9 oz	547	38	19	1355	n/a	1
Bob Evans Country Fried Steak (a la Carte)							
	1 steak	496	33	31	1217	n/a	0
Bob Evans Country Fried Steak with Gravy (a la Carte)							
	1 steak	550	37	37	1510	n/a	0
Bob Evans Country Spinach Salad							
	10.9 oz	479	31	12	1297	n/a	5
Bob Evans Country Spinach Salad, Savor Size							
	8.6 oz	435	30	10	1082	n/a	4
Bob Evans County Fair Cheese Bites							
	11.4 oz	942	66	47	1757	n/a	5
Bob Evans Cranberry Apple Pork Loin							
	1 pork loin	241	12	25	596	n/a	2
Bob Evans Cranberry Apple Pork Loin							
	2 pork loins	390	22	30	1156	n/a	2
Bob Evans Cranberry Pecan Chicken Salad							
	16.3 oz	894	60	45	2338	n/a	5
Bob Evans Cranberry Pecan Chicken Salad, Savor Size							
	10.5 oz	673	45	38	1658	n/a	4
Bob Evans Cranberry Relish							
	1.2 oz	68	0	16	7	n/a	1
Bob Evans Cup of Bean Soup							
	5.4 oz	110	2	15	549	n/a	4
Bob Evans Cup of Cheddar Baked Potato Soup							
	6.2 oz	172	9	15	744	n/a	0

RESTAURANT/ FOOD ITEM SERVING SIZE	CALORIES	FAT	CARBS	SODIUM	PROTEIN	FIBER
Bob Evans Cup of Grits						
5.8 oz	148	6	22	143	n/a	1
Bob Evans Cup of Oatmeal						
5.8 oz	91	2	17	140	n/a	2
Bob Evans Cup of Sausage Chili						
6 oz	215	14	15	550	n/a	6
Bob Evans Cup of Sausage Gravy						
6.8 oz	219	15	14	922	n/a	0
Bob Evans Cup of Vegetable Beef Soup						
6.3 oz	90	2	13	503	n/a	2
Bob Evans Dill Pickle Slices						
0.9 oz	2	0	0	239	n/a	0
Bob Evans Dinner Rolls						
1 roll	201	5	34	268	n/a	1
Bob Evans Earl Grey Hot Decaf Tea						
9.3 oz	1	0	1	8	n/a	0
Bob Evans Eggs (a la Carte)						
1 egg	131	11	1	68	n/a	0
Bob Evans English Breakfast Hot Tea						
9.3 oz	1	0	1	8	n/a	0
Bob Evans English Muffin						
1 muffin	156	4	26	336	n/a	1
Bob Evans Farmer's Market Omelet						
14.2 oz	659	47	14	2245	n/a	1
Bob Evans Farmer's Market Omelet with Bob Evans Egg Lites						
14.1 oz	466	28	13	1888	n/a	1
Bob Evans Farmer's Market Omelet with Egg Whites						
14.2 oz	481	31	13	1800	n/a	1
Bob Evans Fit from the Farm Breakfast with Oatmeal						
14.7 oz	372	9	46	813	n/a	3
Bob Evans Fit from the Farm Breakfast with Parfait						
8.8 oz	281	7	40	489	n/a	3
Bob Evans Fit from the Farm Breakfast with Yogurt Crepe						
16.9 oz	571	23	61	933	n/a	6
Bob Evans French Dressing (Dinner)						
2.8 oz	410	38	18	461	n/a	0
Bob Evans French Dressing (Side)						
1.6 oz	234	22	10	263	n/a	0
Bob Evans French Fries						
4.5 oz	319	13	46	92	n/a	1
Bob Evans French Silk Pie						
5.5 oz	662	44	60	320	n/a	2
Bob Evans French Toast (a la Carte)						
1 piece	164	3	18	283	n/a	1
Bob Evans Fried Chicken Breast (a la Carte)						
1 breast	285	13	13	758	n/a	1
Bob Evans Fried Chicken Club Sandwich						
10.2 oz	637	31	47	1567	n/a	3
Bob Evans Fried Chicken Sandwich						
8.9 oz	489	18	47	1109	n/a	3

RESTAURANT/ FOOD ITEM	SERVING SIZE	CALORIES	FAT	CARBS	SODIUM	PROTEIN	FIBER
Bob Evans Fried Chicken Strips (a la Carte)							
	1 strip	137	8	10	301	n/a	0
Bob Evans Fried Haddock (a la Carte)							
	6.5 oz	363	18	27	608	n/a	2
Bob Evans Fried Haddock Sandwich							
	11.3 oz	732	33	71	1596	n/a	4
Bob Evans Fruit & Yogurt Plate							
	18.5 oz	347	2	82	74	n/a	9
Bob Evans Fruit Cup							
	7.7 oz	148	1	38	8	n/a	4
Bob Evans Fruit Dish							
	3.8 oz	58	0	14	7	n/a	1
Bob Evans Garden Harvest Omelet							
	13.2 oz	542	38	14	1762	n/a	2
Bob Evans Garden Harvest Omelet with Bob Evans Egg Lites							
	13.1 oz	349	19	13	1405	n/a	2
Bob Evans Garden Harvest Omelet with Egg Whites							
	13.2 oz	364	22	13	1317	n/a	2
Bob Evans Garden Salad							
	3.2 oz	58	1	9	132	n/a	1
Bob Evans Garden Vegetables							
	6 oz	119	8	11	234	n/a	4
Bob Evans Garlic Butter Grilled Chicken Breast (a la Carte)							
	1 breast	242	14	1	691	n/a	0
Bob Evans Garlic Butter Salmon (a la Carte)							
	7.9 oz	300	15	1	172	n/a	0
Bob Evans Glazed Carrots							
	3.6 oz	101	5	14	101	n/a	3
Bob Evans Green Beans							
	3.8 oz	47	2	6	515	n/a	2
Bob Evans Green Tea							
	9.3 oz	1	0	1	8	n/a	0
Bob Evans Grilled Cheese Sandwich							
	4.2 oz	350	15	22	729	n/a	2
Bob Evans Grilled Chicken Breast (a la Carte)							
	1 breast	242	14	0	635	n/a	0
Bob Evans Grilled Chicken Club Sandwich							
	9.3 oz	583	31	34	1420	n/a	2
Bob Evans Grilled Chicken Sandwich							
	8.1 oz	441	19	33	971	n/a	2
Bob Evans Grilled Chicken Tenders (a la Carte)							
	1 tender	87	6	0	188	n/a	0
Bob Evans Grilled Mushrooms							
	7 oz	87	5	10	865	n/a	5
Bob Evans Ham & Cheddar Omelet							
	10.2 oz	515	36	4	1808	n/a	0
Bob Evans Ham & Cheddar Omelet with Bob Evans Egg Lites							
	10.1 oz	322	17	3	1451	n/a	0
Bob Evans Ham & Cheddar Omelet with Egg Whites							
	10.2 oz	337	20	3	1363	n/a	0

RESTAURANT/ FOOD ITEM SERVING SIZE	CALORIES	FAT	CARBS	SODIUM	PROTEIN	FIBER
Bob Evans Hamburger						
9.3 oz	542	22	34	776	n/a	2
Bob Evans Hamburger Patty (a la Carte)						
4.5 oz	336	17	0	186	n/a	0
Bob Evans Hardcooked Egg (a la Carte)						
1 egg	57	4	1	52	n/a	0
Bob Evans Heritage Chef Salad						
12.4 oz	398	25	10	1320	n/a	3
Bob Evans Heritage Chef Salad, Savor Size						
8.6 oz	294	18	7	923	n/a	2
Bob Evans Hi-C Fruit Punch						
9.6 oz	127	0	35	11	n/a	0
Bob Evans Hi-C Fruit Punch						
Kids	92	0	25	8	n/a	0
Bob Evans Home Fries						
5.1 oz	183	6	28	685	n/a	3
Bob Evans Honey Mustard Dressing (Dinner)						
2.8 oz	358	33	15	461	n/a	0
Bob Evans Honey Mustard Dressing (Side)						
1.6 oz	205	19	9	263	n/a	0
Bob Evans Hot Bacon Dressing (Dinner)						
2.8 oz	198	6	33	353	n/a	0
Bob Evans Hot Bacon Dressing (Side)						
1.6 oz	113	3	19	202	n/a	0
Bob Evans Hot Cocoa						
8.2 oz	253	10	39	233	n/a	1
Bob Evans Iced Coffee						
9.8 oz	47	4	4	134	n/a	0
Bob Evans Iced Tea						
9.4 oz	0	0	0	8	n/a	0
Bob Evans Itsy Bitsy Sandwich Trio						
16 oz	1134	55	111	1898	n/a	5
Bob Evans Itsy Bitsy Trio, Mini Pot Roast Sandwich (1 to Mix-&-Match)						
3.5 oz	243	11	23	582	n/a	1
Bob Evans Itsy Bitsy Trio, Mini Pulled Pork Sandwich (1 to Mix-&-Match)						
3.6 oz	281	14	22	502	n/a	1
Bob Evans Itsy Bitsy Trio, Mini Sausage Sandwich (1 to Mix-&-Match)						
3.7 oz	298	17	20	767	n/a	1
Bob Evans Kaiser Bun						
1 bun	195	5	31	347	n/a	1
Bob Evans Knife & Fork Bob-B-Q Pulled Pork Sandwich						
15 oz	859	32	91	1176	n/a	7
Bob Evans Knife & Fork Meatloaf Sandwich						
18.6 oz	820	37	51	3182	n/a	3
Bob Evans Knife & Fork Pork Loin Sandwich						
16 oz	771	46	51	2543	n/a	3
Bob Evans Knife & Fork Turkey Sandwich						
15.5 oz	718	37	46	2784	n/a	2
Bob Evans Lemonade						
Kids	100	0	24	8	n/a	0

RESTAURANT/ FOOD ITEM	SERVING SIZE	CALORIES	FAT	CARBS	SODIUM	PROTEIN	FIBER
Bob Evans Lemonade							
	Large	95	0	22	7	n/a	0
Bob Evans Lettuce & Tomato							
	1.7 oz	9	0	2	4	n/a	1
Bob Evans Lettuce, Tomato and Pickle							
	2.6 oz	12	0	2	244	n/a	1
Bob Evans Lite Ranch Dressing (Dinner)							
	2.8 oz	192	18	4	704	n/a	0
Bob Evans Lite Ranch Dressing (Side)							
	1.6 oz	110	11	2	402	n/a	0
Bob Evans Loaded Baked Potato							
	11.8 oz	388	16	53	983	n/a	6
Bob Evans Loaded Potato Bites							
	14 oz	1008	63	93	2180	n/a	6
Bob Evans Mashed Potatoes							
	5.6 oz	192	7	16	428	n/a	1
Bob Evans Meat Lover's BoBurrito							
	13.4 oz	860	56	41	2116	n/a	3
Bob Evans Meat Lover's BoBurrito with Bob Evans Egg Lites							
	13.4 oz	746	45	41	2212	n/a	3
Bob Evans Meat Lover's BoBurrito with Egg Whites							
	13.4 oz	740	45	41	2154	n/a	3
Bob Evans Meatloaf (a la Carte)							
	1 slice	435	22	22	1958	n/a	1
Bob Evans Mini Bun							
	1 bun	126	3	20	233	n/a	1
Bob Evans Monterey Jack Cheese							
	1 slice	71	6	0	340	n/a	0
Bob Evans Multigrain Hotcake, No Topping (a la Carte)							
	1 cake	374	11	61	897	n/a	4
Bob Evans Mush (a la Carte)							
	1 piece	171	7	25	1012	n/a	5
Bob Evans NSA Apple Pie							
	6.8 oz	499	30	56	426	n/a	4
Bob Evans NSA Apple Pie a la Mode							
	9.6 oz	610	36	69	461	n/a	4
Bob Evans Omelet Shell (a la Carte)							
	4 oz	194	14	2	476	n/a	0
Bob Evans Omelet Shell (a la Carte)							
	6 oz	304	22	3	714	n/a	0
Bob Evans Omelet Shell, Bob Evans Egg Lites (a la Carte)							
	6.1 oz	111	3	2	357	n/a	0
Bob Evans Omelet Shell, Egg Whites (a la Carte)							
	6.2 oz	126	6	2	269	n/a	0
Bob Evans Onion Petals							
	4.8 oz	288	14	35	464	n/a	2
Bob Evans Open-Faced Roast Beef							
	9.6 oz	476	24	22	1041	n/a	1
Bob Evans Orange Juice							
	Kids	102	0	25	8	n/a	0

RESTAURANT/ FOOD ITEM	SERVING SIZE	CALORIES	FAT	CARBS	SODIUM	PROTEIN	FIBER
Bob Evans Orange Juice							
	Large	170	0	42	10	n/a	0
Bob Evans Orange Juice							
	Regular	85	0	21	5	n/a	0
Bob Evans Parmesan Crusted Garlic Bread							
	1 piece	195	9	23	430	n/a	1
Bob Evans Plain Crepe (a la Carte)							
	1 piece	353	25	27	297	n/a	1
Bob Evans Pot Roast Beef Stew Deep-Dish Dinner							
	20.1 oz	727	34	67	2900	n/a	3
Bob Evans Pot Roast Hash							
	13.2 oz	701	45	34	1210	n/a	4
Bob Evans Pot Roast Sandwich							
	8.4 oz	556	26	51	1321	n/a	2
Bob Evans Pot Roast Sandwich, Half							
	6.3 oz	371	18	30	829	n/a	2
Bob Evans Pot Roast Stroganoff							
	23.7 oz	1147	56	111	1944	n/a	4
Bob Evans Pot Roast Stroganoff, Savor Size							
	12.2 oz	591	29	56	986	n/a	2
Bob Evans Potato-Crusted Flounder (a la Carte)							
	5 oz	218	12	9	531	n/a	0
Bob Evans Premium Decaf Coffee							
	8.7 oz	0	0	0	7	n/a	0
Bob Evans Premium Regular Coffee							
	8.7 oz	0	0	0	7	n/a	0
Bob Evans Pumpkin Bread							
	1 piece	222	7	37	347	n/a	1
Bob Evans Pumpkin Pie							
	6.7 oz	489	24	64	308	n/a	1
Bob Evans Roasted Caramel Apple Crepe							
	1 piece	376	25	32	302	n/a	1
Bob Evans Roasted Caramel Apple Stuffed French Toast							
	15.8 oz	731	19	91	1011	n/a	4
Bob Evans Rye Bread							
	1 piece	109	1	21	229	n/a	1
Bob Evans Rye Bread, toasted and buttered							
	1 piece	129	3	21	252	n/a	1
Bob Evans Salmon (a la Carte)							
	7.6 oz	294	14	0	101	n/a	0
Bob Evans Sausage & Cheddar Omelet							
	10.1 oz	678	53	4	1574	n/a	0
Bob Evans Sausage & Cheddar Omelet with Bob Evans Egg Lites							
	10 oz	485	34	3	1217	n/a	0
Bob Evans Sausage & Cheddar Omelet with Egg Whites							
	10.1 oz	500	37	3	1128	n/a	0
Bob Evans Sausage Breakfast Patty (a la Carte)							
	1 patty	140	11	0	313	n/a	0
Bob Evans Sausage Link (a la Carte)							
	1 link	133	12	0	184	n/a	0

RESTAURANT/ FOOD ITEM SERVING SIZE	CALORIES	FAT	CARBS	SODIUM	PROTEIN	FIBER
Bob Evans Scrambled Bob Evans Egg Lites (a la Carte)						
1 egg	74	3	5	128	n/a	1
Bob Evans Scrambled Bob Evans Egg Lites (a la Carte)						
2 eggs	103	3	6	247	n/a	1
Bob Evans Scrambled Bob Evans Egg Lites (a la Carte)						
3 eggs	131	3	6	366	n/a	1
Bob Evans Scrambled Egg (a la Carte)						
1 egg	84	5	1	238	n/a	0
Bob Evans Scrambled Egg (a la Carte)						
2 eggs	168	11	2	476	n/a	0
Bob Evans Scrambled Egg (a la Carte)						
3 eggs	253	16	3	714	n/a	0
Bob Evans Scrambled Egg Whites (a la Carte)						
1 egg	50	3	1	90	n/a	0
Bob Evans Scrambled Egg Whites (a la Carte)						
2 eggs	75	3	1	179	n/a	0
Bob Evans Scrambled Egg Whites (a la Carte)						
3 eggs	100	3	2	269	n/a	0
Bob Evans Sirloin Steak (a la Carte)						
1 steak	421	29	3	638	n/a	0
Bob Evans Slow-Roasted Chicken-N-Noodles						
10.9 oz	289	16	23	695	n/a	1
Bob Evans Slow-Roasted Chicken Pot Pie						
18 oz	886	60	66	2710	n/a	5
Bob Evans Slow-Roasted Turkey (a la Carte)						
4 oz	136	5	1	972	n/a	0
Bob Evans Smoked Ham (a la Carte)						
1 piece	99	3	3	1293	n/a	0
Bob Evans Sourdough Bread						
1 piece	130	3	21	258	n/a	1
Bob Evans Spaghetti with Meat Sauce						
22.6 oz	1165	46	142	2307	n/a	8
Bob Evans Spaghetti with Meat Sauce, Savor Size						
13.4 oz	660	29	74	1520	n/a	5
Bob Evans Specialty Garden Salad						
3.7 oz	124	7	10	334	n/a	1
Bob Evans Stacked & Stuffed Blueberry Cream Hotcakes						
19.4 oz	1047	36	165	1852	n/a	6
Bob Evans Stacked & Stuffed Caramel Banana Pecan Hotcakes						
22.7 oz	1493	70	204	2265	n/a	9
Bob Evans Stacked & Stuffed Cinnamon Cream Hotcakes						
16.9 oz	1070	43	155	1911	n/a	4
Bob Evans Stacked & Stuffed Roasted Caramel Apple Cream Hotcakes						
24 oz	1387	54	203	1969	n/a	6
Bob Evans Stacked & Stuffed Strawberry Banana Cream Hotcakes						
26.7 oz	1168	36	197	1837	n/a	12
Bob Evans Strawberry Banana Crepes						
1 piece	412	25	42	297	n/a	3
Bob Evans Strawberry Banana Fruit & Yogurt Crepe						
1 piece	396	17	53	287	n/a	5

RESTAURANT/ FOOD ITEM	SERVING SIZE	CALORIES	FAT	CARBS	SODIUM	PROTEIN	FIBER
Bob Evans Strawberry Banana Mini Fruit & Yogurt Parfait							
	6.6 oz	151	1	33	55	n/a	3
Bob Evans Strawberry Blueberry Fruit & Yogurt Crepe							
	1 piece	378	17	48	292	n/a	5
Bob Evans Strawberry Blueberry Mini Fruit & Yogurt Parfait							
	6.7 oz	158	1	34	62	n/a	3
Bob Evans Strawberry Shortcake							
	12.7 oz	569	22	86	924	n/a	4
Bob Evans Strawberry Sundae							
	11.1 oz	419	20	56	113	n/a	2
Bob Evans Strawberry Supreme Pie							
	8.7 oz	651	47	58	333	n/a	3
Bob Evans Strawberry Yogurt							
	3.2 oz	93	1	18	54	n/a	0
Bob Evans Stuffed French Toast, No Topping							
	12.3 oz	627	19	65	977	n/a	3
Bob Evans Sunshine Skillet							
	14.1 oz	638	41	36	1905	n/a	4
Bob Evans Sweet Cream Waffle, No topping							
	6.3 oz	394	8	66	849	n/a	2
Bob Evans Sweet Iced Tea							
	9.5 oz	68	0	18	8	n/a	0
Bob Evans Sweet Italian Dressing (Dinner)							
	2.8 oz	322	30	15	943	n/a	0
Bob Evans Sweet Italian Dressing (Side)							
	1.6 oz	184	17	9	539	n/a	0
Bob Evans Swiss Bacon Dressing (Dinner)							
	2.8 oz	423	48	3	741	n/a	0
Bob Evans Swiss Bacon Dressing (Side)							
	1.6 oz	242	27	2	423	n/a	0
Bob Evans Texas Toast							
	1 piece	122	3	10	129	n/a	1
Bob Evans Thousand Island Dressing (Dinner)							
	2.8 oz	397	37	13	661	n/a	0
Bob Evans Thousand Island Dressing (Side)							
	1.6 oz	227	21	8	378	n/a	0
Bob Evans Three Cheese Omelet							
	8.3 oz	528	40	5	1451	n/a	0
Bob Evans Three Cheese Omelet with Bob Evans Egg Lites							
	8.2 oz	335	21	3	1094	n/a	0
Bob Evans Three Cheese Omelet with Egg Whites							
	8.3 oz	350	24	3	1005	n/a	0
Bob Evans Tomato Juice							
	Large	69	0	17	1474	n/a	2
Bob Evans Tomato Juice							
	Kids	53	0	13	1126	n/a	1
Bob Evans Tomato Juice							
	Regular	35	0	9	747	n/a	1
Bob Evans Tomato Slices							
	2 pieces	11	0	2	5	n/a	1

RESTAURANT/ FOOD ITEM SERVING SIZE	CALORIES	FAT	CARBS	SODIUM	PROTEIN	FIBER
Bob Evans Turkey and Dressing						
17.4 oz	690	31	52	3065	n/a	2
Bob Evans Turkey & Spinach Omelet						
14.1 oz	618	40	7	2422	n/a	1
Bob Evans Turkey & Spinach Omelet with Bob Evans Egg Lites						
14 oz	425	21	6	2065	n/a	1
Bob Evans Turkey & Spinach Omelet with Egg Whites						
14.1 oz	440	24	6	1976	n/a	1
Bob Evans Turkey Bacon Melt						
10.4 oz	589	28	47	2079	n/a	2
Bob Evans Turkey Bacon Melt, Half						
5.2 oz	292	14	23	1035	n/a	1
Bob Evans Turkey Sausage (a la Carte)						
1 piece	72	4	1	404	n/a	0
Bob Evans Turkey Sausage Breakfast						
11.7 oz	388	9	48	1009	n/a	5
Bob Evans Vanilla Ice Cream						
2.8 oz	111	6	13	36	n/a	0
Bob Evans Vanilla Iced Coffee						
10.6 oz	106	4	19	134	n/a	0
Bob Evans Vinegar & Oil Dressing (Dinner)						
3 oz	54	6	0	0	n/a	0
Bob Evans Vinegar & Oil Dressing (Side)						
1.5 oz	27	3	0	0	n/a	0
Bob Evans Western BoBurrito						
14.6 oz	738	44	42	2081	n/a	3
Bob Evans Western BoBurrito with Bob Evans Egg Lites						
14.6 oz	625	32	42	2178	n/a	3
Bob Evans Western BoBurrito with Egg Whites						
14.6 oz	618	32	42	2119	n/a	3
Bob Evans Western Omelet						
11.8 oz	529	36	8	1809	n/a	1
Bob Evans Western Omelet with Bob Evans Egg Lites						
11.7 oz	336	17	6	1453	n/a	1
Bob Evans Western Omelet with Egg Whites						
11.8 oz	351	20	6	1364	n/a	1
Bob Evans Wheat Bread						
1 piece	77	1	14	164	n/a	2
Bob Evans Wheat Bread, Toasted and Buttered						
1 piece	97	4	14	187	n/a	2
Bob Evans White Bread						
1 piece	83	1	15	168	n/a	1
Bob Evans White Bread, Toasted and Buttered						
1 piece	104	3	15	190	n/a	1
Bob Evans White Milk 2%						
Kids	153	6	14	140	n/a	0
Bob Evans White Milk 2%						
Large	200	8	18	184	n/a	0

RESTAURANT/ FOOD ITEM	SERVING SIZE	CALORIES	FAT	CARBS	SODIUM	PROTEIN	FIBER
Bob Evans White Milk 2%							
	Regular	103	4	9	94	n/a	0
Bob Evans Wild Raspberry Iced Tea							
	10.2 oz	58	0	14	8	n/a	0
Bob Evans Wild Raspberry Lemonade							
	10.8 oz	181	0	43	7	n/a	0
Bob Evans Wildfire Chicken Quesadilla							
	15.2 oz	766	34	55	1581	n/a	6
Bob Evans Wildfire Fried Chicken Salad							
	15 oz	711	34	70	1332	n/a	7
Bob Evans Wildfire Fried Chicken Salad, Savor Size							
	10.6 oz	543	27	54	995	n/a	5
Bob Evans Wildfire Grilled Chicken Breast (a la Carte)							
	1 piece	299	14	15	719	n/a	1
Bob Evans Wildfire Grilled Chicken Salad							
	13.7 oz	440	19	37	963	n/a	6
Bob Evans Wildfire Grilled Chicken Salad, Savor Size							
	10 oz	391	18	35	769	n/a	5
Bob Evans Wildfire Ranch Dressing (Dinner)							
	2.8 oz	225	17	16	573	n/a	0
Bob Evans Wildfire Ranch Dressing (Side)							
	1.6 oz	129	10	9	328	n/a	0
Bob Evans Wildfire Salmon (a la Carte)							
	8.6 oz	357	14	15	200	n/a	1
Boston Market 1 Thigh & 1 Drumstick							
	145 oz	290	17	0	950	37	0
Boston Market Apple Pie							
	1 slice	580	30	74	690	43	3
Boston Market Baked Beans							
	219 g	270	1.5	53	1000	11	11
Boston Market BBQ Brisket							
	184 g	400	20	28	760	26	1
Boston Market BBQ Chicken							
	Half	730	30	28	2360	90	1
Boston Market BBQ Dark Chicken							
	3 pieces	430	13	28	1400	52	1
Boston Market Beef Brisket							
	113 g	280	20	1	260	26	0
Boston Market Boston Chicken Carver							
	321 g	750	29	64	1960	57	3
Boston Market Boston Chicken Carver							
	Half	375	14.5	32	980	28	1
Boston Market Boston Meatloaf Carver							
	448 g	980	46	92	2350	47	4
Boston Market Boston Turkey Carver							
	344 g	700	26	65	1710	50	3
Boston Market Boston Turkey Carver							
	Half	350	13	32	850	25	2

RESTAURANT/ FOOD ITEM	SERVING SIZE	CALORIES	FAT	CARBS	SODIUM	PROTEIN	FIBER
Boston Market Brisket Dip Carver	303 g	890	51	63	1350	43	3
Boston Market Caesar Salad Dressing	71 g	360	38	4	910	2	1
Boston Market Caesar Salad Entrée	227 g	420	38	9	930	12	2
Boston Market Caesar Salad Entrée Add: Roasted Sirloin	3 oz	160	6	0	170	26	0
Boston Market Caesar Salad Entrée Add: Roasted Turkey	3 oz	110	2	0	370	23	0
Boston Market Caesar Salad Entrée Add: Rotisserie Chicken	5 oz	180	3	0	620	39	0
Boston Market Caesar Salad Entrée without Dressing	171 g	140	8	7	270	10	2
Boston Market Caesar Side Salad	93 g	180	17	4	410	4	1
Boston Market Caesar Side Salad without Dressing	64 g	40	2	3	75	3	1
Boston Market Chicken Noodle Soup	414 g	250	8	23	1420	22	2
Boston Market Chicken Tortilla Soup with Toppings	363 g	410	26	30	2100	17	2
Boston Market Chicken Tortilla Soup without Toppings	306 g	160	8	13	1690	10	2
Boston Market Chocolate Cake	145 g	580	34	67	360	5	3
Boston Market Chocolate Chip Fudge Brownie	85 g	320	13	49	220	5	3
Boston Market Chocolate Chunk Cookie	85 g	370	18	50	280	4	2
Boston Market Cinnamon Apples	145 g	210	3	47	15	0	3
Boston Market Classic Chicken Salad Sandwich	363 g	800	41	65	1900	40	4
Boston Market Coleslaw	189 g	300	20	27	280	2	4
Boston Market Cornbread	1 piece	180	5	31	320	2	0
Boston Market Creamed Spinach	191 g	280	23	12	580	9	4
Boston Market Crispy Country Chicken	90 g	220	11	16	480	16	1
Boston Market Dark (2 Thighs & Drumstick) Chicken	3 pieces	490	29	0	1600	60	0
Boston Market Dark Individual Meal Chicken	3 pieces	390	22	1	1270	51	0
Boston Market Dark Skinless (2 Thighs & Drumstick) Chicken	3 pieces	350	15	0	1210	52	0
Boston Market Dark Skinless (Thigh & 2 Drumsticks) Chicken	3 pieces	290	11	0	1010	45	0

RESTAURANT/ FOOD ITEM	SERVING SIZE	CALORIES	FAT	CARBS	SODIUM	PROTEIN	FIBER
Boston Market Fresh Steamed Vegetables							
	136 g	60	2	8	40	2	3
Boston Market Fresh Vegetable Stuffing							
	136 g	190	8	25	580	3	2
Boston Market Garlic Dill New Potatoes							
	156 g	140	3	24	120	3	3
Boston Market Green Beans							
	91 g	60	3.5	7	180	2	3
Boston Market Lite Ranch Dressing							
	1 package	70	4	8	310	1	0
Boston Market Macaroni and Cheese							
	221 g	300	11	35	1100	11	2
Boston Market Market Chopped Salad							
	397 g	480	40	24	1640	9	7
Boston Market Market Chopped Salad Add: Roasted Sirloin							
	3 oz	160	6	0	170	26	0
Boston Market Market Chopped Salad Add: Roasted Turkey							
	3 oz	110	2	0	370	23	0
Boston Market Market Chopped Salad Add: Rotisserie Chicken							
	5 oz	180	3	0	620	39	0
Boston Market Market Chopped Salad Dressing							
	71 g	360	39	2	1710	0	0
Boston Market Mashed Potatoes							
	221 g	270	11	36	820	5	4
Boston Market Mashed Potatoes Add: Beef Gravy							
	3 oz	35	1.5	4	500	1	0
Boston Market Mashed Potatoes Add: Poultry Gravy							
	4 oz	50	2	7	690	0	0
Boston Market Meatloaf							
	218 g	520	36	21	1030	29	0
Boston Market Meatloaf Open-Faced Sandwich							
	374 g	670	38	48	1760	34	1
Boston Market Pastry Top Chicken Pot Pie							
	425 g	800	48	59	1090	32	4
Boston Market Potato Salad							
	200 g	390	29	26	640	3	3
Boston Market Roasted Sirloin Open-Faced Sandwich							
	334 g	410	15	32	1640	35	1
Boston Market Roasted Turkey							
	113 g	150	2.5	0	500	31	0
Boston Market Roasted Turkey							
	142 g	180	3	0	635	38	0
Boston Market Roasted Turkey Open-Faced Sandwich							
	300 g	330	6	43	1480	26	1
Boston Market Rotisserie Chicken							
	Half	610	29	1	1860	89	0
Boston Market Rotisserie Chicken							
	170 g	310	15	0	930	44	0
Boston Market Rotisserie Chicken Open-Faced Sandwich							
	289 g	320	8	34	1630	27	1

RESTAURANT/ FOOD ITEM	SERVING SIZE	CALORIES	FAT	CARBS	SODIUM	PROTEIN	FIBER
Boston Market Seasonal Fresh Fruit Salad							
	142 g	60	0	15	20	1	1
Boston Market Smokehouse BBQ Chicken Sandwich							
	363 g	850	29	101	2810	44	4
Boston Market Sweet Corn							
	176 g	170	4	37	95	6	2
Boston Market Sweet Potato Casserole							
	198 g	460	16	77	270	4	3
Boston Market White BBQ Chicken							
	¼ chicken	430	13	28	1400	52	1
Boston Market White Rotisserie Chicken							
	¼ chicken	320	12	0	900	52	0
Boston Market White Rotisserie Chicken, No Skin							
	¼ chicken	240	4	1	890	50	0
Burger King 3 Cheese Steakhouse XT							
1 sandwich							
		1050	71	52	2150	51	3
Burger King Bacon Egg & Cheese Biscuit							
1 sandwich							
		430	25	34	1400	17	1
Burger King BK Big Fish Sandwich							
1 sandwich							
		640	32	66	1540	23	3
Burger King BK Big Fish Sandwich without Tartar Sauce							
1 sandwich							
		460	13	64	1320	23	3
Burger King BK Breakfast Shots, Bacon and Cheese							
	2 packs	310	20	18	800	14	1
Burger King BK Breakfast Shots, Ham and Cheese							
	2 packs	270	16	18	840	13	1
Burger King BK Breakfast Shots, Sausage and Cheese							
	2 packs	420	31	18	910	18	1
Burger King BK Burger Shots							
	2 packs	220	10	18	420	14	1
Burger King BK Burger Shots							
	6 pieces	650	31	53	1280	40	2
Burger King BK Chicken Fries							
	6 pieces	250	15	16	820	14	1
Burger King BK Chicken Fries							
	9 pieces	380	22	24	1220	21	2
Burger King BK Chicken Fries							
	12 pieces	500	29	32	1630	28	3
Burger King BK Double Stacker							
	1 burger	620	39	32	1100	34	1
Burger King BK Fresh Apple Fries							
	1 serving	25	0	6	0	0	1
Burger King BK Joe Coffee Decaf							
	12 oz	5	0	0	5	0	0
Burger King BK Joe Coffee Decaf							
	16 oz	5	0	1	10	1	0

RESTAURANT/ FOOD ITEM SERVING SIZE	CALORIES	FAT	CARBS	SODIUM	PROTEIN	FIBER
Burger King BK Joe Coffee Decaf						
20 oz	5	0	1	10	1	0
Burger King BK Joe Coffee Regular						
12 oz	5	0	1	15	1	0
Burger King BK Joe Coffee Regular						
16 oz	10	0	1	20	1	0
Burger King BK Joe Coffee Regular						
20 oz	10	0	2	25	1	0
Burger King BK Joe Coffee Turbo						
12 oz	10	0	1	20	1	0
Burger King BK Joe Coffee Turbo						
16 oz	10	0	2	30	1	0
Burger King BK Joe Coffee Turbo						
20 oz	15	0	2	40	2	0
Burger King BK Quad Stacker						
1 burger	1010	70	34	1800	64	1
Burger King BK Triple Stacker						
1 burger	820	55	33	1450	49	1
Burger King BK Veggie Burger						
1 burger	420	16	46	1090	23	7
Burger King BK Veggie Burger with Cheese						
1 burger	470	20	47	1300	25	7
Burger King BK Veggie Burger without Mayo						
1 burger	340	8	46	1030	23	7
Burger King Caramel Sauce						
1 package	45	0.5	10	35	0	0
Burger King Cheeseburger						
1 burger	340	16	31	770	18	1
Burger King Cheesy Tots Potatoes						
6 pieces	220	12	21	630	7	2
Burger King Cheesy Tots Potatoes						
9 pieces	330	18	31	950	11	3
Burger King Cheesy Tots Potatoes						
12 pieces	440	24	41	1270	14	4
Burger King Cheesy Bacon BK Wrapper						
1 burger	390	24	29	1060	14	2
Burger King Chicken Tenders						
4 pieces	180	11	13	310	9	0
Burger King Chicken Tenders						
5 pieces	230	13	16	380	11	0
Burger King Chicken Tenders						
6 pieces	270	16	19	460	14	0
Burger King Chicken Tenders						
8 pieces	360	21	25	610	18	0
Burger King Chocolate Milk Shake						
12 oz	310	11	53	220	6	1
Burger King Chocolate Milk Shake						
16 oz	450	15	79	330	8	1
Burger King Chocolate Milk Shake						
22 oz	670	21	119	510	11	2

RESTAURANT/ FOOD ITEM SERVING SIZE	CALORIES	FAT	CARBS	SODIUM	PROTEIN	FIBER
Burger King Chocolate Milk Shake						
32 oz	990	31	178	750	17	3
Burger King Cini-Minis						
4 pieces	400	18	52	380	7	2
Burger King Croissan'wich Bacon, Egg & Cheese						
1 sandwich	350	19	27	870	15	0
Burger King Croissan'wich Egg & Cheese						
1 sandwich	310	16	27	730	12	0
Burger King Croissan'wich Ham, Egg & Cheese						
1 sandwich	340	17	28	1200	18	0
Burger King Croissan'wich Sausage & Cheese						
1 sandwich	380	24	26	780	14	0
Burger King Croissan'wich Sausage, Egg & Cheese						
1 sandwich	470	31	28	1030	20	0
Burger King Double Cheeseburger						
1 burger	510	29	31	1020	30	1
Burger King Double Croissan'wich Bacon, Egg & Cheese						
1 sandwich	430	26	28	1240	20	0
Burger King Double Croissan'wich Ham, Egg & Cheese						
1 sandwich	420	21	30	1890	26	0
Burger King Double Croissan'wich Ham, Bacon, Egg & Cheese						
1 sandwich	430	24	29	1570	23	0
Burger King Double Croissan'wich Ham, Sausage, Egg & Cheese						
1 sandwich	550	36	30	1730	28	0
Burger King Double Croissan'wich Sausage, Bacon, Egg & Cheese						
1 sandwich	560	38	29	1400	25	0
Burger King Double Croissan'wich Sausage, Egg & Cheese						
1 sandwich	690	50	30	1560	30	0
Burger King Double Hamburger						
1 burger	420	22	30	590	26	1
Burger King Double Whopper						
1 burger	920	58	51	1090	48	3
Burger King Double Whopper without Mayo						
1 burger	760	41	51	950	48	3
Burger King Double Whopper with Cheese						
1 burger	1010	66	53	1530	53	3
Burger King Double Whopper with Cheese without Mayo						
1 burger	850	48	52	1390	53	3

RESTAURANT/ FOOD ITEM SERVING SIZE	CALORIES	FAT	CARBS	SODIUM	PROTEIN	FIBER
Burger King Dutch Apple Pie						
1 pie	320	13	47	290	2	1
Burger King French Fries						
Value	220	11	28	380	2	2
Burger King French Fries						
Small	340	17	44	590	4	4
Burger King French Fries						
Medium	480	23	61	820	5	5
Burger King French Fries						
Large	580	28	74	990	6	6
Burger King French Fries (no salt)						
Value	220	11	28	240	2	2
Burger King French Fries (no salt)						
Small	340	17	44	380	4	4
Burger King French Fries (no salt)						
Medium	480	23	61	530	5	5
Burger King French Fries (no salt)						
Large	580	28	74	640	6	6
Burger King French Toast Sticks						
3 pieces	230	11	29	260	3	1
Burger King French Toast Sticks						
5 pieces	380	18	49	430	5	2
Burger King Garden Salad (no chicken)						
1 salad	70	4	7	100	4	3
Burger King Garlic Parmesan Crouton						
1 serving	60	2	9	120	1	0
Burger King Ham Omelet Sandwich						
1 sandwich						
	290	12	33	870	13	1
Burger King Ham, Egg & Cheese Biscuit						
1 sandwich						
	410	23	34	1490	17	1
Burger King Hamburger						
1 burger	290	12	30	550	15	1
Burger King Hash Browns						
Value	250	16	24	410	2	3
Burger King Hash Browns						
Small	420	27	40	680	3	6
Burger King Hash Browns						
Medium	610	39	58	980	5	8
Burger King Hershey's 1% Low Fat Chocolate Milk						
8 oz	180	2.5	31	140	9	1
Burger King Hershey's Fat Free Milk						
8 oz	100	0	14	150	9	0
Burger King Hershey's Sundae Pie						
1 pie	310	19	32	220	3	1
Burger King Ken's Creamy Caesar Dressing						
4 oz	210	21	4	610	3	0
Burger King Ken's Honey Mustard Dressing						
5 oz	270	23	15	510	1	0

RESTAURANT/ FOOD ITEM	SERVING SIZE	CALORIES	FAT	CARBS	SODIUM	PROTEIN	FIBER
Burger King Ken's Light Italian Dressing	2 oz	120	11	5	440	0	0
Burger King Ken's Ranch Dressing	3 oz	190	20	2	550	1	0
Burger King Kraft Macaroni and Cheese	1 serving	160	5	22	340	7	1
Burger King Mocha BK Joe Iced Coffee	1 serving	360	10	66	290	6	1
Burger King Mushroom and Swiss Steakhouse XT	1 serving	870	49	54	1890	43	4
Burger King Onion Rings	Value	150	8	17	230	2	1
Burger King Onion Rings	Small	310	17	36	490	4	3
Burger King Onion Rings	Medium	450	24	52	700	6	5
Burger King Onion Rings	Large	510	27	60	810	7	5
Burger King Oreo BK Sundae Shake, Chocolate	16 oz	700	26	116	530	11	2
Burger King Oreo BK Sundae Shake, Chocolate	22 oz	1010	35	171	800	15	3
Burger King Oreo BK Sundae Shake, Strawberry	16 oz	680	25	114	430	10	1
Burger King Oreo BK Sundae Shake, Strawberry	22 oz	980	34	168	620	14	2
Burger King Original Chicken Sandwich	1 sandwich	630	39	46	1390	24	3
Burger King Original Chicken Sandwich without Mayo	1 sandwich	420	16	46	1210	24	3
Burger King Sausage Biscuit	1 sandwich	420	27	32	1090	13	1
Burger King Sausage Egg & Cheese Biscuit	1 sandwich	560	37	35	1560	21	1
Burger King Side Salad	1 salad	40	2	2	45	3	1
Burger King Spicy Chick'n Crisp	1 serving	450	30	34	810	12	2
Burger King Spicy Chick'n Crisp without Mayo	1 serving	290	12	34	670	12	2
Burger King Steakhouse Burger	1 burger	950	59	55	1950	40	4
Burger King Steakhouse XT	1 serving	970	61	55	1930	42	4
Burger King Strawberry Milk Shake	12 oz	310	11	52	190	6	0

RESTAURANT/ FOOD ITEM SERVING SIZE	CALORIES	FAT	CARBS	SODIUM	PROTEIN	FIBER
Burger King Strawberry Milk Shake						
16 oz	440	15	77	260	8	0
Burger King Strawberry Milk Shake						
22 oz	650	20	116	350	11	0
Burger King Strawberry Milk Shake						
32 oz	960	29	173	530	16	1
Burger King Tendercrisp Chicken Garden Salad						
1 salad	410	23	27	1060	27	4
Burger King Tendercrisp Chicken Sandwich						
1 sandwich						
	800	46	68	1640	32	3
Burger King Tendercrisp Chicken Sandwich without Mayo						
1 sandwich						
	590	22	68	1450	31	3
Burger King Tendergrill Chicken Garden Salad						
1 salad	210	7	8	780	29	3
Burger King Tendergrill Chicken Sandwich						
1 sandwich						
	490	21	51	1220	26	3
Burger King Tendergrill Chicken Sandwich without Mayo						
1 sandwich						
	380	9	51	1130	25	3
Burger King Triple Whopper						
1 burger	1160	76	51	1170	68	3
Burger King Triple Whopper without Mayo						
1 burger	1000	59	51	1030	68	3
Burger King Triple Whopper with Cheese						
1 burger	1250	84	52	1600	73	3
Burger King Triple Whopper with Cheese without Mayo						
1 burger	1090	66	52	1460	73	3
Burger King Vanilla Icing for Cini-Minis						
1 serving	90	0	22	25	0	0
Burger King Vanilla Milk Shake						
12 oz	270	11	42	180	6	0
Burger King Vanilla Milk Shake						
16 oz	360	15	57	240	8	0
Burger King Vanilla Milk Shake						
22 oz	480	20	76	320	11	0
Burger King Vanilla Milk Shake						
32 oz	720	29	113	480	16	1
Burger King Whopper						
1 burger	670	40	51	1020	29	3
Burger King Whopper Jr						
1 burger	370	21	31	560	16	2
Burger King Whopper Jr without Mayo						
1 burger	290	12	31	500	16	2
Burger King Whopper Jr with Cheese						
1 burger	420	25	31	780	18	2
Burger King Whopper Jr with Cheese without Mayo						
1 burger	340	16	31	710	18	2

RESTAURANT/ FOOD ITEM	SERVING SIZE	CALORIES	FAT	CARBS	SODIUM	PROTEIN	FIBER
Burger King Whopper with Cheese							
	1 burger	770	48	52	1450	33	3
Burger King Whopper with Cheese without Mayo							
	1 burger	610	30	52	1310	33	3
Burger King Whopper without Mayo							
	1 burger	520	23	51	880	28	3
Carl's Jr. Bacon & Egg Burrito							
	208 g	550	32	37	990	29	1
Carl's Jr. Bacon Cheese Six Dollar Burger							
	364 g	950	62	49	1980	51	3
Carl's Jr. Bacon Swiss Crispy Chicken Sandwich							
	310 g	750	40	62	1990	36	4
Carl's Jr. Big Hamburger							
	209 g	460	17	54	1090	24	3
Carl's Jr. Blue Cheese Dressing							
	57 g	320	34	1	410	2	0
Carl's Jr. Breakfast Burger							
	291 g	780	41	64	1460	38	3
Carl's Jr. Carl's Catch Fish Sandwich							
	291 g	710	37	74	1280	20	4
Carl's Jr. Charbroiled BBQ Chicken Sandwich							
	239 g	380	7	49	1010	34	2
Carl's Jr. Charbroiled Chicken Club Sandwich							
	262 g	560	27	44	1280	39	2
Carl's Jr. Charbroiled Chicken Salad							
	410 g	250	9	14	590	29	4
Carl's Jr. Charbroiled Santa Fe Chicken Sandwich							
	266 g	630	35	44	1410	36	2
Carl's Jr. Chicken Stars							
	4 pieces	210	16	10	310	8	1
Carl's Jr. Chicken Stars							
	6 pieces	320	24	14	460	12	2
Carl's Jr. Chicken Stars							
	9 pieces	480	36	21	690	18	2
Carl's Jr. Chicken Strips							
	3 pieces	370	26	19	620	14	2
Carl's Jr. Chicken Strips							
	5 pieces	610	43	32	1030	23	3
Carl's Jr. Chili Cheese Fries							
	349 g	990	56	89	2380	28	8
Carl's Jr. Chili Cheeseburger							
	315 g	780	41	58	1650	41	4
Carl's Jr. Chocolate Cake							
	85 g	300	12	48	350	3	1
Carl's Jr. Chocolate Chip Cookie							
	71 g	370	19	48	350	3	2
Carl's Jr. Chocolate Malt							
	414 g	780	34	100	370	15	1
Carl's Jr. Chocolate Shake							
	397 g	710	33	86	300	14	1

RESTAURANT/ FOOD ITEM	SERVING SIZE	CALORIES	FAT	CARBS	SODIUM	PROTEIN	FIBER
Carl's Jr. CrissCut Fries	139 g	450	29	42	900	5	4
Carl's Jr. Double Western Bacon Cheeseburger	319 g	960	52	70	1750	52	3
Carl's Jr. Famous Star with Cheese	278 g	660	39	53	1300	27	3
Carl's Jr. Fish & Chips	284 g	730	39	72	1630	22	6
Carl's Jr. French Toast Dips	5 pc	460	21	60	570	9	3
Carl's Jr. Fried Zucchini	139 g	330	18	36	610	6	2
Carl's Jr. Green Burrito Taco Salad	594 g	970	58	76	1850	42	17
Carl's Jr. Guacamole Six Dollar Burger	411 g	1040	70	53	2240	49	4
Carl's Jr. Hash Brown Nuggets	108 g	350	23	32	440	3	3
Carl's Jr. House Dressing	57 g	220	22	3	440	1	0
Carl's Jr. Jalapeño Burger	287 g	720	46	50	1340	27	3
Carl's Jr. Jalapeño Six Dollar Burger	384 g	930	61	52	2190	45	3
Carl's Jr. Loaded Breakfast Burrito	312 g	780	49	51	1480	36	3
Carl's Jr. Low Carb Six Dollar Burger	300 g	570	43	7	1480	38	1
Carl's Jr. Low Fat Balsamic Dressing	57 g	35	1.5	5	480	0	0
Carl's Jr. Natural-Cut Fries	82 g	220	11	29	580	3	2
Carl's Jr. Natural-Cut Fries	119 g	320	15	42	830	4	4
Carl's Jr. Natural-Cut Fries	169 g	460	22	60	1180	5	5
Carl's Jr. Natural-Cut Fries	184 g	500	24	65	1290	6	5
Carl's Jr. Onion Rings	128 g	530	28	61	590	8	3
Carl's Jr. Oreo Cookie Malt	414 g	790	38	95	440	17	1
Carl's Jr. Oreo Cookie Shake	397 g	730	38	81	360	15	1
Carl's Jr. Side Salad	139 g	50	2.5	4	55	3	2
Carl's Jr. Sourdough Breakfast Sandwich	196 g	450	21	38	1470	29	1
Carl's Jr. Spicy Chicken Sandwich	156 g	420	27	33	930	12	2

RESTAURANT/ FOOD ITEM SERVING SIZE	CALORIES	FAT	CARBS	SODIUM	PROTEIN	FIBER
Carl's Jr. Steak & Egg Burrito						
311 g	650	36	43	1750	41	1
Carl's Jr. Strawberry Malt						
414 g	770	34	99	320	15	0
Carl's Jr. Strawberry Shake						
397 g	700	33	85	250	14	0
Carl's Jr. Strawberry Swirl Cheesecake						
99 g	290	16	32	230	6	0
Carl's Jr. Sunrise Croissant Sandwich						
172 g	590	44	27	810	20	1
Carl's Jr. Super Star with Cheese						
383 g	920	58	54	1640	47	3
Carl's Jr. The Original Six Dollar Burger						
384 g	890	54	58	2040	45	3
Carl's Jr. Thousand Island Dressing						
57 g	240	23	7	460	0	0
Carl's Jr. Vanilla Malt						
414 g	780	34	101	320	15	0
Carl's Jr. Vanilla Shake						
397 g	710	33	86	240	14	0
Carl's Jr. Western Bacon Cheeseburger						
236 g	710	33	69	1410	32	3
Carl's Jr. Western Six Dollar Burger						
340 g	1020	53	81	2520	53	3
Cheesecake Factory* Adam's Peanut Butter Cup Fudge Ripple						
1 serving	1326	n/a	136	700	n/a	n/a
Cheesecake Factory* Ahi Carpaccio						
serves 2	260	n/a	11	1223	n/a	n/a
Cheesecake Factory* Avocado Eggrolls						
serves 2–4						
	958	n/a	104	1131	n/a	n/a
Cheesecake Factory* B.B.Q. Chicken Pizza						
serves 2–4						
	1559	n/a	177	2982	n/a	n/a
Cheesecake Factory* B.B.Q. Pulled Pork Sandwich						
1 serving	1438	n/a	107	2608	n/a	n/a
Cheesecake Factory* B.L.T. Salad						
1 serving	465	n/a	15	1405	n/a	n/a
Cheesecake Factory* Baja Chicken Hash						
1 serving	1496	n/a	64	1945	n/a	n/a
Cheesecake Factory* Baja Chicken Tacos						
1 serving	1188	n/a	113	2118	n/a	n/a
Cheesecake Factory* Bang-Bang Chicken and Shrimp						
1 serving	1383	n/a	159	1936	n/a	n/a
Cheesecake Factory* Barbeque Ranch Chicken Lunch Salad						
1 serving	704	n/a	79	444	n/a	n/a
Cheesecake Factory* Barbeque Ranch Chicken Salad						
1 serving	959	n/a	112	741	n/a	n/a

*From the Cheesecake Factory website: "At this point, we do not provide nutritional information for our menu selections." (Data obtained from CalorieLab.com.)

RESTAURANT/ FOOD ITEM SERVING SIZE	CALORIES	FAT	CARBS	SODIUM	PROTEIN	FIBER
Cheesecake Factory* Beef Ribs						
1 serving	2306	n/a	110	1613	n/a	n/a
Cheesecake Factory* Beer Battered Fish & Chips						
1 serving	2160	n/a	152	1816	n/a	n/a
Cheesecake Factory* Bistro Shrimp Pasta						
1 serving	2285	n/a	196	824	n/a	n/a
Cheesecake Factory* Black-Out Cake						
1 serving	1289	n/a	178	900	n/a	n/a
Cheesecake Factory* Blackened Chicken Sandwich						
1 serving	1341	n/a	83	2443	n/a	n/a
Cheesecake Factory* Boston House Salad						
1 serving	305	n/a	11	713	n/a	n/a
Cheesecake Factory* Brioche Breakfast Sandwich						
1 serving	1025	n/a	54	2221	n/a	n/a
Cheesecake Factory* Brownie Sundae Cheesecake						
1 serving	1265	n/a	137	245	n/a	n/a
Cheesecake Factory* Buffalo Blasts serves 2–4						
	1088	n/a	100	4058	n/a	n/a
Cheesecake Factory* Buffalo Wings serves 2–4						
	933	n/a	32	4416	n/a	n/a
Cheesecake Factory* Caesar Lunch Salad						
1 serving	860	n/a	18	861	n/a	n/a
Cheesecake Factory* Caesar Salad						
1 serving	1279	n/a	23	1330	n/a	n/a
Cheesecake Factory* Cajun Chicken "Littles"						
1 serving	907	n/a	43	1009	n/a	n/a
Cheesecake Factory* Cajun Jambalaya Pasta						
1 serving	1071	n/a	97	1058	n/a	n/a
Cheesecake Factory* California Cheesesteak						
1 serving	853	n/a	58	1675	n/a	n/a
Cheesecake Factory* California Omelette						
1 serving	916	n/a	13	1340	n/a	n/a
Cheesecake Factory* Carrot Cake						
1 serving	1549	n/a	183	490	n/a	n/a
Cheesecake Factory* Cheese Pizza serves 2–4						
	1355	n/a	148	2514	n/a	n/a
Cheesecake Factory* Cherry Cheesecake						
1 serving	862	n/a	100	425	n/a	n/a
Cheesecake Factory* Chicken and Biscuits						
1 serving	2262	n/a	164	2866	n/a	n/a
Cheesecake Factory* Chicken Madeira						
1 serving	1424	n/a	78	2038	n/a	n/a
Cheesecake Factory* Chicken Madeira and Steak Diane						
1 serving	1591	n/a	71	2477	n/a	n/a

*From the Cheesecake Factory website: "At this point, we do not provide nutritional information for our menu selections." (Data obtained from CalorieLab.com.)

RESTAURANT/ FOOD ITEM	SERVING SIZE	CALORIES	FAT	CARBS	SODIUM	PROTEIN	FIBER
Cheesecake Factory* Chicken Marsala and Mushrooms							
	1 serving	1475	n/a	148	850	n/a	n/a
Cheesecake Factory* Chicken Parmesan Sandwich							
	1 serving	1568	n/a	87	2937	n/a	n/a
Cheesecake Factory* Chicken Piccata							
	1 serving	1385	n/a	72	734	n/a	n/a
Cheesecake Factory* Chicken Pot Stickers							
	serves 2–4	377	n/a	43	2341	n/a	n/a
Cheesecake Factory* Chicken Salad Sandwich							
	1 serving	1228	n/a	68	1909	n/a	n/a
Cheesecake Factory* Chinese Chicken Lunch Salad							
	1 serving	535	n/a	63	506	n/a	n/a
Cheesecake Factory* Chinese Chicken Salad							
	1 serving	962	n/a	119	874	n/a	n/a
Cheesecake Factory* Chocolate Chip Cookie-Dough Cheesecake							
	1 serving	1114	n/a	106	580	n/a	n/a
Cheesecake Factory* Chocolate Coconut Cream Cheesecake							
	1 serving	1054	n/a	118	318	n/a	n/a
Cheesecake Factory* Chocolate Mousse Cheesecake							
	1 serving	939	n/a	79	340	n/a	n/a
Cheesecake Factory* Chocolate Oreo Mudslide Cheesecake							
	1 serving	1076	n/a	104	280	n/a	n/a
Cheesecake Factory* Chocolate Raspberry Truffle							
	1 serving	1079	n/a	104	350	n/a	n/a
Cheesecake Factory* Chocolate Tower Truffle Cake							
	1 serving	1679	n/a	206	970	n/a	n/a
Cheesecake Factory* Chocolate Tuxedo Cream Cheesecake							
	1 serving	934	n/a	98	388	n/a	n/a
Cheesecake Factory* Chris' Outrageous Chocolate Cake							
	1 serving	1507	n/a	183	580	n/a	n/a
Cheesecake Factory* Cobb Lunch Salad							
	1 serving	569	n/a	14	1143	n/a	n/a
Cheesecake Factory* Cobb Salad							
	1 serving	927	n/a	24	1890	n/a	n/a
Cheesecake Factory* Corn Succotash							
	1 serving	284	n/a	38	171	n/a	n/a
Cheesecake Factory* Crab Hash							
	1 serving	940	n/a	29	1245	n/a	n/a
Cheesecake Factory* Crabcake Sandwich							
	1 serving	1157	n/a	71	2069	n/a	n/a
Cheesecake Factory* Crabcakes							
	serves 2–4	980	n/a	31	1487	n/a	n/a
Cheesecake Factory* Craig's Crazy Carrot Cake Cheesecake							
	1 serving	986	n/a	102	330	n/a	n/a

*From the Cheesecake Factory website: "At this point, we do not provide nutritional information for our menu selections." (Data obtained from CalorieLab.com.)

RESTAURANT/ FOOD ITEM	SERVING SIZE	CALORIES	FAT	CARBS	SODIUM	PROTEIN	FIBER
Cheesecake Factory* Crispy Chicken Costoletta							
	1 serving	1238	n/a	62	1835	n/a	n/a
Cheesecake Factory* Crispy Crab Wontons							
	serves 2–4						
		667	n/a	83	1562	n/a	n/a
Cheesecake Factory* Crispy Spicy Beef							
	1 serving	1528	n/a	236	3380	n/a	n/a
Cheesecake Factory* Crispy Taquitos							
	serves 2–4						
		1141	n/a	77	1162	n/a	n/a
Cheesecake Factory* Crusted Chicken Romano							
	1 serving	1610	n/a	159	1820	n/a	n/a
Cheesecake Factory* Cuban Sandwich							
	1 serving	1135	n/a	76	2786	n/a	n/a
Cheesecake Factory* Double B.B.Q. Bacon Cheeseburger							
	1 serving	1583	n/a	110	2987	n/a	n/a
Cheesecake Factory* Dulce de Leche Caramel Cheesecake							
	1 serving	1079	n/a	91	406	n/a	n/a
Cheesecake Factory* Dutch Apple Caramel Struesel							
	1 serving	871	n/a	100	362	n/a	n/a
Cheesecake Factory* Edamame							
	serves 2–4						
		323	n/a	31	1261	n/a	n/a
Cheesecake Factory* Eggs Benedict with Fresh Spinach, Bacon, Tomato							
	1 serving	1418	n/a	55	1730	n/a	n/a
Cheesecake Factory* Endive, Pecan and Blue Cheese							
	1 serving	333	n/a	16	464	n/a	n/a
Cheesecake Factory* Energy Breakfast							
	1 serving	638	n/a	9	1261	n/a	n/a
Cheesecake Factory* Evelyn's Favorite Pasta							
	1 serving	1192	n/a	163	1406	n/a	n/a
Cheesecake Factory* Factory Appetizer Favorites							
	serves 2–4						
		3218	n/a	297	6703	n/a	n/a
Cheesecake Factory* Factory Burrito Grande							
	1 serving	1839	n/a	165	3776	n/a	n/a
Cheesecake Factory* Factory Chopped Salad							
	1 serving	518	n/a	28	995	n/a	n/a
Cheesecake Factory* Factory Huevos Rancheros							
	1 serving	1223	n/a	71	2183	n/a	n/a
Cheesecake Factory* Factory Mud Pie							
	serves 2	2065	n/a	251	950	n/a	n/a
Cheesecake Factory* Factory Nachos							
	serves 2–4						
		1665	n/a	100	2408	n/a	n/a
Cheesecake Factory* Famous Factory Meatloaf							
	1 serving	1079	n/a	68	3569	n/a	n/a

*From the Cheesecake Factory website: "At this point, we do not provide nutritional information for our menu selections." (Data obtained from CalorieLab.com.)

RESTAURANT/ FOOD ITEM SERVING SIZE	CALORIES	FAT	CARBS	SODIUM	PROTEIN	FIBER
Cheesecake Factory* Farfalle with Chicken and Roasted Garlic						
1 serving	2193	n/a	164	1833	n/a	n/a
Cheesecake Factory* Fettucini with Chicken and Sun-Dried Tomatoes						
1 serving	1832	n/a	83	876	n/a	n/a
Cheesecake Factory* Filet Mignon						
1 serving	992	n/a	24	1705	n/a	n/a
Cheesecake Factory* Fire-Roasted Fresh Artichoke						
serves 2–4						
	1028	n/a	62	787	n/a	n/a
Cheesecake Factory* Firecracker Salmon Rolls						
serves 2–4						
	630	n/a	62	1791	n/a	n/a
Cheesecake Factory* Four Cheese Pasta						
1 serving	1238	n/a	134	1929	n/a	n/a
Cheesecake Factory* French Country Salad						
1 serving	389	n/a	27	668	n/a	n/a
Cheesecake Factory* French Fries						
1 serving	689	n/a	84	448	n/a	n/a
Cheesecake Factory* French Toast						
1 serving	1369	n/a	98	1314	n/a	n/a
Cheesecake Factory* French Toast Napoleon						
1 serving	1696	n/a	160	1270	n/a	n/a
Cheesecake Factory* French Toast with Bacon						
1 serving	1849	n/a	98	3114	n/a	n/a
Cheesecake Factory* French Toast with Grilled Ham						
1 serving	1569	n/a	98	3095	n/a	n/a
Cheesecake Factory* Fresh Asparagus						
1 serving	43	n/a	7	1	n/a	n/a
Cheesecake Factory* Fresh Banana Cream Cheesecake						
1 serving	925	n/a	84	360	n/a	n/a
Cheesecake Factory* Fresh Broccoli						
1 serving	102	n/a	15	76	n/a	n/a
Cheesecake Factory* Fresh Fish Tacos						
1 serving	1221	n/a	130	2164	n/a	n/a
Cheesecake Factory* Fresh Grilled Mahi Mahi						
1 serving	466	n/a	3	394	n/a	n/a
Cheesecake Factory* Fresh Strawberry Cheesecake						
1 serving	733	n/a	66	425	n/a	n/a
Cheesecake Factory* Fresh Strawberry Shortcake						
1 serving	878	n/a	105	904	n/a	n/a
Cheesecake Factory* Fried Calamari						
serves 2–4						
	777	n/a	52	1196	n/a	n/a
Cheesecake Factory* Fried Macaroni and Cheese						
serves 2–4						
	1528	n/a	77	1761	n/a	n/a
Cheesecake Factory* Garlic Noodles						
1 serving	1499	n/a	176	1797	n/a	n/a

*From the Cheesecake Factory website: "At this point, we do not provide nutritional information for our menu selections." (Data obtained from CalorieLab.com.)

RESTAURANT/ FOOD ITEM	SERVING SIZE	CALORIES	FAT	CARBS	SODIUM	PROTEIN	FIBER
Cheesecake Factory* Giant Belgian Waffle							
	1 serving	424	n/a	62	911	n/a	n/a
Cheesecake Factory* Goblet of Fresh Strawberries							
	1 serving	108	n/a	15	0	n/a	n/a
Cheesecake Factory* Godiva Chocolate Brownie Sundae							
serves 2							
		1018	n/a	103	206	n/a	n/a
Cheesecake Factory* Godiva Chocolate Cheesecake							
	1 serving	1109	n/a	105	210	n/a	n/a
Cheesecake Factory* Green Beans							
	1 serving	114	n/a	12	224	n/a	n/a
Cheesecake Factory* Grilled Cheese							
	1 serving	719	n/a	51	1301	n/a	n/a
Cheesecake Factory* Grilled Chicken Medallions							
	1 serving	1409	n/a	121	1241	n/a	n/a
Cheesecake Factory* Grilled Chicken Tostada Salad							
	1 serving	1131	n/a	93	2152	n/a	n/a
Cheesecake Factory* Grilled Pork Chops							
	1 serving	1375	n/a	75	1218	n/a	n/a
Cheesecake Factory* Grilled Portabella on a Bun							
	1 serving	1133	n/a	65	1279	n/a	n/a
Cheesecake Factory* Grilled Shrimp and Bacon Club							
	1 serving	1643	n/a	124	2690	n/a	n/a
Cheesecake Factory* Grilled Turkey Burger							
	1 serving	1373	n/a	65	1628	n/a	n/a
Cheesecake Factory* Guacamole Made-to-Order							
serves 2–4							
		1608	n/a	134	1171	n/a	n/a
Cheesecake Factory* Hawaiian Pizza							
serves 2–4							
		1444	n/a	160	2973	n/a	n/a
Cheesecake Factory* Herb Crusted Filet of Salmon							
	1 serving	1195	n/a	92	676	n/a	n/a
Cheesecake Factory* Herb Crusted Salmon and Shrimp Scampi							
	1 serving	1827	n/a	71	1420	n/a	n/a
Cheesecake Factory* Herb Crusted Salmon Salad							
	1 serving	559	n/a	28	660	n/a	n/a
Cheesecake Factory* Hibachi Steak							
	1 serving	1533	n/a	110	3724	n/a	n/a
Cheesecake Factory* Hot Fudge Sundae							
	1 serving	1534	n/a	162	416	n/a	n/a
Cheesecake Factory* Hot Spinach and Cheese Dip							
serves 2–4							
		1031	n/a	93	1269	n/a	n/a
Cheesecake Factory* Jamaican Black Pepper Shrimp							
	1 serving	1142	n/a	146	2058	n/a	n/a
Cheesecake Factory* Joe's Special							
	1 serving	785	n/a	15	1940	n/a	n/a

*From the Cheesecake Factory website: "At this point, we do not provide nutritional information for our menu selections." (Data obtained from CalorieLab.com.)

RESTAURANT/ FOOD ITEM	SERVING SIZE	CALORIES	FAT	CARBS	SODIUM	PROTEIN	FIBER
Cheesecake Factory* Kahlua Cocoa Coffee Cheesecake							
	1 serving	879	n/a	83	240	n/a	n/a
Cheesecake Factory* Key Lime Cheesecake							
	1 serving	869	n/a	78	370	n/a	n/a
Cheesecake Factory* Kobe Burger							
	1 serving	990	n/a	61	1673	n/a	n/a
Cheesecake Factory* Lemon Raspberry Cream Cheesecake							
	1 serving	734	n/a	75	330	n/a	n/a
Cheesecake Factory* Lemon-Herb Roasted Chicken							
	1 serving	1249	n/a	30	2320	n/a	n/a
Cheesecake Factory* Lemoncello Cream Torte							
	1 serving	1034	n/a	114	490	n/a	n/a
Cheesecake Factory* Linda's Fudge Cake							
	1 serving	1369	n/a	280	1080	n/a	n/a
Cheesecake Factory* Louisiana Chicken Pasta							
	1 serving	2052	n/a	168	1943	n/a	n/a
Cheesecake Factory* Low Carb Cheesecake							
	1 serving	570	n/a	37	310	n/a	n/a
Cheesecake Factory* Low Carb Cheesecake with Strawberries							
	1 serving	602	n/a	39	310	n/a	n/a
Cheesecake Factory* Luau Salad							
	1 serving	801	n/a	85	1527	n/a	n/a
Cheesecake Factory* Luau Santa Fe Lunch Salad							
	1 serving	509	n/a	51	973	n/a	n/a
Cheesecake Factory* Macaroni & Cheese							
	1 serving	1309	n/a	92	768	n/a	n/a
Cheesecake Factory* Mashed Potatoes							
	1 serving	564	n/a	44	851	n/a	n/a
Cheesecake Factory* Miso Salmon							
	1 serving	1673	n/a	131	2416	n/a	. n/a
Cheesecake Factory* Monte Cristo Sandwich							
	1 serving	1618	n/a	92	2775	n/a	n/a
Cheesecake Factory* Morning Quesadilla							
	1 serving	2015	n/a	91	4347	n/a	n/a
Cheesecake Factory* Old Fashioned Hamburger							
	1 serving	958	n/a	55	1800	n/a	n/a
Cheesecake Factory* Orange Chicken							
	1 serving	1791	n/a	298	2850	n/a	n/a
Cheesecake Factory* Oreo Cheesecake							
	1 serving	869	n/a	78	480	n/a	n/a
Cheesecake Factory* Pasta Carbonara							
	1 serving	2134	n/a	144	1246	n/a	n/a
Cheesecake Factory* Pasta Da Vinci							
	1 serving	1524	n/a	132	576	n/a	n/a
Cheesecake Factory* Pepperoni Pizza							
	serves 2–4						
		1565	n/a	148	3219	n/a	n/a

*From the Cheesecake Factory website: "At this point, we do not provide nutritional information for our menu selections." (Data obtained from CalorieLab.com.)

RESTAURANT/ FOOD ITEM SERVING SIZE	CALORIES	FAT	CARBS	SODIUM	PROTEIN	FIBER
Cheesecake Factory* Petite Filet						
1 serving	704	n/a	23	948	n/a	n/a
Cheesecake Factory* Popcorn Shrimp						
serves 2–4	812	n/a	69	1391	n/a	n/a
Cheesecake Factory* Pumpkin Cheesecake						
1 serving	739	n/a	95	370	n/a	n/a
Cheesecake Factory* Pumpkin Pecan Cheesecake						
1 serving	1079	n/a	95	370	n/a	n/a
Cheesecake Factory* Quesadilla						
serves 2–4	931	n/a	54	1928	n/a	n/a
Cheesecake Factory* Ranch House Burger						
1 serving	1887	n/a	61	2831	n/a	n/a
Cheesecake Factory* Road Side Sliders						
serves 2–4	731	n/a	69	1464	n/a	n/a
Cheesecake Factory* Roasted Vegetables and Goat Cheese Pizza						
serves 2–4	1481	n/a	156	2896	n/a	n/a
Cheesecake Factory* Sante Fe Salad						
1 serving	871	n/a	76	871	n/a	n/a
Cheesecake Factory* Sautéed Snow Peas and Vegetables						
1 serving	155	n/a	15	1701	n/a	n/a
Cheesecake Factory* Sautéed Spinach						
1 serving	170	n/a	10	517	n/a	n/a
Cheesecake Factory* Seared Tuna Tataki Salad						
1 serving	442	n/a	24	1386	n/a	n/a
Cheesecake Factory* Shepherd's Pie						
1 serving	1677	n/a	83	4209	n/a	n/a
Cheesecake Factory* Shrimp and Chicken Gumbo						
1 serving	1527	n/a	99	2217	n/a	n/a
Cheesecake Factory* Shrimp Scampi and Chicken Madeira						
1 serving	1121	n/a	42	1053	n/a	n/a
Cheesecake Factory* Shrimp Scampi and Steak Diane						
1 serving	1769	n/a	74	2115	n/a	n/a
Cheesecake Factory* Shrimp with Angel Hair						
1 serving	845	n/a	106	1586	n/a	n/a
Cheesecake Factory* Smoked Salmon Platter						
1 serving	745	n/a	73	1867	n/a	n/a
Cheesecake Factory* Snickers Bar Chunks and Cheesecake						
1 serving	1057	n/a	99	466	n/a	n/a
Cheesecake Factory* Southern Fried Chicken Sliders						
serves 2–4	1379	n/a	92	2819	n/a	n/a
Cheesecake Factory* Spicy Ahi Tempura Roll						
serves 2–4	678	n/a	55	2361	n/a	n/a

*From the Cheesecake Factory website: "At this point, we do not provide nutritional information for our menu selections." (Data obtained from CalorieLab.com.)

RESTAURANT/ FOOD ITEM	SERVING SIZE	CALORIES	FAT	CARBS	SODIUM	PROTEIN	FIBER
Cheesecake Factory* Spicy Cashew Chicken							
	1 serving	1809	n/a	252	4450	n/a	n/a
Cheesecake Factory* Spicy Chicken Chipotle Pasta							
	1 serving	1749	n/a	149	1541	n/a	n/a
Cheesecake Factory* Spicy Crispy Chicken Sandwich with Buffalo Sauce							
	1 serving	1184	n/a	87	2714	n/a	n/a
Cheesecake Factory* Spicy Crispy Chicken Sandwich with Chipotle Mayo							
	1 serving	1384	n/a	86	2174	n/a	n/a
Cheesecake Factory* Spinach, Mushroom, Cheese and Bacon Omelette							
	1 serving	832	n/a	6	2092	n/a	n/a
Cheesecake Factory* Steak and Eggs							
	1 serving	815	n/a	3	1062	n/a	n/a
Cheesecake Factory* Steak Diane							
	1 serving	964	n/a	10	1580	n/a	n/a
Cheesecake Factory* Steak Diane and Herb Crusted Salmon							
	1 serving	1734	n/a	57	1993	n/a	n/a
Cheesecake Factory* Stuffed Chicken Tortillas							
	1 serving	1797	n/a	114	2847	n/a	n/a
Cheesecake Factory* Sunrise Fiesta Burrito							
	1 serving	1720	n/a	128	4600	n/a	n/a
Cheesecake Factory* Sweet Corn Tamale Cakes							
	serves 2–4						
		1495	n/a	106	1378	n/a	n/a
Cheesecake Factory* Teriyaki Chicken							
	1 serving	1403	n/a	210	2793	n/a	n/a
Cheesecake Factory* Tex Mex Eggrolls							
	serves 2–4						
		778	n/a	79	1751	n/a	n/a
Cheesecake Factory* Thai Chicken Pasta							
	1 serving	1531	n/a	135	2175	n/a	n/a
Cheesecake Factory* Thai Lettuce Wraps							
	serves 2–4						
		1025	n/a	114	2347	n/a	n/a
Cheesecake Factory* The Classic Burger							
	1 serving	1375	n/a	55	1592	n/a	n/a
Cheesecake Factory* The Club							
	1 serving	1433	n/a	115	3263	n/a	n/a
Cheesecake Factory* The Factory Burger							
	1 serving	737	n/a	53	1018	n/a	n/a
Cheesecake Factory* The Incredible Grilled Eggplant Sandwich							
	1 serving	1015	n/a	72	1749	n/a	n/a
Cheesecake Factory* The Navajo							
	1 serving	1278	n/a	91	1439	n/a	n/a
Cheesecake Factory* The Original							
	1 serving	707	n/a	62	425	n/a	n/a
Cheesecake Factory* Tiramisu							
	1 serving	932	n/a	74	301	n/a	n/a

*From the Cheesecake Factory website: "At this point, we do not provide nutritional information for our menu selections." (Data obtained from CalorieLab.com.)

RESTAURANT/ FOOD ITEM SERVING SIZE	CALORIES	FAT	CARBS	SODIUM	PROTEIN	FIBER
Cheesecake Factory* Tiramisu Cheesecake						
1 serving	798	n/a	68	351	n/a	n/a
Cheesecake Factory* Tomato, Basil and Cheese						
serves 2–4						
	1346	n/a	152	2526	n/a	n/a
Cheesecake Factory* Tons of Fun Burger						
1 serving	1399	n/a	58	2033	n/a	n/a
Cheesecake Factory* Tossed Green Salad						
1 serving	189	n/a	21	173	n/a	n/a
Cheesecake Factory* Vanilla Bean Cheesecake						
1 serving	869	n/a	72	320	n/a	n/a
Cheesecake Factory* Vietnamese Shrimp Summer Rolls						
serves 2–4						
	663	n/a	98	1680	n/a	n/a
Cheesecake Factory* Warm Apple Crisp						
1 serving	1305	n/a	193	176	n/a	n/a
Cheesecake Factory* Wasabi Crusted Ahi Tuna						
1 serving	1750	n/a	113	1302	n/a	n/a
Cheesecake Factory* Weight Management Grilled Chicken						
1 serving	583	n/a	28	1921	n/a	n/a
Cheesecake Factory* White Chicken Chili						
1 serving	880	n/a	67	2124	n/a	n/a
Cheesecake Factory* White Chocolate Caramel Macadamia Nut Cheesecake						
1 serving	1222	n/a	114	444	n/a	n/a
Cheesecake Factory* White Chocolate Raspberry Truffle Cheesecake						
1 serving	929	n/a	85	370	n/a	n/a
Chick-fil-A Bacon, Egg & Cheese Biscuit						
172 g	490	26	43	1350	21	2
Chick-fil-A Biscuit						
86 g	310	13	41	700	5	2
Chick-fil-A Chargrilled & Fruit Salad						
347 g	220	6	21	860	22	4
Chick-fil-A Chargrilled Chicken Club Sandwich						
250 g	380	12	34	1650	36	7
Chick-fil-A Chargrilled Chicken Cool Wrap						
291 g	410	12	49	1510	33	9
Chick-fil-A Chargrilled Chicken Garden Salad						
298 g	170	6	10	860	22	4
Chick-fil-A Chargrilled Chicken Sandwich						
220 g	260	3	33	1300	27	7
Chick-fil-A Cheesecake						
91 g	310	23	22	280	5	1
Chick-fil-A Chick-n-Minis						
94 g	260	10	29	590	13	1
Chick-fil-A Chick-n-Strips						
215g	470	23	22	1390	44	3

*From the Cheesecake Factory website: "At this point, we do not provide nutritional information for our menu selections." (Data obtained from CalorieLab.com.)

RESTAURANT/ FOOD ITEM	SERVING SIZE	CALORIES	FAT	CARBS	SODIUM	PROTEIN	FIBER
Chick-fil-A Chick-n-Strips Salad	388g	450	22	26	1160	39	6
Chick-fil-A Chicken Biscuit	150g	450	20	48	1310	19	3
Chick-fil-A Chicken Breakfast Burrito	184g	420	18	41	890	22	4
Chick-fil-A Chicken Caesar Cool Wrap	232g	460	15	46	1720	39	8
Chick-fil-A Chicken, Egg & Cheese Bagel	213g	500	20	49	1280	30	3
Chick-fil-A Chicken Salad Sandwich	233g	500	20	53	1220	29	4
Chick-fil-A Chicken Sandwich	179g	430	17	39	1370	31	3
Chick-fil-A Chocolate Milkshake	517g	740	28	112	520	16	1
Chick-fil-A Cookies & Cream Milkshake	510g	700	33	98	550	17	1
Chick-fil-A Fudge Nut Brownie	79g	370	19	45	180	5	3
Chick-fil-A Hearty Breast of Chicken Soup	439g	240	7	30	1670	15	2
Chick-fil-A Icedream	135g	170	4	31	115	5	0
Chick-fil-A Lemon Pie	120g	360	13	58	290	6	1
Chick-fil-A Nuggets	170g	400	19	15	1250	40	3
Chick-fil-A Peach Milkshake	595g	850	21	153	540	15	1
Chick-fil-A Sausage Breakfast Burrito	184g	480	27	38	870	21	4
Chick-fil-A Spicy Chicken Cool Wrap	277g	400	12	47	1320	35	9
Chick-fil-A Strawberry Milkshake	567g	760	28	117	520	16	1
Chick-fil-A Vanilla Milkshake	482g	660	27	90	510	16	0
Chili's Bacon Burger	1 serving	1140	72	61	2150	59	3
Chili's Baked Potato Soup	1 cup	230	16	12	820	8	1
Chili's Baked Potato Soup	1 bowl	470	32	24	1630	17	2
Chili's Big Mouth Bites with Jalapeno Ranch	1 serving	1780	120	103	3020	64	6
Chili's Black Bean Soup	1 cup	150	4	19	670	8	5
Chili's Black Bean Soup	1 bowl	290	8	38	1340	16	11

RESTAURANT/ FOOD ITEM	SERVING SIZE	CALORIES	FAT	CARBS	SODIUM	PROTEIN	FIBER
Chili's Boneless Buffalo Chicken Salad							
	1 serving	1070	77	46	4380	44	5
Chili's Boneless Buffalo Wings with Bleu Cheese							
	1 serving	1200	91	48	3750	44	1
Chili's Boneless Sweet Chile Glazed Wings with Ranch							
	1 serving	1300	80	95	2880	46	2
Chili's Bottomless Tostada Chips with Hot Sauce							
	1 serving	470	39	26	2790	4	5
Chili's Broccoli Cheese Soup							
	1 cup	120	8	9	650	5	1
Chili's Buffalo Chicken							
	1 serving	1110	78	53	5350	48	6
Chili's Cajun Chicken Pasta							
	1 serving	1340	68	106	3650	67	6
Chili's Cajun Ribeye							
	1 serving	910	70	19	1570	50	3
Chili's Cheesecake							
	1 serving	710	42	68	460	12	0
Chili's Chicken Caesar Salad							
	1 serving	900	71	28	1740	37	6
Chili's Chicken Club Tacos							
	3 tacos	1430	70	137	4770	62	12
Chili's Chicken Crispers							
	1 serving	1750	121	104	2910	65	9
Chili's Chicken Enchilada Soup							
	1 cup	200	12	9	630	13	1
Chili's Chicken Enchilada Soup							
	1 bowl	400	25	18	1260	27	1
Chili's Chicken Noodle Soup							
	1 cup	60	0.5	10	580	3	1
Chili's Chicken Noodle Soup							
	1 bowl	120	1.5	20	1150	7	1
Chili's Chicken Tacos							
	3 tacos	1200	45	144	4430	61	16
Chili's Chicken Tortilla Soup							
	1 cup	130	7	10	1030	7	1
Chili's Chicken Tortilla Soup							
	1 bowl	260	15	20	2060	14	3
Chili's Chocolate Chip Molten Cake							
	1 serving	1140	56	150	690	14	3
Chili's Chocolate Chip Paradise Pie							
	1 serving	1290	68	163	680	16	5
Chili's Classic Chicken							
	1 serving	380	12	28	2110	39	4
Chili's Classic Combo							
	1 serving	440	19	28	2370	43	4
Chili's Classic Sirloin							
	1 serving	460	29	19	1200	33	2
Chili's Classic Steak							
	1 serving	490	26	27	2630	46	4

RESTAURANT/ FOOD ITEM	SERVING SIZE	CALORIES	FAT	CARBS	SODIUM	PROTEIN	FIBER
Chili's Country-Fried Chicken Crispers No Sauce							
	1 serving	1490	90	110	3010	60	8
Chili's Country-Fried Steak with Sides							
	1 serving	1470	84	127	3390	53	9
Chili's Crispy Chicken Crisper Tacos							
	3 tacos	1990	104	194	5790	72	13
Chili's Crispy Honey-Chipotle Chicken Crispers							
	1 serving	1930	108	181	4400	61	8
Chili's Crispy Sweet Chile Glazed Chicken Crispers							
	1 serving	1860	108	158	4170	63	8
Chili's Fajita Condiments							
	1 serving	230	19	7	360	10	2
Chili's Fajita Trio							
	1 serving	560	27	31	3120	52	5
Chili's Fire Grilled Bacon Chicken Ranch Quesadilla with Salsa Ranch							
	1 serving	1750	122	95	4270	77	5
Chili's Fire Grilled Chicken Fajita Quesadilla							
	1 serving	1480	96	99	3510	69	6
Chili's Fire Grilled Jalapeno Beef Quesadilla with Ancho Chile Ranch							
	1 serving	1790	126	99	4720	68	7
Chili's Flame-Grilled Ribeye							
	1 serving	910	70	19	1450	50	2
Chili's Flour Tortillas							
	3 tortillas	380	10	62	1000	10	3
Chili's Flour Tortillas							
	6 tortillas	750	19	125	1990	20	6
Chili's Frosty Chocolate Shake							
	1 serving	740	35	100	210	8	0
Chili's Grilled Salmon with Garlic & Herbs							
	1 serving	630	29	50	1060	47	5
Chili's Grilled Shrimp Alfredo							
	1 serving	1310	76	105	3500	49	6
Chili's Guiltless Black Bean Burger							
	1 serving	610	11	91	1790	37	18
Chili's Guiltless Buffalo Chicken Sandwich							
	1 serving	390	7	46	2300	36	9
Chili's Guiltless Carne Asada Steak							
	1 serving	370	10	11	1440	46	6
Chili's Guiltless Cedar Plank Tilapia							
	1 serving	200	4	8	690	34	5
Chili's Guiltless Chicken Platter							
	1 serving	370	2	49	1940	39	7
Chili's Guiltless Grilled Chicken Sandwich							
	1 serving	360	5	44	1390	36	9
Chili's Guiltless Grilled Salmon							
	1 serving	400	20	8	420	51	3
Chili's Guiltless Honey-Mustard Glazed Salmon							
	1 serving	420	20	13	610	50	2
Chili's Hot Spinach & Artichoke Dip with Chips							
	1 serving	1040	85	40	3320	31	3

RESTAURANT/ FOOD ITEM SERVING SIZE	CALORIES	FAT	CARBS	SODIUM	PROTEIN	FIBER
Chili's Kickin' Jack Nachos						
12 nachos 1200		90	62	2680	54	8
Chili's Kickin' Jack Nachos						
8 nachos 820		62	42	1820	37	6
Chili's Kickin' Jack Nachos w/Fajita Chicken						
12 nachos 1340		92	64	3610	82	8
Chili's Kickin' Jack Nachos w/Fajita Chicken						
8 nachos 960		64	45	2740	65	6
Chili's Kickin' Jack Nachos w/Fajita Steak						
12 nachos 1380		94	63	3620	81	8
Chili's Kickin' Jack Nachos w/Fajita Steak						
8 nachos 1010		66	44	2760	63	6
Chili's Margarita Grilled Chicken						
1 serving 660		14	80	2340	52	8
Chili's Memphis Dry Rub Ribs						
½ rack 610		43	23	2480	29	2
Chili's Memphis Dry Rub Ribs						
1 serving 1170		87	33	4410	58	4
Chili's Mesquite Chicken Salad						
1 serving 920		57	45	2680	54	10
Chili's Molten Chocolate Cake						
1 serving 1070		51	143	820	11	5
Chili's Monterey Chicken						
1 serving 860		44	56	3160	62	9
Chili's Mushroom Jack						
1 serving 740		41	39	3490	58	6
Chili's Onion String & Crispy Jalapeno Stack with Jalapeno Ranch						
1 serving 1030		87	49	1790	8	6
Chili's Original Ribs						
1 serving 1110		81	33	4100	57	2
Chili's Original Ribs						
½ rack 560		41	17	2050	28	1
Chili's Quesadilla Explosion Salad						
1 serving 1390		89	86	2710	61	10
Chili's Shiner Bock BBQ Ribs						
1 serving 1340		82	84	4330	59	1
Chili's Shiner Bock BBQ Ribs						
½ rack 650		41	38	2090	29	0
Chili's Side Salad Caesar						
1 serving 350		31	13	550	6	2
Chili's Side Salad House, No Dressing						
1 serving 210		12	17	310	10	3
Chili's Skillet Queso w/Chips						
1 serving 920		73	46	4770	30	9
Chili's Southwest Cedar Plank Tilapia						
1 serving 610		31	55	1730	30	7
Chili's Southwestern Cobb Salad						
1 serving 1080		71	57	2650	55	9
Chili's Southwestern Eggrolls with Avocado Ranch						
1 serving 910		57	72	1960	27	7

RESTAURANT/ FOOD ITEM SERVING SIZE	CALORIES	FAT	CARBS	SODIUM	PROTEIN	FIBER
Chili's Southwestern Vegetable Soup						
1 cup	100	4	13	630	4	2
Chili's Southwestern Vegetable Soup						
1 bowl	210	8	26	1250	9	5
Chili's Spicy Garlic & Lime Grilled Shrimp Salad						
1 serving	580	37	43	1740	24	9
Chili's Steak & Portobello						
1 serving	800	57	36	3370	47	7
Chili's Sweet Shot Double Chocolate Fudge Brownie						
1 serving	420	24	51	25	1	1
Chili's Sweet Shot Key Lime Pie						
1 serving	240	12	30	75	4	0
Chili's Sweet Shot Red Velvet Cake						
1 serving	250	9	39	200	3	1
Chili's Sweet Shot Warm Cinnamon Roll						
1 serving	280	13	38	95	3	1
Chili's Terlingua Chili with Toppings						
1 cup	230	15	11	580	12	2
Chili's Terlingua Chili with Toppings						
1 bowl	450	30	23	1170	24	3
Chili's Texas Cheese Fries with Jalapeno Ranch						
½ rack	1400	111	41	2510	64	4
Chili's Texas Cheese Fries with Jalapeno Ranch						
1 serving	1920	147	67	3580	84	7
Chili's Triple Dipper Big Mouth Bites with Jalapeno Ranch						
1 serving	790	52	46	1410	30	2
Chili's Triple Dipper Boneless Buffalo Wings with Bleu Cheese						
1 serving	740	60	26	2070	24	1
Chili's Triple Dipper Boneless Sweet Chile Glazed Wings with Ranch						
1 serving	760	50	49	1640	25	1
Chili's Triple Dipper Buffalo Chicken Crisper Bites with Bleu Cheese						
1 serving	820	55	55	2630	24	2
Chili's Triple Dipper Chicken Crisper Bites with Ancho Chile Ranch						
1 serving	690	40	58	1970	20	2
Chili's Triple Dipper Chicken Crispers, No Dressing						
1 serving	600	42	20	1300	34	2
Chili's Triple Dipper Hot Spinach & Artichoke Dip with Chips						
1 serving	520	43	20	1660	16	2
Chili's Triple Dipper Southwestern Eggrolls with Avocado Ranch						
1 serving	640	42	48	1370	18	5
Chili's Triple Dipper Wings Over Buffalo with Bleu Cheese						
1 serving	800	72	1	1730	34	0
Chili's White Chocolate Molten Cake						
1 serving	1250	65	150	460	15	0
Chili's Wings Over Buffalo with Bleu Cheese						
1 serving	1330	116	2	1880	66	0
Denny's All-American Slam						
10 oz	820	69	5	1520	42	1
Denny's Bacon Strips						
4 strips	180	13	2	700	14	0

RESTAURANT/ FOOD ITEM SERVING SIZE	CALORIES	FAT	CARBS	SODIUM	PROTEIN	FIBER
Denny's Biscuits & Sausage Gravy						
8 oz	580	34	57	1660	9	0
Denny's BLT						
6 oz	570	37	36	850	20	2
Denny's Boca Burger						
11 oz	500	15	62	1320	30	10
Denny's Broccoli & Cheddar Soup						
12 oz	374	29	16	1568	10	4
Denny's Cherry Cherry Limeade						
12 oz	180	0	45	30	0	0
Denny's Chicken Deluxe Salad-Chicken Strip						
18 oz	590	29	44	1180	42	4
Denny's Chicken Noodle Soup						
12 oz	166	4	19	1304	12	1
Denny's Chicken Ranch Melt						
12 oz	920	42	79	2800	53	4
Denny's Chicken Sausage Patty						
1 patty	110	9	0	260	7	0
Denny's Clam Chowder						
12 oz	266	17	24	1822	5	2
Denny's Classic Cheeseburger						
13 oz	930	58	56	2190	49	5
Denny's Club Sandwich						
11 oz	660	34	55	1640	29	4
Denny's Country-Fried Potatoes						
5 oz	550	37	48	780	6	10
Denny's Country-Fried Steak & Eggs						
11 oz	660	42	29	1620	39	3
Denny's Cranberry Pecan Salad with Chicken						
9 oz	250	8	11	830	32	1
Denny's Eggs						
1 egg	120	10	0	120	6	0
Denny's Egg Whites						
4 oz	50	0	1	180	11	0
Denny's Fit Fare Boca Burger						
10 oz	410	8	60	770	25	17
Denny's Fit Fare Grilled Chicken Breast						
17 oz	290	10	15	770	36	4
Denny's Fit Fare Grilled Tilapia						
17 oz	600	11	66	1560	58	3
Denny's French Toast Slam						
15 oz	940	53	68	1820	47	4
Denny's Grand Slam Burrito						
16 oz	1160	62	106	2730	43	6
Denny's Grand Slamwich						
12 oz	1030	66	68	2330	37	3
Denny's Grilled Chicken						
17 oz	290	10	15	770	36	4
Denny's Grilled Honey Ham Slice						
3 oz	110	5	1	810	14	0

RESTAURANT/ FOOD ITEM SERVING SIZE	CALORIES	FAT	CARBS	SODIUM	PROTEIN	FIBER
Denny's Grits						
12 oz	260	5	47	840	5	1
Denny's Ham & Cheddar Omelette						
10 oz	590	44	4	1330	40	0
Denny's Hash Browns						
5 oz	210	12	26	650	2	2
Denny's Hash Browns with Cheese						
5 oz	310	19	26	780	8	2
Denny's Heartland Scramble						
20 oz	1150	66	97	2800	40	7
Denny's Island Fizz						
12 oz	190	0	47	20	0	0
Denny's Lemon Pepper Tilapia						
13 oz	640	27	41	1520	55	2
Denny's Lemon Tea Chiller						
16 oz	100	0	26	0	0	0
Denny's Lumberjack Slam						
15 oz	850	46	60	2770	45	3
Denny's Mango Tea Chiller						
16 oz	160	0	40	0	0	0
Denny's Meat Lover's Scramble						
19 oz	1130	66	80	3180	51	6
Denny's Moons Over My Hammy						
13 oz	780	42	50	2580	46	2
Denny's Oatmeal with 8 oz milk						
16 oz	270	7	37	290	14	4
Denny's OJ						
Small	140	0	0	34	0	30
Denny's OJ Mango Juicy Fusion						
16 oz	240	0	60	5	0	0
Denny's Pancakes, Buttermilk						
3 cakes	510	6	102	1770	12	3
Denny's Pancakes, Wheat						
2 cakes	310	1.5	64	950	10	8
Denny's Pineapple Dream						
12 oz	190	0	50	40	0	1
Denny's Prime Rib Sizzlin' Breakfast Skillet						
21 oz	850	40	77	2110	41	6
Denny's Razzdango						
12 oz	190	0	49	30	0	1
Denny's Ruby Red Grapefruit Juice						
Small	164	0	40	41	1	0
Denny's Sausage Links						
4 links	370	34	4	660	9	3
Denny's Slamburger						
9 oz	750	60	13	1560	41	2
Denny's Southwestern Sizzlin' Skillet						
17 oz	990	61	71	2140	35	6
Denny's Spicy Buffalo Chicken Melt						
14 oz	940	46	81	3870	46	4

RESTAURANT/ FOOD ITEM SERVING SIZE	CALORIES	FAT	CARBS	SODIUM	PROTEIN	FIBER
Denny's Strawberry Mango Pucker						
12 oz	220	0	56	10	0	1
Denny's Super Grand Slamwich						
16 oz	1320	89	71	3060	53	4
Denny's T-Bone Steak						
12 oz	740	56	0	740	59	0
Denny's T-Bone Steak & Eggs						
16 oz	780	36	4	1210	110	0
Denny's Top Sirloin Steak						
6 oz	220	6	1	600	41	0
Denny's Top Sirloin Steak & Eggs						
10 oz	420	21	1	920	54	0
Denny's Turkey Bacon						
2 slices	76	4	0	304	8	0
Denny's Two Eggs Breakfast						
4 oz	200	15	1	330	13	0
Denny's Ultimate Omelette						
12 oz	670	54	8	740	36	2
Denny's Vegetable Beef Soup						
12 oz	124	1	18	1457	10	3
Denny's Veggie Cheese Omelette						
13 oz	500	37	10	940	29	2
Denny's Very Double Berry Juicy Fusion						
16 oz	280	0.5	69	10	0	0
Denny's Western Burger						
17 oz	1300	82	83	2700	58 -	6
Domino's Amazin' Greens Garden Fresh Salad						
1 salad	130	8	10	160	8	4
Domino's Amazin' Greens Grilled Chicken Caesar Salad						
1 salad	170	7	10	560	19	4
Domino's Breadsticks						
1 piece	870	50	89	780	17	3
Domino's Brooklyn Style, Alfredo Sauce, no toppings						
1 lg slice	200	8	24	380	8	1
Domino's Brooklyn Style, BBQ Sauce, no toppings						
1 lg slice	195	6.5	27	390	8	1
Domino's Brooklyn Style, Cheddar Sauce, no toppings						
1 lg slice	195	7.5	25	415	9	1
Domino's Brooklyn Style, Garlic Parm Sauce, no toppings						
1 lg slice	210	10	24	395	8	1
Domino's Brooklyn Style, Hearty Marinara Sauce, no toppings						
1 lg slice	190	6.5	25	430	8	1
Domino's Brooklyn Style, New Pizza Sauce, no toppings						
1 lg slice	190	6.5	26	415	8	1
Domino's Buffalo Chicken with Blue Cheese Sandwich						
1 sandwich						
	841	41	74	2660	44	3
Domino's Cheesy Bread						
1 piece	930	52	92	1170	28	3

RESTAURANT/ FOOD ITEM	SERVING SIZE	CALORIES	FAT	CARBS	SODIUM	PROTEIN	FIBER
Domino's Chicken Alfredo Pasta in a Bread Bowl							
	½ bowl	701	25	93	1070	26	3
Domino's Chicken Bacon Ranch Sandwich							
	1 sandwich						
		889	45	72	2210	49	2
Domino's Chicken Carbonara Pasta in a Bread Bowl							
	½ bowl	740	28	94	1140	28	3
Domino's Chicken Parm Sandwich							
	1 sandwich						
		766	30	73	2130	51	3
Domino's Chocolate Lava Crunch Cake							
	1 cake	700	34	94	340	8	2
Domino's Cinna Stix							
	1 piece	940	49	109	690	16	4
Domino's Crunchy Thin, Alfredo Sauce, no toppings							
	¼ sm pizza						
		200	12.5	17	285	7	1
Domino's Crunchy Thin, BBQ Sauce, no toppings							
	¼ sm pizza						
		185	9	20	280	7	1
Domino's Crunchy Thin, Cheddar Sauce, no toppings							
	¼ sm pizza						
		185	10	18	305	8	1
Domino's Crunchy Thin, Garlic Parm Sauce, no toppings							
	¼ sm pizza						
		200	12.5	17	285	7	1
Domino's Crunchy Thin, Hearty Marinara Sauce, no toppings							
	¼ sm pizza						
		180	9	18	320	7	1
Domino's Crunchy Thin, New Pizza Sauce, no toppings							
	¼ sm pizza						
		180	9	19	305	7	1
Domino's Deep Dish, Alfredo Sauce, no toppings							
	1 med slice						
		240	11	26	500	8	3
Domino's Deep Dish, BBQ Sauce, no toppings							
	1 med slice						
		235	9.5	29	510	8	3
Domino's Deep Dish, Cheddar Sauce, no toppings							
	1 med slice						
		235	10.5	27	535	9	3
Domino's Deep Dish, Garlic Parm Sauce, no toppings							
	1 med slice						
		250	13	26	515	8	3
Domino's Deep Dish, Hearty Marinara Sauce, no toppings							
	1 med slice						
		230	9.5	27	550	8	3
Domino's Deep Dish, New Pizza Sauce, no toppings							
	1 med slice						
		230	9.5	28	535	8	3
Domino's Hand Tossed Crust, Alfredo Sauce, no toppings							
	1 sm slice	200	7.5	23	375	8	1

RESTAURANT/ FOOD ITEM SERVING SIZE	CALORIES	FAT	CARBS	SODIUM	PROTEIN	FIBER
Domino's Hand Tossed Crust, BBQ Sauce, no toppings						
1 sm slice	195	6	26	385	8	1
Domino's Hand Tossed Crust, Cheddar Sauce, no toppings						
1 sm slice	195	7	24	410	9	1
Domino's Hand Tossed Crust, Garlic Parm Sauce, no toppings						
1 sm slice	210	9.5	23	390	8	1
Domino's Hand Tossed Crust, Hearty Marinara Sauce, no toppings						
1 sm slice	190	6	24	425	8	1
Domino's Hand Tossed Crust, New Pizza Sauce, no toppings						
1 sm slice	190	6	25	410	8	1
Domino's Italian Sandwich						
1 sandwich	877	45	71	2560	47	3
Domino's Italian Sausage & Peppers Sandwich						
1 sandwich	879	47	71	2110	43	4
Domino's Italian Sausage Marinara Pasta in a Bread Bowl						
½ bowl	726	26	97	1410	26	4
Domino's Mac-N-Cheese in a Bread Bowl						
½ bowl	740	28	95	1420	27	3
Domino's Mediterranean Veggie Sandwich						
1 sandwich	668	28	71	1990	33	4
Domino's Pasta Primavera in a Bread Bowl						
½ bowl	672	24	94	910	20	4
Domino's Philly Cheese Steak Sandwich						
1 sandwich	695	27	72	2080	41	3
Domino's Sweet & Spicy Chicken Habanero Sandwich						
1 sandwich	817	33	82	2130	48	3
Dunkin' Donuts Apple 'n Spice Donut						
1 donut	240	11	32	320	3	1
Dunkin' Donuts Apple Cheese Danish						
1 danish	330	16	41	270	4	1
Dunkin' Donuts Apple Crumb Donut						
1 donut	460	14	80	330	4	2
Dunkin' Donuts Apple Fritter						
1 fritter	400	15	63	530	5	2
Dunkin' Donuts Bacon, Egg & Cheese on Bagel						
1 sandwich	530	18	76	1370	26	3
Dunkin' Donuts Bacon, Egg & Cheese on Biscuit						
1 sandwich	470	29	36	1200	16	1
Dunkin' Donuts Bacon, Egg & Cheese on Croissant						
1 sandwich	510	31	39	930	18	1
Dunkin' Donuts Bacon, Egg & Cheese on English Muffin						
1 sandwich	360	16	35	920	18	2

RESTAURANT/ FOOD ITEM SERVING SIZE	CALORIES	FAT	CARBS	SODIUM	PROTEIN	FIBER
Dunkin' Donuts Bavarian Kreme Donut						
1 donut	250	12	31	330	3	1
Dunkin' Donuts Biscuit						
1 biscuit	280	14	32	620	5	1
Dunkin' Donuts Blueberry Bagel						
1 bagel	370	4	73	710	13	5
Dunkin' Donuts Blueberry Cake Donut						
1 donut	330	18	38	460	3	1
Dunkin' Donuts Blueberry Crumb Donut						
1 donut	470	14	84	330	4	2
Dunkin' Donuts Blueberry Muffin						
1 muffin	510	16	87	490	6	3
Dunkin' Donuts Boston Kreme Donut						
1 donut	280	12	38	350	3	1
Dunkin' Donuts Bow Tie Donut						
1 donut	310	15	39	400	4	1
Dunkin' Donuts Broccoli Cheddar Soup						
8 oz	190	11	14	990	10	2
Dunkin' Donuts Brownie						
1 brownie	430	23	56	260	3	1
Dunkin' Donuts Caesar Salad						
7.3 oz	320	29	11	790	6	3
Dunkin' Donuts Cheese Danish						
1 danish	330	17	39	270	5	1
Dunkin' Donuts Chicken Bruschetta Sandwich						
1 sandwich						
	580	26	49	1200	37	2
Dunkin' Donuts Chicken Caesar Salad						
10.4 oz	440	33	11	1020	25	3
Dunkin' Donuts Chicken Noodle Soup						
8 oz	130	3	19	970	7	1
Dunkin' Donuts Chicken Parmesan Flatbread						
1 sandwich						
	500	24	49	1270	24	3
Dunkin' Donuts Chipotle Chicken Sandwich						
1 sandwich						
	600	25	50	1380	43	3
Dunkin' Donuts Chocolate Chip Muffin						
1 muffin	630	23	98	520	8	5
Dunkin' Donuts Chocolate Chunk Cookie						
1 cookie	540	23	80	550	7	3
Dunkin' Donuts Chocolate Coconut Cake Donut						
1 donut	340	18	42	400	3	2
Dunkin' Donuts Chocolate Frosted Cake Donut						
1 donut	340	19	38	330	3	1
Dunkin' Donuts Chocolate Frosted Coffee Roll						
1 roll	380	19	50	530	5	2
Dunkin' Donuts Chocolate Frosted Donut						
1 donut	230	10	32	330	3	1

RESTAURANT/ FOOD ITEM SERVING SIZE	CALORIES	FAT	CARBS	SODIUM	PROTEIN	FIBER
Dunkin' Donuts Chocolate Glazed Cake Donut						
1 donut	280	15	33	400	3	1
Dunkin' Donuts Chocolate Iced Bismark						
1 bismark	350	14	53	460	4	1
Dunkin' Donuts Chocolate Kreme Filled Donut						
1 donut	310	16	37	340	4	1
Dunkin' Donuts Cinnamon Cake Donut						
1 donut	290	18	30	310	3	1
Dunkin' Donuts Cinnamon Cake Munchkin						
1 Munchkin						
	60	3	6	60	1	0
Dunkin' Donuts Cinnamon Cake Stick						
1 stick	310	20	30	300	3	1
Dunkin' Donuts Cinnamon Raisin Bagel						
1 bagel	370	4	72	530	13	3
Dunkin' Donuts Coffee						
Extra large/24 oz						
	15	0	2	15	1	0
Dunkin' Donuts Coffee						
Large/20 oz						
	10	0	2	15	1	0
Dunkin' Donuts Coffee						
Medium/14 oz						
	10	0	1	10	1	0
Dunkin' Donuts Coffee						
Small/10 oz						
	5	0	1	5	0	0
Dunkin' Donuts Coffee Cake Muffin						
1 muffin	660	26	98	530	7	2
Dunkin' Donuts Coffee Coolatta with Cream						
24 oz	490	35	73	95	5	0
Dunkin' Donuts Coffee Coolatta with Cream						
32 oz	650	46	97	125	6	0
Dunkin' Donuts Coffee Coolatta with Milk						
16 oz	170	4	50	75	4	0
Dunkin' Donuts Coffee Coolatta with Milk						
24 oz	250	6	75	115	6	0
Dunkin' Donuts Coffee Coolatta with Milk						
32 oz	330	8	101	150	8	0
Dunkin' Donuts Coffee Coolatta with Skim Milk						
16 oz	140	0	51	75	4	0
Dunkin' Donuts Coffee Coolatta with Skim Milk						
24 oz	210	0	76	115	7	0
Dunkin' Donuts Coffee Coolatta with Skim Milk						
32 oz	270	0	102	150	9	0
Dunkin' Donuts Coffee Roll						
1 roll	370	18	49	510	5	2
Dunkin' Donuts Coffee with Cream						
Small/10 oz						
	60	6	2	20	1	0

RESTAURANT/ FOOD ITEM	SERVING SIZE	CALORIES	FAT	CARBS	SODIUM	PROTEIN	FIBER
Dunkin' Donuts Coffee with Cream and Sugar							
	Small/10 oz	120	6	19	20	1	0
Dunkin' Donuts Coffee with Milk							
	Small/10 oz	25	1	2	20	1	0
Dunkin' Donuts Coffee with Milk and Sugar							
	Small/10 oz	80	1	20	20	1	0
Dunkin' Donuts Coffee with Skim Milk							
	Small/10 oz	15	0	3	25	2	0
Dunkin' Donuts Coffee with Skim Milk and Splenda							
	Large/20 oz	45	0	8	45	3	0
Dunkin' Donuts Coffee with Skim Milk and Splenda							
	Medium/14 oz	30	0	6	35	2	0
Dunkin' Donuts Coffee with Skim Milk and Splenda							
	Small/10 oz	25	0	5	25	2	0
Dunkin' Donuts Coffee with Skim Milk and Sugar							
	Small/10 oz	70	0	20	25	2	0
Dunkin' Donuts Coffee with Splenda							
	Large/20 oz	25	0	5	15	1	0
Dunkin' Donuts Coffee with Splenda							
	Medium/14 oz	15	0	3	10	1	0
Dunkin' Donuts Coffee with Splenda							
	Small/10 oz	15	0	3	5	0	0
Dunkin' Donuts Coffee with Sugar							
	Small/10 oz	60	0	18	5	0	0
Dunkin' Donuts Corn Muffin							
	1 muffin	510	17	84	860	6	2
Dunkin' Donuts Double Chocolate Cake Donut							
	1 donut	290	16	34	410	3	1
Dunkin' Donuts Eclair							
	1 eclair	350	14	53	460	4	1
Dunkin' Donuts Egg & Cheese on Bagel							
	1 sandwich	480	15	75	1180	22	3
Dunkin' Donuts Egg & Cheese on Biscuit							
	1 sandwich	430	26	36	1010	13	1
Dunkin' Donuts Egg & Cheese on Croissant							
	1 sandwich	470	28	39	750	15	1

RESTAURANT/ FOOD ITEM SERVING SIZE	CALORIES	FAT	CARBS	SODIUM	PROTEIN	FIBER
Dunkin' Donuts Egg & Cheese on English Muffin						
1 sandwich						
	320	13	34	730	14	2
Dunkin' Donuts Egg White Turkey Sausage Flatbread						
1 sandwich						
	280	6	37	820	19	3
Dunkin' Donuts Egg White Veggie Flatbread						
1 sandwich						
	290	9	39	680	11	3
Dunkin' Donuts English Muffin						
1 muffin	160	1.5	31	340	6	2
Dunkin' Donuts Everything Bagel						
1 bagel	360	5	74	780	15	3
Dunkin' Donuts French Cruller						
1 donut	250	20	18	105	2	0
Dunkin' Donuts Garden Salad						
12.3 oz	180	6	21	500	8	4
Dunkin' Donuts Garlic Bagel						
1 bagel	350	3.5	76	780	15	4
Dunkin' Donuts Glazed Cake Donut						
1 donut	320	18	37	310	3	1
Dunkin' Donuts Glazed Cake Munchkin						
1 Munchkin						
	60	3	8	65	1	0
Dunkin' Donuts Glazed Cake Stick						
1 stick	340	20	38	300	3	1
Dunkin' Donuts Glazed Chocolate Cake Munchkin						
1 Munchkin						
	60	3	8	90	1	0
Dunkin' Donuts Glazed Chocolate Cake Stick						
1 stick	390	25	40	540	3	2
Dunkin' Donuts Glazed Donut						
1 donut	220	9	31	320	3	1
Dunkin' Donuts Glazed Fritter						
1 fritter	400	15	63	530	5	2
Dunkin' Donuts Glazed Munchkin						
1 Munchkin						
	50	2.5	7	65	1	0
Dunkin' Donuts Grape Coolatta						
Large/32 oz						
	500	0	121	115	0	0
Dunkin' Donuts Grape Coolatta						
Medium/24 oz						
	370	0	88	85	0	0
Dunkin' Donuts Grape Coolatta						
Small/16 oz						
	240	0	59	55	0	0
Dunkin' Donuts Grilled Cheese Flatbread						
1 sandwich						
	370	18	33	830	17	1

RESTAURANT/ FOOD ITEM SERVING SIZE	CALORIES	FAT	CARBS	SODIUM	PROTEIN	FIBER
Dunkin' Donuts Ham & Swiss Flatbread						
1 sandwich	340	12	36	1030	21	1
Dunkin' Donuts Ham, Egg & Cheese on Bagel						
1 sandwich	520	17	75	1480	28	3
Dunkin' Donuts Ham, Egg & Cheese on Biscuit						
1 sandwich	470	28	36	1320	19	1
Dunkin' Donuts Ham, Egg & Cheese on Croissant						
1 sandwich	510	30	39	1050	21	1
Dunkin' Donuts Ham, Egg & Cheese on English Muffin						
1 sandwich	350	15	35	1040	21	2
Dunkin' Donuts Hash Browns						
9 pieces	200	11	22	730	2	3
Dunkin' Donuts Honey Bran Raisin Muffin						
1 muffin	500	14	86	450	7	9
Dunkin' Donuts Iced Caramel Swirl Latte						
Small/16 oz	220	6	35	150	8	0
Dunkin' Donuts Iced Caramel Swirl Latte with Skim Milk						
Small/16 oz	180	0	36	150	9	0
Dunkin' Donuts Iced Coffee						
Large/32 oz	20	0	3	15	1	0
Dunkin' Donuts Iced Coffee						
Medium/24 oz	15	0	2	10	1	0
Dunkin' Donuts Iced Coffee						
Small/16 oz	10	0	2	5	1	0
Dunkin' Donuts Iced Coffee with Cream						
Small/16 oz	70	6	3	20	1	0
Dunkin' Donuts Iced Coffee with Cream and Sugar						
Small/16 oz	120	6	20	20	1	0
Dunkin' Donuts Iced Coffee with Milk						
Small/16 oz	30	1	3	20	2	0
Dunkin' Donuts Iced Coffee with Milk and Sugar						
Small/16 oz	90	1	21	20	2	0
Dunkin' Donuts Iced Coffee with Skim Milk						
Small/16 oz	20	0	3	25	2	0

RESTAURANT/ FOOD ITEM / SERVING SIZE	CALORIES	FAT	CARBS	SODIUM	PROTEIN	FIBER
Dunkin' Donuts Iced Coffee with Skim Milk and Splenda Large/32 oz	60	0	10	45	3	0
Dunkin' Donuts Iced Coffee with Skim Milk and Splenda Small/16 oz	30	0	5	25	2	0
Dunkin' Donuts Iced Coffee with Skim Milk and Sugar Small/16 oz	80	0	21	25	2	0
Dunkin' Donuts Iced Coffee with Sugar Small/16 oz	70	0	19	5	1	0
Dunkin' Donuts Iced Latte Small/16 oz	120	6	10	105	6	0
Dunkin' Donuts Iced Latte Lite Large/32 oz	160	0	25	220	14	0
Dunkin' Donuts Iced Latte Lite Medium/24 oz	120	0	19	170	10	0
Dunkin' Donuts Iced Latte Lite Small/16 oz	80	0	13	110	7	0
Dunkin' Donuts Iced Latte with Skim Milk Small/16 oz	70	0	11	110	7	0
Dunkin' Donuts Iced Latte with Skim Milk and Sugar Small/16 oz	130	0	28	110	7	0
Dunkin' Donuts Iced Latte with Sugar Small/16 oz	170	6	27	100	6	0
Dunkin' Donuts Iced Mocha Raspberry Latte Large/32 oz	450	12	73	220	13	2
Dunkin' Donuts Iced Mocha Raspberry Latte Medium/24 oz	340	9	54	160	10	2
Dunkin' Donuts Iced Mocha Raspberry Latte Small/16 oz	230	6	36	110	7	1
Dunkin' Donuts Iced Mocha Swirl Latte Small/16 oz	220	6	35	115	7	1
Dunkin' Donuts Iced Mocha Swirl Latte with Skim Milk Small/16 oz	180	0	36	125	8	1
Dunkin' Donuts Iced Vanilla Latte Lite 16 oz	90	0	14	110	7	0

RESTAURANT/ FOOD ITEM SERVING SIZE	CALORIES	FAT	CARBS	SODIUM	PROTEIN	FIBER
Dunkin' Donuts Jelly Filled Donut						
1 donut	260	11	36	330	3	1
Dunkin' Donuts Jelly Filled Munchkin						
1 Munchkin						
	60	2.5	8	65	1	0
Dunkin' Donuts Jelly Stick						
1 stick	400	20	54	320	3	1
Dunkin' Donuts Low Fat Apple Caramel Muffin						
1 muffin	430	3	94	520	8	3
Dunkin' Donuts Maple Frosted Coffee Roll						
1 roll	380	18	50	520	5	2
Dunkin' Donuts Maple Frosted Donut						
1 donut	230	10	33	330	3	1
Dunkin' Donuts Multigrain Bagel						
1 bagel	400	9	65	600	18	10
Dunkin' Donuts Oatmeal Raisin Cookie						
1 cookie	480	14	83	310	8	5
Dunkin' Donuts Old Fashioned Cake Donut						
1 donut	280	18	27	310	3	1
Dunkin' Donuts Onion Bagel						
1 bagel	340	3.5	65	660	12	3
Dunkin' Donuts Pastrami Supreme Sandwich						
1 sandwich						
	750	39	51	2060	48	3
Dunkin' Donuts Plain Bagel						
1 bagel	330	3	71	780	14	3
Dunkin' Donuts Plain Cake Munchkin						
1 Munchkin						
	50	3	5	60	1	0
Dunkin' Donuts Plain Cake Stick						
1 stick	300	20	26	300	3	1
Dunkin' Donuts Plain Cream Cheese						
50 g	150	15	3	250	3	0
Dunkin' Donuts Plain Croissant						
1 croissant						
	310	16	35	350	7	1
Dunkin' Donuts Poppy Seed Bagel						
1 bagel	370	6	73	780	15	3
Dunkin' Donuts Powdered Cake Donut						
1 donut	300	18	30	310	3	1
Dunkin' Donuts Powdered Cake Munchkin						
1 Munchkin						
	60	3.5	6	60	1	0
Dunkin' Donuts Powdered Cake Stick						
1 stick	320	20	31	300	3	1
Dunkin' Donuts Pressed Cuban Sandwich						
1 sandwich						
	680	33	50	2000	46	2
Dunkin' Donuts Pumpkin Coffee						
Extra large/24 oz						
	270	0	63	120	5	0

RESTAURANT/ FOOD ITEM SERVING SIZE	CALORIES	FAT	CARBS	SODIUM	PROTEIN	FIBER
Dunkin' Donuts Pumpkin Coffee Large/20 oz	220	0	51	100	4	0
Dunkin' Donuts Pumpkin Coffee Medium/14 oz	170	0	38	75	3	0
Dunkin' Donuts Pumpkin Coffee Small/10 oz	110	0	25	50	2	0
Dunkin' Donuts Pumpkin Coffee with Cream Extra large/24 oz	420	15	66	150	7	0
Dunkin' Donuts Pumpkin Coffee with Cream Large/20 oz	340	12	53	120	6	0
Dunkin' Donuts Pumpkin Coffee with Cream Medium/14 oz	250	9	40	90	4	0
Dunkin' Donuts Pumpkin Coffee with Cream Small/10 oz	170	6	26	60	3	0
Dunkin' Donuts Pumpkin Donut 1 donut	300	16	35	240	3	1
Dunkin' Donuts Pumpkin Muffin 1 muffin	630	28	88	510	8	3
Dunkin' Donuts Reduced Fat Blueberry Cream Cheese 50 g	150	9	15	210	2	0
Dunkin' Donuts Reduced Fat Blueberry Muffin 1 muffin	450	10	86	670	6	3
Dunkin' Donuts Reduced Fat Cream Cheese 50 g	100	8	5	250	4	0
Dunkin' Donuts Reduced Fat Onion & Chive Cream Cheese 50 g	130	11	6	250	3	0
Dunkin' Donuts Reduced Fat Smoked Salmon Cream Cheese 50 g	140	11	6	260	4	0
Dunkin' Donuts Reduced Fat Strawberry Cream Cheese 50 g	150	10	15	200	2	0
Dunkin' Donuts Reduced Fat Veggie Cream Cheese 50 g	120	10	6	240	2	0
Dunkin' Donuts Salt Bagel 1 bagel	330	3	71	3540	14	3
Dunkin' Donuts Sausage Biscuit 1 sandwich	450	28	33	1020	12	1
Dunkin' Donuts Sausage, Egg & Cheese on Bagel 1 sandwich	660	29	76	1590	30	3
Dunkin' Donuts Sausage, Egg & Cheese on Biscuit 1 sandwich	600	40	37	1410	20	1

RESTAURANT/ FOOD ITEM SERVING SIZE	CALORIES	FAT	CARBS	SODIUM	PROTEIN	FIBER
Dunkin' Donuts Sausage, Egg & Cheese on Croissant						
1 sandwich	640	42	40	1150	22	1
Dunkin' Donuts Sausage, Egg & Cheese on English Muffin						
1 sandwich	490	28	35	1130	22	2
Dunkin' Donuts Sesame Bagel						
1 bagel	370	7	72	780	16	3
Dunkin' Donuts Spiced Apple Twist						
1 twist	210	10	28	230	3	1
Dunkin' Donuts Steak and Cheese Sandwich						
1 sandwich	470	16	50	2040	31	2
Dunkin' Donuts Strawberry Cheese Danish						
1 danish	320	16	40	260	4	1
Dunkin' Donuts Strawberry Frosted Donut						
1 donut	230	10	33	330	3	1
Dunkin' Donuts Strawberry Fruit Coolatta						
Large/32 oz	590	0	145	80	1	0
Dunkin' Donuts Strawberry Fruit Coolatta						
Medium/24 oz	440	0	108	60	1	0
Dunkin' Donuts Strawberry Fruit Coolatta						
Small/16 oz	300	0	72	40	0	0
Dunkin' Donuts Sugar Raised Donut						
1 donut	190	9	22	320	3	1
Dunkin' Donuts Sugar Raised Munchkin						
1 Munchkin	40	2.5	5	65	1	0
Dunkin' Donuts Toasted Italian Sandwich						
1 sandwich	560	25	52	2630	33	3
Dunkin' Donuts Toffee for Your Coffee Donut						
1 donut	400	24	42	330	4	1
Dunkin' Donuts Tropicana Orange Coolatta						
Large/32 oz	430	0	105	75	2	0
Dunkin' Donuts Tropicana Orange Coolatta						
Medium/24 oz	330	0	79	55	2	0
Dunkin' Donuts Tropicana Orange Coolatta						
Small/16 oz	220	0	52	35	1	0
Dunkin' Donuts Tuna (Albacore) Sandwich						
1 sandwich	660	19	56	1280	31	3
Dunkin' Donuts Tuna Melt Sandwich						
1 sandwich	770	30	57	1560	36	3

RESTAURANT/ FOOD ITEM SERVING SIZE	CALORIES	FAT	CARBS	SODIUM	PROTEIN	FIBER
Dunkin' Donuts Turkey and Bacon Club Sandwich						
1 sandwich	440	13	51	1800	35	3
Dunkin' Donuts Turkey and Cheese Sandwich						
1 sandwich	450	13	52	1500	35	3
Dunkin' Donuts Turkey, Cheddar & Bacon Flatbread						
1 sandwich	390	19	34	1090	21	1
Dunkin' Donuts Vanilla Bean Coolatta						
Large/32 oz	860	11	181	340	6	0
Dunkin' Donuts Vanilla Bean Coolatta						
Medium/24 oz	650	9	136	260	4	0
Dunkin' Donuts Vanilla Bean Coolatta						
Small/16 oz	430	6	90	170	3	0
Dunkin' Donuts Vanilla Frosted Coffee Roll						
1 roll	380	18	50	520	5	2
Dunkin' Donuts Vanilla Kreme Filled Donut						
1 donut	320	17	37	340	3	1
Dunkin' Donuts WakeUp Wrap						
1 wrap	170	10	14	450	7	1
Dunkin' Donuts WakeUp Wrap with Bacon						
1 wrap	190	12	14	540	9	1
Dunkin' Donuts Watermelon Coolatta						
Large/32 oz	500	0	121	110	0	0
Dunkin' Donuts Watermelon Coolatta						
Medium/24 oz	370	0	91	85	0	0
Dunkin' Donuts Watermelon Coolatta						
Small/16 oz	250	0	60	55	0	0
Dunkin' Donuts Wheat Bagel						
1 bagel	350	4	66	650	13	5
KFC Apple Turnover						
1 turnover	260	13	35	170	2	1
KFC BBQ Baked Beans						
130 g	200	1.5	39	680	8	9
KFC Biscuit						
54 g	180	8	23	530	4	1
KFC Boneless Fiery Buffalo Wings						
1 wing	80	3.5	6	390	5	1
KFC Boneless HBBQ Wings						
1 wing	80	3.5	7	340	5	1
KFC Brownie Bites						
1 pack	280	16	31	180	3	1
KFC Caesar Side Salad without Dressing & Croutons						
76 g	35	2	2	90	3	1

RESTAURANT/ FOOD ITEM	SERVING SIZE	CALORIES	FAT	CARBS	SODIUM	PROTEIN	FIBER
KFC Café Valley Bakery Chocolate Chip Cake							
	1 slice	280	9	47	160	3	1
KFC Chicken Little							
	1 serving	190	10	20	390	6	1
KFC Chicken Pot Pie							
	369 g	690	40	57	1760	27	3
KFC Cole Slaw							
	130 g	180	10	22	270	1	3
KFC Cookie Dough Pie Slice							
	68 g	240	12	31	190	3	1
KFC Cornbread Muffin							
	52 g	210	9	28	240	3	1
KFC Corn on the Cob							
	3 inches	70	0.5	16	0	2	2
KFC Corn on the Cob							
	5.5 inches	140	1	33	5	5	4
KFC Country Fried Steak with Peppered White Gravy							
	155 g	390	26	23	1200	16	2
KFC Country Fried Steak without Peppered White Gravy							
	111 g	360	24	19	1040	16	2
KFC Creamy Parmesan Caesar Dressing							
	1 package	260	26	4	540	2	0
KFC Creamy Ranch Dipping Sauce							
	25 g	140	15	1	230	0	0
KFC Crispy Chicken BLT Salad without Dressing							
	315 g	340	19	14	840	30	3
KFC Crispy Chicken Caesar Salad without Dressing & Croutons							
	262 g	320	19	12	660	28	3
KFC Crispy Strips							
	2 strips	250	15	8	480	22	1
KFC Crispy Strips							
	3 strips	380	22	12	720	33	1
KFC Crispy Twister with Crispy Strip							
	238 g	580	30	49	1250	28	3
KFC Crispy Twister with Crispy Strip without Sauce							
	216 g	480	20	48	1100	28	2
KFC Crispy Twister with Original Recipe Strip							
	235 g	540	26	48	1430	28	4
KFC Crispy Twister with Original Recipe Strip without Sauce							
	212 g	440	15	47	1280	28	3
KFC Double Crunch Sandwich with Crispy Strip							
	214 g	510	27	36	840	27	1
KFC Double Crunch Sandwich with Crispy Strip without Sauce							
	191 g	410	16	34	690	27	1
KFC Double Crunch Sandwich with Original Recipe Strip							
	211 g	470	23	35	1020	27	2
KFC Double Crunch Sandwich with Original Recipe Strip without Sauce							
	187 g	360	12	33	870	27	2
KFC Dutch Apple Pie Slice							
	108 g	320	14	47	300	2	1

RESTAURANT/ FOOD ITEM SERVING SIZE	CALORIES	FAT	CARBS	SODIUM	PROTEIN	FIBER
KFC EC Chicken Breast						
181 g	490	31	17	1080	38	0
KFC EC Chicken Drumstick						
58 g	150	9	6	360	11	0
KFC EC Chicken Thigh						
113 g	370	27	12	840	18	0
KFC EC Chicken Whole Wing						
48 g	150	10	6	320	11	1
KFC EC Drumstick Value Box						
171 g	440	23	42	1180	15	3
KFC EC Thigh Value Box						
226 g	660	42	49	1670	22	3
KFC Famous Bowls—Mashed Potato with Gravy						
525 g	700	32	77	2260	26	6
KFC Famous Bowls—Rice and Gravy						
505 g	790	28	106	2690	29	5
KFC Fiery Buffalo Dipping Sauce						
25 g	25	0	6	530	0	0
KFC Fiery Buffalo Hot Wings						
1 wing	80	5	5	280	4	1
KFC Fiery Buffalo Hot Wings Value Box						
190 g	500	27	46	1580	16	4
KFC Fiery Buffalo Wings						
1 wing	80	5	4	230	4	1
KFC Garlic Parmesan Dipping Sauce						
25 g	130	13	2	220	0	0
KFC Gizzards						
55 g	200	11	15	800	11	1
KFC Green Beans						
98 g	25	0	5	380	1	2
KFC Grilled Chicken Breast						
119 g	180	4	0	440	35	0
KFC Grilled Chicken Drumstick						
39 g	70	4	0	200	10	0
KFC Grilled Chicken Thigh						
65 g	140	9	0	320	15	0
KFC Grilled Chicken Whole Wing						
33 g	80	4	0	160	10	0
KFC Grilled Drumstick Value Box						
152 g	360	18	37	1040	14	3
KFC Grilled Thigh Value Box						
178 g	430	23	37	1140	19	3
KFC HBBQ Dipping Sauce						
25 g	40	0	9	310	0	0
KFC HBBQ Hot Wings						
1 wing	90	5	7	260	4	0
KFC HBBQ Hot Wings Value Box						
195 g	520	27	53	1530	16	4
KFC HBBQ Wings						
1 wing	80	5	5	170	4	1

RESTAURANT/ FOOD ITEM	SERVING SIZE	CALORIES	FAT	CARBS	SODIUM	PROTEIN	FIBER
KFC Heinz Buttermilk Ranch Dressing							
	28 g	160	17	1	220	0	0
KFC Hidden Valley The Original Ranch Fat Free Dressing							
	1 package	35	0	8	410	1	0
KFC Honey BBQ Sandwich							
	162 g	310	4	42	810	23	1
KFC Honey Mustard Dipping Sauce							
	25 g	120	10	6	110	0	0
KFC Hot & Spicy Breast							
	179 g	470	28	15	1310	38	4
KFC Hot & Spicy Drumstick							
	60 g	160	10	5	400	12	1
KFC Hot & Spicy Thigh							
	128 g	380	28	11	810	22	2
KFC Hot & Spicy Whole Wing							
	55 g	160	8	10	460	12	1
KFC Hot Wings							
	1 wing	70	5	3	150	4	0
KFC Hot Wings Value Box							
	169 g	470	27	41	1190	16	4
KFC House Side Salad without Dressing							
	87 g	15	0	2	10	1	1
KFC Jalapeno Peppers							
	32 g	20	1.5	1	480	0	1
KFC Kentucky Nuggets							
	1 nugget	45	3	2	135	3	0
KFC Lemon Meringue Pie Slice							
	81 g	250	7	42	210	4	0
KFC Lil' Bucket Chocolate Crème Parfait Cup							
	113 g	280	14	37	220	2	1
KFC Lil' Bucket Lemon Crème Parfait Cup							
	127 g	390	14	60	220	7	0
KFC Lil' Bucket Strawberry Shortcake Parfait Cup							
	99 g	230	8	39	220	2	1
KFC Livers							
	55 g	180	10	11	620	11	0
KFC Macaroni and Cheese							
	137 g	180	9	20	880	6	2
KFC Macaroni Salad							
	107 g	180	9	20	400	3	1
KFC Marzetti Light Italian Dressing							
	28 g	10	0.5	2	510	0	0
KFC Mashed Potatoes with Gravy							
	153 g	130	4.5	20	550	2	1
KFC Mashed Potatoes without Gravy							
	109 g	100	3	16	350	2	1
KFC Mean Greens							
	128 g	30	0	4	400	3	2
KFC Mini Melt							
	108 g	250	7	31	690	15	2

RESTAURANT/ FOOD ITEM SERVING SIZE	CALORIES	FAT	CARBS	SODIUM	PROTEIN	FIBER
KFC Original Recipe Chicken BLT Salad without Dressing						
311 g	300	15	13	1020	29	4
KFC Original Recipe Chicken Breast						
166 g	370	21	7	1050	38	0
KFC Original Recipe Chicken Caesar Salad without Dressing & Croutons						
258 g	280	14	11	840	28	4
KFC Original Recipe Chicken Drumstick						
50 g	110	7	2	290	10	0
KFC Original Recipe Chicken Thigh						
98 g	260	19	6	670	16	0
KFC Original Recipe Chicken Whole Wing						
42 g	110	7	3	310	9	0
KFC Original Recipe Chicken Breast without Skin or Breading						
108 g	140	2	1	510	29	0
KFC Original Recipe Drumstick Value Box						
163 g	400	21	38	1120	15	3
KFC Original Recipe Filet Sandwich						
215 g	480	23	38	1230	25	2
KFC Original Recipe Filet Sandwich without Sauce						
191 g	370	12	36	1080	25	2
KFC Original Recipe Strips						
2 strips	200	10	7	660	21	1
KFC Original Recipe Strips						
3 strips	310	15	11	990	32	2
KFC Original Recipe Thigh Value Box						
211 g	550	33	43	1500	20	3
KFC Parmesan Garlic Croutons Pouch						
1 pouch	70	3	8	140	2	1
KFC Pecan Pie						
1 slice	410	21	52	220	4	1
KFC Popcorn Chicken						
Kids	290	19	16	850	16	2
KFC Popcorn Chicken						
Large	550	35	30	1600	29	3
KFC Popcorn Chicken						
Individual	400	26	22	1160	21	3
KFC Popcorn Chicken Value Box						
218 g	660	38	55	1900	25	5
KFC Potato Salad						
128 g	200	10	24	540	2	3
KFC Potato Wedges						
102 g	260	13	33	740	4	3
KFC Red Beans with Sausage and Rice						
144 g	160	2.5	26	340	24	4
KFC Roasted Chicken BLT Salad without Dressing						
304 g	200	7	7	720	30	3
KFC Roasted Chicken Caesar Salad without Dressing & Croutons						
251 g	190	6	5	530	29	2
KFC Sara Lee Apple Pie						
1 slice	310	13	48	290	2	1

RESTAURANT/ FOOD ITEM	SERVING SIZE	CALORIES	FAT	CARBS	SODIUM	PROTEIN	FIBER
KFC Sara Lee Pecan Pie							
	1 slice	450	22	61	460	5	1
KFC Sara Lee Sweet Potato Pie							
	1 slice	340	16	46	330	5	0
KFC Seasoned Rice							
	99 g	140	0.5	31	560	3	1
KFC Snacker with Crispy Strip							
	115 g	300	14	28	470	15	2
KFC Snacker with Crispy Strip without Sauce							
	105 g	250	9	27	410	15	2
KFC Snacker with Crispy Strip, Buffalo							
	115 g	260	9	30	580	15	2
KFC Snacker with Crispy Strip, Ultimate Cheese							
	114 g	280	11	29	560	16	2
KFC Snacker with Original Recipe Strip							
	113 g	270	12	28	560	15	2
KFC Snacker with Original Recipe Strip without Sauce							
	103 g	230	7	27	500	15	2
KFC Snacker with Original Recipe Strip, Buffalo							
	113 g	240	7	29	670	15	2
KFC Snacker with Original Recipe Strip, Ultimate Cheese							
	113 g	260	9	29	650	15	2
KFC Snacker, Fish							
	116 g	320	14	31	640	16	2
KFC Snacker, Fish without Sauce							
	105 g	290	12	29	550	16	1
KFC Snacker, Honey BBQ							
	98 g	210	3	32	470	13	2
KFC Snack-Size Bowl							
	232 g	320	15	34	990	12	3
KFC Strawberry Cream Cheese Pie							
	1 slice	270	15	31	220	3	0
KFC Sweet and Sour Dipping Sauce							
	25 g	45	0	12	95	0	0
KFC Sweet Kernel Corn							
	102 g	110	0.5	23	0	4	2
KFC Sweet Life Chocolate Chip Cookie							
	35 g	170	8	23	90	2	1
KFC Sweet Life Oatmeal Raisin Cookie							
	35 g	150	6	23	130	2	1
KFC Sweet Life Sugar Cookie							
	35 g	160	7	22	125	2	0
KFC Teddy Grahams, Graham Snacks, Cinnamon							
	21 g	90	3	15	95	1	1
KFC Tender Roast Sandwich							
	228 g	400	15	29	810	34	1
KFC Tender Roast Sandwich without Sauce							
	204 g	300	4	28	660	34	0
KFC Tender Roast Twister							
	228 g	440	18	42	1120	29	2

RESTAURANT/ FOOD ITEM / SERVING SIZE	CALORIES	FAT	CARBS	SODIUM	PROTEIN	FIBER
KFC Tender Roast Twister without Sauce						
205 g	340	7	41	980	29	2
KFC Three Bean Salad						
87 g	70	0	14	170	3	3
KFC Toasted Wrap with Crispy Strip						
133 g	360	20	27	730	17	2
KFC Toasted Wrap with Crispy Strip without Sauce						
119 g	300	14	27	640	17	1
KFC Toasted Wrap with Original Recipe Strip						
131 g	340	18	27	820	17	2
KFC Toasted Wrap with Original Recipe Strip without Sauce						
117 g	270	11	26	730	17	2
KFC Toasted Wrap with Tender Roast Filet						
146 g	310	14	24	740	22	1
KFC Toasted Wrap with Tender Roast Filet without Sauce						
132 g	250	8	24	650	22	1
Krispy Kreme Apple Fritter						
101 g	380	20	47	220	4	2
Krispy Kreme Berries & Kreme Chiller						
12 oz	620	28	92	220	3	<1
Krispy Kreme Berries & Kreme Chiller						
20 oz	960	40	150	330	3	<1
Krispy Kreme Caramel Kreme Crunch						
98 g	380	19	49	170	4	<1
Krispy Kreme Chocolate Glazed Cruller						
69 g	290	15	37	240	2	<1
Krispy Kreme Chocolate Iced Cake						
71 g	280	14	36	320	3	<1
Krispy Kreme Chocolate Iced Custard Filled						
86 g	300	17	35	150	3	<1
Krispy Kreme Chocolate Iced Glazed						
66 g	250	12	33	100	3	<1
Krispy Kreme Chocolate Iced Kreme Filled						
86 g	350	20	39	140	3	<1
Krispy Kreme Chocolate Iced with Sprinkles						
71 g	270	12	38	100	3	<1
Krispy Kreme Chocolate, Chocolate Chiller						
12 oz	670	29	104	320	4	2
Krispy Kreme Chocolate, Chocolate Chiller						
20 oz	1050	42	170	490	6	4
Krispy Kreme Cinnamon Apple Filled						
81 g	290	16	32	150	3	<1
Krispy Kreme Cinnamon Bun						
67 g	260	16	28	125	3	<1
Krispy Kreme Cinnamon Twist						
59 g	240	15	23	130	3	<1
Krispy Kreme Dulce De Leche						
75 g	300	18	31	160	3	<1
Krispy Kreme Glazed Blueberry Doughnut Holes						
56 g (4 holes)						
	220	12	27	280	3	<1

RESTAURANT/ FOOD ITEM SERVING SIZE	CALORIES	FAT	CARBS	SODIUM	PROTEIN	FIBER
Krispy Kreme Glazed Cake Doughnut Holes						
56 g (4 holes)	210	10	29	240	2	<1
Krispy Kreme Glazed Chocolate Cake						
80 g	300	15	42	250	3	2
Krispy Kreme Glazed Chocolate Cake Doughnut Holes						
56 g (4 holes)	210	10	29	240	2	<1
Krispy Kreme Glazed Cinnamon						
54 g	210	12	24	100	2	<1
Krispy Kreme Glazed Cruller						
54 g	240	14	26	240	2	<1
Krispy Kreme Glazed Kreme Filled						
86 g	340	20	39	140	3	<1
Krispy Kreme Glazed Lemon Filled						
85 g	290	16	35	135	3	<1
Krispy Kreme Glazed Pumpkin Spice						
80 g	300	14	42	250	2	<1
Krispy Kreme Glazed Pumpkin Spice Doughnut Holes						
56 g (4 holes)	210	10	29	240	2	<1
Krispy Kreme Glazed Raspberry Filled						
85 g	300	16	36	125	3	<1
Krispy Kreme Glazed Sour Cream						
80 g	300	13	43	250	2	<1
Krispy Kreme Lemon Sherbert Chiller						
12 oz	630	28	95	220	3	<1
Krispy Kreme Lemon Sherbert Chiller						
20 oz	980	40	155	330	3	<1
Krispy Kreme Lotta Latte Chiller						
12 oz	670	28	49	380	4	<1
Krispy Kreme Lotta Latte Chiller						
20 oz	1050	40	79	580	5	<1
Krispy Kreme Maple Iced Glazed						
66 g	240	12	32	100	2	<1
Krispy Kreme Mocha Dream Chiller						
12 oz	670	28	105	320	3	1
Krispy Kreme Mocha Dream Chiller						
20 oz	1050	41	171	490	5	2
Krispy Kreme New York Cheesecake						
90 g	340	20	34	200	4	<1
Krispy Kreme Orange You Glad Chiller						
12 oz	180	0	43	10	0	0
Krispy Kreme Orange You Glad Chiller						
20 oz	300	0	71	10	0	0
Krispy Kreme Oranges & Kreme Chiller						
12 oz	630	28	92	220	3	<1
Krispy Kreme Oranges & Kreme Chiller						
20 oz	970	40	150	330	3	<1
Krispy Kreme Original Glazed						
52 g	200	12	22	95	2	<1

RESTAURANT/ FOOD ITEM SERVING SIZE	CALORIES	FAT	CARBS	SODIUM	PROTEIN	FIBER
Krispy Kreme Original Glazed Doughnut Holes						
54 g (4 holes)	200	11	25	90	2	<1
Krispy Kreme Powdered Cake						
71 g	290	14	37	320	3	<1
Krispy Kreme Powdered Strawberry Filled						
81 g	290	16	33	135	3	<1
Krispy Kreme Sugar						
49 g	200	12	21	95	2	0
Krispy Kreme Traditional Cake						
57 g	230	13	25	320	3	<1
Krispy Kreme Very Berry Chiller						
12 oz	170	0	43	10	0	0
Krispy Kreme Very Berry Chiller						
20 oz	290	0	71	10	0	0
McDonald's Angus Bacon & Cheese						
10.2 oz	790	39	63	2070	45	4
McDonald's Angus Deluxe						
11.1 oz	750	39	61	1700	40	4
McDonald's Angus Mushroom & Swiss						
10 oz	770	40	59	1170	44	4
McDonald's Apple Dippers						
1 package 35	0	0	8	0	0	0
McDonald's Bacon, Egg & Cheese Biscuit						
Regular	420	23	37	1160	15	2
McDonald's Bacon, Egg & Cheese Biscuit						
Large	480	27	43	1270	15	3
McDonald's Bacon, Egg & Cheese McGriddles						
3.2 oz	420	18	48	1110	15	2
McDonald's Baked Hot Apple Pie						
2.7 oz	250	13	32	170	2	4
McDonald's BBQ Sauce						
1 package 50	0	12	260	0	0	
McDonald's Big Breakfast						
Regular	740	48	51	1560	28	3
McDonald's Big Breakfast						
Large	800	52	56	1680	28	4
McDonald's Big Mac						
7.5 oz	540	29	45	1040	25	3
McDonald's Big N' Tasty						
7.2 oz	460	24	37	720	24	3
McDonald's Big N' Tasty with Cheese						
7.7 oz	510	28	38	960	27	3
McDonald's Biscuit						
Medium	260	12	33	740	5	2
McDonald's Biscuit						
Large	320	16	39	850	5	3
McDonald's Breakfast Egg McMuffin						
7.1 oz	300	12	30	820	18	2
McDonald's Butter Garlic Croutons						
0.5 oz	60	1.5	10	140	2	1

RESTAURANT/ FOOD ITEM	SERVING SIZE	CALORIES	FAT	CARBS	SODIUM	PROTEIN	FIBER
McDonald's Cappuccino with Sugar Free Vanilla Syrup with Whole Milk							
	12 oz	100	5	15	105	5	0
McDonald's Cappuccino with Sugar Free Vanilla Syrup with Whole Milk							
	16 oz	120	6	18	130	6	0
McDonald's Cappuccino with Sugar Free Vanilla Syrup with Whole Milk							
	20 oz	150	8	22	160	8	0
McDonald's Cappuccino with Whole Milk							
	12 oz	120	7	9	85	6	0
McDonald's Cappuccino with Whole Milk							
	16 oz	140	8	11	105	8	0
McDonald's Cappuccino with Whole Milk							
	20 oz	180	10	13	130	9	0
McDonald's Caramel Cappuccino with Whole Milk							
	12 oz	200	5	32	125	5	0
McDonald's Caramel Cappuccino with Whole Milk							
	16 oz	240	6	41	150	6	0
McDonald's Caramel Cappuccino with Whole Milk							
	20 oz	290	8	49	190	8	0
McDonald's Caramel Latte with Whole Milk							
	12 oz	230	7	35	140	7	0
McDonald's Caramel Latte with Whole Milk							
	16 oz	280	8	43	170	8	0
McDonald's Caramel Latte with Whole Milk							
	20 oz	330	9	52	210	9	0
McDonald's Cheeseburger							
	4 oz	300	12	33	750	15	2
McDonald's Chicken McNuggets							
	4 pieces	190	12	11	400	10	0
McDonald's Chicken McNuggets							
	6 pieces	280	17	16	600	14	0
McDonald's Chicken McNuggets							
	10 pieces	460	29	27	1000	24	0
McDonald's Chicken Selects Premium Breast Strips							
	3 pieces	400	24	23	1010	23	0
McDonald's Chicken Selects Premium Breast Strips							
	5 pieces	660	40	39	1680	38	0
McDonald's Chipotle BBQ Snack Wrap (Crispy)							
	4.2 oz	330	15	35	810	14	1
McDonald's Chipotle BBQ Snack Wrap (Grilled)							
	4.2 oz	260	9	28	830	18	1
McDonald's Chocolate Chip Cookie							
	1 cookie	160	8	21	90	2	1
McDonald's Chocolate Triple Thick Shake							
	12 oz	440	10	76	190	10	1
McDonald's Chocolate Triple Thick Shake							
	16 oz	580	14	102	250	13	1
McDonald's Chocolate Triple Thick Shake							
	21 oz	770	18	134	330	18	1
McDonald's Chocolate Triple Thick Shake							
	32 oz	1160	27	203	510	27	2

RESTAURANT/ FOOD ITEM	SERVING SIZE	CALORIES	FAT	CARBS	SODIUM	PROTEIN	FIBER
McDonald's Cinnamon Melts							
	4 oz	460	19	66	370	6	3
McDonald's Coffee							
	Small	0	0	0	0	0	0
McDonald's Coffee							
	Large	0	0	0	0	0	0
McDonald's Creamy Ranch Sauce							
	1.5 oz	200	22	2	320	0	0
McDonald's Deluxe Breakfast without Syrup & Margarine							
	Regular	1090	56	111	2150	36	6
McDonald's Deluxe Breakfast without Syrup & Margarine							
	Large	1150	60	116	2260	36	7
McDonald's Double Cheeseburger							
	5.8 oz	440	23	34	1150	25	2
McDonald's Double Quarter Pounder with Cheese							
	9.8 oz	740	42	40	1380	48	3
McDonald's Filet-O-Fish							
	5 oz	380	18	38	640	15	2
McDonald's Fruit 'n Yogurt Parfait							
	7 oz	160	2	31	85	4	1
McDonald's Fruit 'n Yogurt Parfait (without Granola)							
	7 oz	130	2	25	55	4	0
McDonald's Grape Jam							
	0.5 oz	35	0	9	0	0	0
McDonald's Hamburger							
	3.5 oz	250	9	31	520	12	2
McDonald's Hash Browns							
	2 oz	150	9	15	310	1	2
McDonald's Hazelnut Cappuccino with Whole Milk							
	12 oz	200	5	34	70	5	0
McDonald's Hazelnut Cappuccino with Whole Milk							
	16 oz	240	6	42	85	6	0
McDonald's Hazelnut Cappuccino with Whole Milk							
	20 oz	290	8	51	105	7	0
McDonald's Hazelnut Latte with Whole Milk							
	12 oz	230	7	36	90	7	0
McDonald's Hazelnut Latte with Whole Milk							
	16 oz	280	8	45	110	8	0
McDonald's Hazelnut Latte with Whole Milk							
	20 oz	330	9	53	130	9	0
McDonald's Honey							
	2 packages						
		50	0	12	0	0	0
McDonald's Honey Mustard Snack Wrap (Crispy)							
	4.2 oz	330	16	34	780	14	1
McDonald's Honey Mustard Snack Wrap (Grilled)							
	4.4 oz	260	9	27	800	18	1
McDonald's Hot Caramel Sundae							
	6.4 oz	340	8	60	160	7	1
McDonald's Hotcake Syrup							
	1 package	180	0	45	20	0	0

RESTAURANT/ FOOD ITEM / SERVING SIZE	CALORIES	FAT	CARBS	SODIUM	PROTEIN	FIBER
McDonald's Hotcakes and Sausage without Syrup & Margarine						
6.8 oz	520	24	61	930	15	3
McDonald's Hotcakes without Syrup & Margarine						
5.3 oz	350	9	60	590	8	3
McDonald's Hot Chocolate with Nonfat Milk						
12 oz	250	5	43	140	8	0
McDonald's Hot Chocolate with Nonfat Milk						
16 oz	310	6	55	190	11	0
McDonald's Hot Chocolate with Nonfat Milk						
20 oz	390	6	68	250	16	0
McDonald's Hot Chocolate with Whole Milk						
12 oz	300	12	41	135	8	0
McDonald's Hot Chocolate with Whole Milk						
16 oz	380	15	53	170	10	0
McDonald's Hot Chocolate with Whole Milk						
20 oz	460	18	63	220	13	0
McDonald's Hot Fudge Sundae						
6.3 oz	330	10	54	180	8	2
McDonald's Hot Mustard Sauce						
3 packages						
	60	2.5	9	250	1	2
McDonald's Iced Caramel Latte with Whole Milk						
12 oz	160	3	29	100	3	0
McDonald's Iced Caramel Latte with Whole Milk						
16 oz	180	4.5	31	120	4	0
McDonald's Iced Caramel Latte with Whole Milk						
20 oz	230	6	40	150	6	0
McDonald's Iced Coffee, Caramel						
Small	130	5	21	80	1	0
McDonald's Iced Coffee, Caramel						
Medium	190	8	27	115	2	0
McDonald's Iced Coffee, Caramel						
Large	270	11	41	160	2	0
McDonald's Iced Coffee, Hazelnut						
Small	130	5	21	40	1	0
McDonald's Iced Coffee, Hazelnut						
Medium	190	8	29	60	2	0
McDonald's Iced Coffee, Hazelnut						
Large	270	11	43	85	2	0
McDonald's Iced Coffee, Regular						
Small	140	5	22	40	1	0
McDonald's Iced Coffee, Regular						
Medium	200	8	30	60	2	0
McDonald's Iced Coffee, Regular						
Large	280	11	45	85	2	0
McDonald's Iced Coffee, Sugar Free Vanilla Syrup						
Small	60	5	8	70	1	0
McDonald's Iced Coffee, Sugar Free Vanilla Syrup						
Medium	90	8	11	100	2	0
McDonald's Iced Coffee, Sugar Free Vanilla Syrup						
Large	120	11	16	140	2	0

RESTAURANT/ FOOD ITEM SERVING SIZE	CALORIES	FAT	CARBS	SODIUM	PROTEIN	FIBER
McDonald's Iced Coffee, Vanilla						
Small	130	5	21	40	1	0
McDonald's Iced Coffee, Vanilla						
Medium	190	8	29	60	2	0
McDonald's Iced Coffee, Vanilla						
Large	270	11	43	80	2	0
McDonald's Iced Hazelnut Latte with Whole Milk						
12 oz	160	3	31	45	3	0
McDonald's Iced Hazelnut Latte with Whole Milk						
16 oz	180	4.5	33	65	4	0
McDonald's Iced Hazelnut Latte with Whole Milk						
20 oz	230	6	41	85	6	0
McDonald's Iced Latte with Sugar Free Vanilla Syrup with Whole Milk						
12 oz	60	3	12	80	3	0
McDonald's Iced Latte with Sugar Free Vanilla Syrup with Whole Milk						
16 oz	90	5	14	105	5	0
McDonald's Iced Latte with Sugar Free Vanilla Syrup with Whole Milk						
20 oz	110	6	19	130	6	0
McDonald's Iced Latte with Whole Milk						
12 oz	80	4.5	6	65	4	0
McDonald's Iced Latte with Whole Milk						
16 oz	100	6	8	80	6	0
McDonald's Iced Latte with Whole Milk						
20 oz	140	8	10	105	7	0
McDonald's Iced Mocha with Nonfat Milk						
12 oz	270	8	43	140	7	0
McDonald's Iced Mocha with Whole Milk						
12 oz	310	13	42	140	7	0
McDonald's Iced Nonfat Caramel Latte						
12 oz	140	0	30	105	3	0
McDonald's Iced Nonfat Caramel Latte						
16 oz	150	0	32	120	5	0
McDonald's Iced Nonfat Caramel Latte						
20 oz	190	0	40	150	6	0
McDonald's Iced Nonfat Hazelnut Latte						
12 oz	140	0	32	50	3	0
McDonald's Iced Nonfat Hazelnut Latte						
16 oz	150	0	33	70	5	0
McDonald's Iced Nonfat Hazelnut Latte						
20 oz	190	0	42	80	6	0
McDonald's Iced Nonfat Latte						
12 oz	50	0	7	70	5	0
McDonald's Iced Nonfat Latte						
16 oz	60	0	9	90	6	0
McDonald's Iced Nonfat Latte						
20 oz	70	0	11	105	7	0
McDonald's Iced Nonfat Latte with Sugar Free Vanilla Syrup						
12 oz	40	0	13	85	4	0
McDonald's Iced Nonfat Latte with Sugar Free Vanilla Syrup						
16 oz	50	0	14	100	5	0

RESTAURANT/ FOOD ITEM SERVING SIZE	CALORIES	FAT	CARBS	SODIUM	PROTEIN	FIBER
McDonald's Iced Nonfat Latte with Sugar Free Vanilla Syrup						
20 oz	60	0	19	130	6	0
McDonald's Iced Nonfat Vanilla Latte						
12 oz	140	0	31	50	3	0
McDonald's Iced Nonfat Vanilla Latte						
16 oz	150	0	33	70	5	0
McDonald's Iced Nonfat Vanilla Latte						
20 oz	190	0	41	85	6	0
McDonald's Iced Tea						
Medium	0	0	0	15	0	0
McDonald's Iced Tea						
Large	0	0	1	20	0	0
McDonald's Iced Vanilla Latte with Whole Milk						
12 oz	160	3	31	45	3	0
McDonald's Iced Vanilla Latte with Whole Milk						
16 oz	190	4.5	33	70	5	0
McDonald's Iced Vanilla Latte with Whole Milk						
20 oz	230	6	41	85	6	0
McDonald's Kiddie Cone						
1 oz	45	1	8	20	1	0
McDonald's Large Fries						
5.4 oz	500	25	63	350	6	6
McDonald's Latte with Sugar Free Vanilla Syrup with Whole Milk						
12 oz	130	7	17	125	7	0
McDonald's Latte with Sugar Free Vanilla Syrup with Whole Milk						
16 oz	160	8	21	150	8	0
McDonald's Latte with Sugar Free Vanilla Syrup with Whole Milk						
20 oz	180	10	25	180	10	0
McDonald's Latte with Whole Milk						
12 oz	150	8	11	105	8	0
McDonald's Latte with Whole Milk						
16 oz	180	10	13	130	10	0
McDonald's Latte with Whole Milk						
20 oz	210	11	16	150	11	0
McDonald's Low Fat Caramel Dip						
0.8 oz	70	0.5	15	35	0	0
McDonald's McChicken						
5 oz	360	16	40	830	14	2
McDonald's McDonaldland Cookies						
2 oz	260	8	43	300	4	1
McDonald's McDouble						
5.3 oz	390	19	33	920	22	2
McDonald's McFlurry with M&M's Candies						
12 oz	620	20	96	190	14	1
McDonald's McFlurry with Oreo Cookies						
12 oz	550	17	88	250	13	1
McDonald's McRib						
7.4 oz	500	26	44	980	22	3
McDonald's McSkillet Burrito with Sausage						
8.4 oz	610	36	44	1390	27	3

RESTAURANT/ FOOD ITEM SERVING SIZE	CALORIES	FAT	CARBS	SODIUM	PROTEIN	FIBER
McDonald's McSkillet Burrito with Steak						
9.8 oz	570	30	44	1470	32	3
McDonald's Medium Fries						
4.1 oz	380	19	48	270	4	5
McDonald's Mocha with Nonfat Milk						
12 oz	240	5	41	130	7	0
McDonald's Mocha with Nonfat Milk						
16 oz	280	6	50	160	8	0
McDonald's Mocha with Nonfat Milk						
20 oz	330	6	58	190	10	0
McDonald's Mocha with Whole Milk						
12 oz	280	11	40	125	6	0
McDonald's Mocha with Whole Milk						
16 oz	330	12	48	150	7	0
McDonald's Mocha with Whole Milk						
20 oz	400	14	58	190	10	0
McDonald's Newman's Own Creamy Caesar Dressing						
2 oz	190	18	4	500	2	0
McDonald's Newman's Own Creamy Southwest Dressing						
1.5 oz	100	6	11	340	1	0
McDonald's Newman's Own Low Fat Balsamic Vinaigrette						
1.5 oz	40	3	4	730	0	0
McDonald's Newman's Own Low Fat Family Recipe Italian Dressing						
1.5 oz	60	2.5	8	730	1	0
McDonald's Newman's Own Ranch Dressing						
2 oz	170	15	9	530	1	0
McDonald's Nonfat Cappuccino						
12 oz	60	0	9	85	6	0
McDonald's Nonfat Cappuccino						
16 oz	80	0	12	110	8	0
McDonald's Nonfat Cappuccino						
20 oz	90	0	13	130	9	0
McDonald's Nonfat Cappuccino with Sugar Free Vanilla Syrup						
12 oz	50	0	15	100	5	0
McDonald's Nonfat Cappuccino with Sugar Free Vanilla Syrup						
16 oz	70	0	19	130	7	0
McDonald's Nonfat Cappuccino with Sugar Free Vanilla Syrup						
20 oz	80	0	22	150	8	0
McDonald's Nonfat Caramel Cappuccino						
12 oz	150	0	33	120	5	0
McDonald's Nonfat Caramel Cappuccino						
16 oz	190	0	41	150	6	0
McDonald's Nonfat Caramel Cappuccino						
20 oz	230	0	49	180	7	0
McDonald's Nonfat Caramel Latte						
12 oz	170	0	36	150	7	0
McDonald's Nonfat Caramel Latte						
16 oz	220	0	45	180	9	0
McDonald's Nonfat Caramel Latte						
20 oz	260	0	53	220	10	0

RESTAURANT/ FOOD ITEM SERVING SIZE	CALORIES	FAT	CARBS	SODIUM	PROTEIN	FIBER
McDonald's Nonfat Hazelnut Cappuccino						
12 oz	150	0	34	70	5	0
McDonald's Nonfat Hazelnut Cappuccino						
16 oz	190	0	43	90	6	0
McDonald's Nonfat Hazelnut Cappuccino						
20 oz	230	0	51	100	7	0
McDonald's Nonfat Hazelnut Latte						
12 oz	180	0	37	95	7	0
McDonald's Nonfat Hazelnut Latte						
16 oz	220	0	46	115	9	0
McDonald's Nonfat Hazelnut Latte						
20 oz	260	0	55	135	10	0
McDonald's Nonfat Latte						
12 oz	90	0	13	115	9	0
McDonald's Nonfat Latte						
16 oz	110	0	15	140	10	0
McDonald's Nonfat Latte						
20 oz	120	0	18	160	12	0
McDonald's Nonfat Latte with Sugar Free Vanilla Syrup						
12 oz	80	0	18	130	7	0
McDonald's Nonfat Latte with Sugar Free Vanilla Syrup						
16 oz	90	0	22	160	9	0
McDonald's Nonfat Latte with Sugar Free Vanilla Syrup						
20 oz	110	0	27	190	11	0
McDonald's Nonfat Vanilla Cappuccino						
12 oz	150	0	34	70	5	0
McDonald's Nonfat Vanilla Cappuccino						
16 oz	190	0	42	90	6	0
McDonald's Nonfat Vanilla Cappuccino						
20 oz	230	0	51	100	7	0
McDonald's Nonfat Vanilla Latte						
12 oz	180	0	37	95	7	0
McDonald's Nonfat Vanilla Latte						
16 oz	220	0	46	115	9	0
McDonald's Nonfat Vanilla Latte						
20 oz	260	0	55	135	10	0
McDonald's Oatmeal Raisin Cookie						
1 cookie	150	6	22	135	2	1
McDonald's Premium Bacon Ranch Salad with Crispy Chicken						
11.4 oz	370	20	20	970	29	3
McDonald's Premium Bacon Ranch Salad with Grilled Chicken						
11.3 oz	260	9	12	1010	33	3
McDonald's Premium Bacon Ranch Salad without Chicken						
7.8 g	140	7	10	300	9	3
McDonald's Premium Caesar Salad with Crispy Chicken						
11.1 oz	330	17	20	840	26	3
McDonald's Premium Caesar Salad with Grilled Chicken						
11 oz	220	6	12	890	30	3
McDonald's Premium Caesar Salad without Chicken						
7.5 oz	90	4	9	180	7	3

RESTAURANT/ FOOD ITEM SERVING SIZE	CALORIES	FAT	CARBS	SODIUM	PROTEIN	FIBER
McDonald's Premium Crispy Chicken Classic Sandwich						
8.1 oz	530	20	59	1150	28	3
McDonald's Premium Crispy Chicken Club Sandwich						
9 oz	630	28	60	1360	35	4
McDonald's Premium Crispy Chicken Ranch BLT Sandwich						
8.5 oz	580	23	62	1400	31	3
McDonald's Premium Grilled Chicken Classic Sandwich						
8 oz	420	10	51	1190	32	3
McDonald's Premium Grilled Chicken Club Sandwich						
8.8 oz	530	17	52	1410	39	4
McDonald's Premium Grilled Chicken Ranch BLT Sandwich						
8.3 oz	470	12	54	1440	36	3
McDonald's Premium Southwest Salad with Crispy Chicken						
12.5 oz	430	20	38	920	26	6
McDonald's Premium Southwest Salad with Grilled Chicken						
12.3 oz	320	9	30	960	30	6
McDonald's Premium Southwest Salad without Chicken						
8.1 oz	140	4.5	20	150	6	6
McDonald's Quarter Pounder						
6 oz	410	19	37	730	24	2
McDonald's Quarter Pounder with Cheese						
7 oz	510	26	40	1190	29	3
McDonald's Ranch Snack Wrap (Crispy)						
4.1 oz	340	17	33	810	14	1
McDonald's Ranch Snack Wrap (Grilled)						
4.3 oz	270	10	26	830	18	1
McDonald's Sausage Biscuit						
Regular	430	27	34	1080	11	2
McDonald's Sausage Biscuit						
Large	480	31	39	1190	11	3
McDonald's Sausage Biscuit with Egg						
Regular	510	33	36	1170	18	2
McDonald's Sausage Biscuit with Egg						
Large	570	37	42	1280	18	3
McDonald's Sausage Burrito						
3.9 oz	300	16	26	830	12	1
McDonald's Sausage, Cheese McGriddles						
7.6 oz	560	32	48	1360	20	2
McDonald's Sausage McGriddles						
5 oz	420	22	44	1030	11	2
McDonald's Sausage McMuffin						
6.2 oz	370	22	29	850	14	2
McDonald's Sausage McMuffin with Egg						
8 oz	450	27	30	920	21	2
McDonald's Sausage Patty						
1.4 oz	170	15	1	340	7	0
McDonald's Scrambled Eggs						
2 eggs	170	11	1	180	15	0
McDonald's Side Salad						
3.1 oz	20	0	4	10	1	1

RESTAURANT/ FOOD ITEM SERVING SIZE	CALORIES	FAT	CARBS	SODIUM	PROTEIN	FIBER
McDonald's Small Fries						
2.5 oz	230	11	29	160	3	3
McDonald's Snack Size Fruit and Walnut Salad						
1 package	210	8	31	60	4	2
McDonald's Southern Style Chicken Biscuit						
Regular	410	20	41	1180	17	2
McDonald's Southern Style Chicken Biscuit						
Large	470	24	46	1290	17	3
McDonald's Southern Style Crispy Chicken Sandwich						
8.7 oz	400	17	39	1030	24	1
McDonald's Southwestern Chipotle Sauce						
1.5 oz	70	0	18	260	0	1
McDonald's Spicy Buffalo Sauce						
1.5 oz	70	7	1	960	0	2
McDonald's Strawberry Preserves						
0.5 oz	35	0	9	0	0	0
McDonald's Strawberry Sundae						
6.3 oz	280	6	49	95	6	1
McDonald's Strawberry Triple Thick Shake						
12 oz	420	10	73	130	10	0
McDonald's Strawberry Triple Thick Shake						
16 oz	560	13	97	170	13	0
McDonald's Strawberry Triple Thick Shake						
21 oz	740	18	128	230	17	0
McDonald's Strawberry Triple Thick Shake						
32 oz	1110	26	194	350	25	0
McDonald's Sugar Cookie						
1 cookie	160	7	21	120	2	0
McDonald's Sweet 'n Sour Sauce 4 packages						
	50	0	12	150	0	0
McDonald's Tangy Honey Mustard Sauce						
1.5 oz	70	2.5	13	170	1	0
McDonald's Vanilla Cappuccino with Whole Milk						
12 oz	200	5	34	70	5	0
McDonald's Vanilla Cappuccino with Whole Milk						
16 oz	240	6	42	85	6	0
McDonald's Vanilla Cappuccino with Whole Milk						
20 oz	290	8	51	105	7	0
McDonald's Vanilla Latte with Whole Milk						
12 oz	230	7	36	90	7	0
McDonald's Vanilla Latte with Whole Milk						
16 oz	280	8	44	110	8	0
McDonald's Vanilla Latte with Whole Milk						
20 oz	330	9	53	130	9	0
McDonald's Vanilla Reduced Fat Ice Cream Cone						
3.2 oz	150	3.5	24	60	4	0
McDonald's Vanilla Triple Thick Shake						
12 oz	420	10	72	140	9	0
McDonald's Vanilla Triple Thick Shake						
16 oz	550	13	96	190	13	0

RESTAURANT/ FOOD ITEM SERVING SIZE	CALORIES	FAT	CARBS	SODIUM	PROTEIN	FIBER
McDonald's Vanilla Triple Thick Shake						
21 oz	740	18	128	250	17	0
McDonald's Vanilla Triple Thick Shake						
32 oz	1110	26	193	370	25	0
McDonald's Whipped Margarine						
6 g	40	4.5	0	55	0	0
Olive Garden Berry Sangria						
1 serving	230	0	35	15	n/a	0
Olive Garden Black Tie Mousse Cake						
1 serving	760	48	73	270	n/a	8
Olive Garden Braised Beef & Tortelloni						
1 serving	1020	53	82	2060	n/a	10
Olive Garden Breadstick with Garlic Butter Spread						
1 serving	150	2	28	400	n/a	2
Olive Garden Bruschetta						
1 serving	610	13	100	1760	n/a	10
Olive Garden Caesar Salad without Croutons						
1 serving	800	61	8	1750	n/a	3
Olive Garden Calamari						
1 serving	890	54	64	2340	n/a	2
Olive Garden Calamari Sampler						
1 serving	440	27	32	1160	n/a	0
Olive Garden Capellini Pomodoro						
1 serving	840	17	141	1250	n/a	19
Olive Garden Caprese Flatbread						
1 serving	600	36	46	1520	n/a	5
Olive Garden Cheese Ravioli with Marinara Sauce						
1 serving	660	22	84	1440	n/a	7
Olive Garden Cheese Ravioli with Meat Sauce						
1 serving	790	28	88	1510	n/a	12
Olive Garden Chianti Braised Short Ribs						
1 serving	1060	71	71	2970	n/a	17
Olive Garden Chicken Alfredo						
1 serving	1440	82	103	2070	n/a	5
Olive Garden Chicken Alfredo Pizza						
1 serving	1180	40	144	3330	n/a	11
Olive Garden Chicken & Gnocchi Veronese						
1 serving	1030	58	72	2580	n/a	8
Olive Garden Chicken & Shrimp Carbonara						
1 serving	1440	88	80	3000	n/a	9
Olive Garden Chicken Fingers						
1 serving	330	16	22	930	n/a	0
Olive Garden Chicken Marsala						
1 serving	770	37	59	1800	n/a	16
Olive Garden Chicken Parmigiana						
1 serving	1090	49	79	3380	n/a	27
Olive Garden Chicken Scampi						
1 serving	1020	53	84	1880	n/a	17
Olive Garden Chocolate Almond Amore						
1 serving	600	21	82	135	n/a	0

RESTAURANT/ FOOD ITEM	SERVING SIZE	CALORIES	FAT	CARBS	SODIUM	PROTEIN	FIBER
Olive Garden Chocolate Gelato							
	1 serving	620	25	89	150	n/a	6
Olive Garden Chocolate Martini							
	1 serving	260	3.5	36	45	n/a	0
Olive Garden Chocolate Milkshake							
	1 serving	520	22	72	230	n/a	7
Olive Garden Create Your Own Pizza: Add Bell Peppers							
	1 serving	10	0	2	0	n/a	1
Olive Garden Create Your Own Pizza: Add Black Olives							
	1 serving	45	4	3	350	n/a	1
Olive Garden Create Your Own Pizza: Add Italian Sausage							
	1 serving	130	11	1	360	n/a	0
Olive Garden Create Your Own Pizza: Add Mushrooms							
	1 serving	5	0	1	0	n/a	0
Olive Garden Create Your Own Pizza: Add Onions							
	1 serving	15	0	4	0	n/a	1
Olive Garden Create Your Own Pizza: Add Pepperoni							
	1 serving	120	11	0	460	n/a	0
Olive Garden Create Your Own Pizza: Add Roma Tomatoes							
	1 serving	10	0	2	0	n/a	1
Olive Garden Create Your Own Pizza: with Cheese and Sauce Only							
	1 serving	910	28	129	2970	n/a	8
Olive Garden Eggplant Parmigiana							
	1 serving	850	35	98	1900	n/a	19
Olive Garden Fettuccine Alfredo							
	1 serving	1220	75	99	1350	n/a	5
Olive Garden Five Cheese Ziti al Formo							
	1 serving	1050	48	112	2370	n/a	9
Olive Garden Fried Mozzarella							
	1 serving	370	22	26	800	n/a	2
Olive Garden Fried Zucchini							
	1 serving	370	20	42	630	n/a	4
Olive Garden Frozen Tiramisu							
	1 serving	410	14	54	95	n/a	0
Olive Garden Garden-Fresh Salad							
	1 serving	350	26	22	1930	n/a	3
Olive Garden Garden-Fresh Salad without Croutons							
	1 serving	300	24	16	1860	n/a	3
Olive Garden Garden-Fresh Salad without Dressing							
	1 serving	120	3.5	17	550	n/a	3
Olive Garden Garlic-Herb Chicken con Broccoli							
	1 serving	960	41	90	2180	n/a	12
Olive Garden Grilled Chicken Caesar Salad							
	1 serving	850	64	14	1880	n/a	4
Olive Garden Grilled Chicken Flatbread							
	1 serving	760	44	47	1500	n/a	5
Olive Garden Grilled Shrimp Caprese							
	1 serving	900	40	82	3490	n/a	0
Olive Garden Herb-Grilled Salmon							
	1 serving	510	26	5	760	n/a	2

RESTAURANT/ FOOD ITEM	SERVING SIZE	CALORIES	FAT	CARBS	SODIUM	PROTEIN	FIBER
Olive Garden Hot Artichoke-Spinach Dip							
	1 serving	650	31	68	1430	n/a	6
Olive Garden Italian Margarita Cocktail							
	1 serving	240	0	32	10	n/a	0
Olive Garden Lasagna Classico							
	1 serving	850	47	39	2830	n/a	19
Olive Garden Lasagna Fritta							
	1 serving	1030	63	82	1590	n/a	9
Olive Garden Lemon Cream Cake							
	1 serving	610	35	69	430	n/a	2
Olive Garden Lime-Mint Fresco							
	1 serving	230	0	29	45	n/a	0
Olive Garden Limoncello Lemonade							
	1 serving	260	0	42	5	n/a	0
Olive Garden Linguine alla Marinara							
	1 serving	430	6	76	900	n/a	9
Olive Garden Mango Daiquiri							
	1 serving	240	0	43	10	n/a	0
Olive Garden Mango Martini							
	1 serving	180	0	31	0	n/a	0
Olive Garden Manicotti Formaggio							
	1 serving	940	46	81	2530	n/a	8
Olive Garden Minestrone							
	1 serving	100	1	18	1020	n/a	3
Olive Garden Mixed Grill							
	1 serving	770	24	48	1980	n/a	13
Olive Garden Mixed Grill (All Chicken)							
	1 serving	630	20	27	1255	n/a	7
Olive Garden Mussels di Napoli							
	1 serving	180	8	13	1770	n/a	0
Olive Garden Parmesan Crusted Tilapia							
	1 serving	590	25	42	910	n/a	6
Olive Garden Pasta e Fagioli							
	1 serving	130	2.5	17	680	n/a	6
Olive Garden Peach Bellini							
	1 serving	170	0	33	0	n/a	0
Olive Garden Peach Daiquiri							
	1 serving	270	0	51	10	n/a	0
Olive Garden Peach Fresco							
	1 serving	200	1	22	10	n/a	0
Olive Garden Peach Sangria							
	1 serving	250	0	40	50	n/a	0
Olive Garden Penne Rigate							
	1 serving	561	19	90	693	n/a	8
Olive Garden Pomegranate Margarita Martini							
	1 serving	290	0	44	5	n/a	0
Olive Garden Pork Milanese							
	1 serving	1510	87	118	3100	n/a	11
Olive Garden Ravioli di Portobello							
	1 serving	670	30	74	1400	n/a	15

RESTAURANT/ FOOD ITEM SERVING SIZE	CALORIES	FAT	CARBS	SODIUM	PROTEIN	FIBER
Olive Garden Seafood Alfredo						
1 serving	1020	52	88	2430	n/a	9
Olive Garden Seafood Portofino						
1 serving	800	33	85	1880	n/a	16
Olive Garden Shrimp & Asparagus Risotto						
1 serving	620	30	44	2530	n/a	19
Olive Garden Shrimp Primavera						
1 serving	730	12	110	1620	n/a	14
Olive Garden Sicilian Citrus Fresco						
1 serving	210	0	25	10	n/a	0
Olive Garden Sicilian Scampi						
1 serving	500	22	43	1850	n/a	7
Olive Garden Smoked Mozzarella Fonduta						
1 serving	940	48	72	1940	n/a	7
Olive Garden Sour Apple Martini						
1 serving	210	0	22	0	n/a	0
Olive Garden Spaghetti & Italian Sausage						
1 serving	1270	67	97	3090	n/a	15
Olive Garden Spaghetti & Meatballs						
1 serving	1110	50	103	2180	n/a	9
Olive Garden Spaghetti with Meat Sauce						
1 serving	710	22	94	1340	n/a	9
Olive Garden Steak Gorgonzola-Alfredo						
1 serving	1310	73	82	2190	n/a	9
Olive Garden Steak Toscano						
1 serving	880	43	45	1700	n/a	12
Olive Garden Steak Toscano, gluten-free						
1 serving	760	46	9	1370	n/a	4
Olive Garden Strawberry Bellini						
1 serving	220	0	46	0	n/a	0
Olive Garden Strawberry Daiquiri						
1 serving	250	0	47	15	n/a	0
Olive Garden Strawberry Fresco						
1 serving	230	0	31	5	n/a	0
Olive Garden Strawberry Frozen Margarita						
1 serving	340	0	67	25	n/a	0
Olive Garden Strawberry Milkshake						
1 serving	500	24	62	160	n/a	10
Olive Garden Strawberry Siciliano						
1 serving	360	10	46	50	n/a	0
Olive Garden Strawberry-Limoncello Martini						
1 serving	300	0	42	15	n/a	0
Olive Garden Strawberry-Mango Frozen Margarita						
1 serving	350	0	68	20	n/a	0
Olive Garden Stuffed Chicken Marsala						
1 serving	800	36	40	2830	n/a	6
Olive Garden Stuffed Mushrooms						
1 serving	410	28	19	980	n/a	3
Olive Garden Sundae						
1 serving	180	9	21	45	n/a	0

RESTAURANT/ FOOD ITEM SERVING SIZE	CALORIES	FAT	CARBS	SODIUM	PROTEIN	FIBER
Olive Garden Tangerine Palermo						
1 serving	410	12	56	50	n/a	0
Olive Garden Tiramisu						
1 serving	510	32	48	75	n/a	2
Olive Garden Toasted Beef & Pork Ravioli						
1 serving	360	16	39	780	n/a	2
Olive Garden Torta di Chocolate						
1 serving	800	51	75	125	n/a	4
Olive Garden Tour of Italy						
1 serving	1450	74	97	3830	n/a	10
Olive Garden Tropical Sangria						
1 serving	220	0	31	10	n/a	0
Olive Garden Vanilla Milkshake						
1 serving	530	23	73	170	n/a	16
Olive Garden Venetian Apricot Chicken						
1 serving	380	4	32	1420	n/a	8
Olive Garden Venetian Sunset Cocktail						
1 serving	190	1	38	10	n/a	0
Olive Garden White Chocolate Raspberry Cheesecake						
1 serving	890	62	70	490	n/a	6
Olive Garden Wild Berry Bellini						
1 serving	160	0	31	10	n/a	0
Olive Garden Wild Berry Daiquiri						
1 serving	270	0	50	5	n/a	0
Olive Garden Wild Berry Frozen Margarita						
1 serving	290	0	55	20	n/a	0
Olive Garden Zeppoli						
1 serving	920	35	131	590	n/a	4
Olive Garden Zeppoli Chocolate Sauce						
1 serving	210	2.5	44	75	n/a	2
Olive Garden Zuppa Toscana						
1 serving	170	4	24	960	n/a	2
Outback Steakhouse Alice Springs Chicken						
1 serving	1303.5	93.6	31.1	2146.9	84.9	2.4
Outback Steakhouse Atlantic Salmon						
1 serving	584.7	46.1	2.4	517.3	39.4	0.8
Outback Steakhouse Aussie Cheese Fries						
Small	414.7	30.2	25.8	734.4	10.8	3
Outback Steakhouse Aussie Fries						
1 serving	375.2	21.4	43.4	539	4.4	5.4
Outback Steakhouse Baby Back Ribs						
Full rack	3020.9	242.4	30.3	4647.5	165.9	1
Outback Steakhouse Bacon Cheese Burger						
1 serving	1112.8	71.8	44.4	2127.4	69.4	3.2
Outback Steakhouse Baked Potato Soup						
1 bowl	772.7	48.4	73	3841	13.8	8
Outback Steakhouse Baked Potato Soup						
1 cup	546.3	35.2	48.8	2613.7	10.4	5.4
Outback Steakhouse Bloomin' Onion						
⅙ onion	260	14	30.9	918.4	4.6	4.1

RESTAURANT/ FOOD ITEM SERVING SIZE	CALORIES	FAT	CARBS	SODIUM	PROTEIN	FIBER
Outback Steakhouse Carrot Cake						
¼ plate	296.5	7	56.7	403.4	3.6	0.3
Outback Steakhouse Chicken Caesar Salad						
1 serving	907.6	60.6	25.6	1438.1	65.1	6
Outback Steakhouse Chocolate Thunder from Down Under Sample						
1 serving	955.7	76.9	67.5	200.7	13.4	6.5
Outback Steakhouse Classic Cheesecake Sample						
1 serving	991.1	34.1	171	353.5	8.7	2
Outback Steakhouse Classic Roasted Filet Wedge Salad						
1 serving	562.5	29.7	27.3	1982.2	42.6	2.3
Outback Steakhouse Crab Stuffed Shrimp						
½ plate	256.9	17.3	14.2	389.9	11.9	1.8
Outback Steakhouse Cream of Broccoli Soup						
1 bowl	412.9	30.3	25.3	1747	11.1	3.1
Outback Steakhouse Cream of Broccoli Soup						
1 cup	284.4	20.9	16.9	1178.4	8	2.1
Outback Steakhouse Filet Tenderloin & Stuffed Shrimp						
1 serving	759.5	50.7	29.8	1562.8	46.3	4
Outback Steakhouse Fresh Steamed Green Beans						
1 serving	228.8	11.4	25.5	396.7	7.3	9.4
Outback Steakhouse Fresh Tilapia with Pure Lump Crab Meat						
1 serving	509.8	28.9	9.1	557.7	54.7	2.1
Outback Steakhouse Garlic Mashed Potatoes						
1 serving	373.8	25	33.2	1063	7.6	6.4
Outback Steakhouse Gold Coast Coconut Shrimp						
¼ plate	130.4	4.9	22.2	154.7	1.1	2.1
Outback Steakhouse Grilled Chicken & Swiss Sandwich						
1 serving	695.9	33.3	50.2	1322.6	47.5	2.7
Outback Steakhouse Grilled Chicken on the Barbie						
1 serving	444.3	15.4	21.2	1159.6	52	0.5
Outback Steakhouse Kookaburra Wings						
¼ plate	427	32.1	6.9	865.9	26.3	1.1
Outback Steakhouse Lobster Tails						
1 serving	639.5	47.8	6	1179.4	47	1.5
Outback Steakhouse New York Strip Steak						
14 oz	712.5	36.8	0.7	693.9	89.5	0.2
Outback Steakhouse New Zealand Rack of Lamb						
1 serving	1304	113	4.9	1373.6	61.4	1.1
Outback Steakhouse No Rules Parmesan Pasta						
1 serving	920.7	53.1	91.2	1093.3	21.2	5.2
Outback Steakhouse No Rules Parmesan Pasta with Chicken						
1 serving	1364.6	77.3	93.2	1639.4	73.4	5.6
Outback Steakhouse No Rules Parmesan Pasta with Shrimp						
1 serving	1288.3	77.3	94.5	1652.4	54.4	5.6
Outback Steakhouse Nutter Butter Peanut Butter Pie Sample						
1 serving	880.2	56.4	88.9	673.3	12.5	2.5
Outback Steakhouse Onion Soup						
1 bowl	436.1	31.9	28.2	1782.8	101	2.8
Outback Steakhouse Onion Soup						
1 cup	299.9	22	18.8	1202.2	7.3	1.9

RESTAURANT/ FOOD ITEM SERVING SIZE	CALORIES	FAT	CARBS	SODIUM	PROTEIN	FIBER
Outback Steakhouse Outback Chicken & Filet Griller						
1 serving	1108.6	46	114.5	2690.9	67.8	12.3
Outback Steakhouse Outback Chicken & Shrimp Griller						
1 serving	1108.6	46.8	116.7	3523.1	64.5	12.8
Outback Steakhouse Outback Chicken Griller						
1 serving	1021.6	39.5	112.2	1452.5	62.5	11.5
Outback Steakhouse Outback Filet Griller						
1 serving	1109.4	51.1	112	1420.1	58.9	11.5
Outback Steakhouse Outback Shrimp & Filet Griller						
1 serving	1108.6	46	114.5	2690.9	67.8	12.3
Outback Steakhouse Outback Shrimp Griller						
1 serving	949.5	39.5	114.2	1565.1	43.9	11.9
Outback Steakhouse Outback Special Steak						
6 oz	331.7	19.3	0.7	562.3	37	0.2
Outback Steakhouse Outback Special Steak						
9 oz	445.1	23.2	0.7	610.2	55.5	0.2
Outback Steakhouse Outback Steak & Shrimp Griller						
1 serving	1108.6	46.8	116.7	3523.1	64.5	12.8
Outback Steakhouse Potato Boats						
1 serving	164.6	2.2	32.4	1149.1	4	3.5
Outback Steakhouse Prime Rib Steak						
8 oz	537.2	44.9	1.7	888.3	28.9	0.2
Outback Steakhouse Prime Rib Steak						
14 oz	1018.3	84.1	11.1	1122.6	50.9	1.3
Outback Steakhouse Queensland Salad without Dressing						
1 serving	1125.3	82.4	40.4	3094.6	57.2	6.9
Outback Steakhouse Ribeye Steak						
14 oz	1193.4	99.2	0.7	689	69.8	0.2
Outback Steakhouse Ribs and Alice Springs Chicken						
1 serving	1615.3	125.9	11.1	3535.5	104.9	1.9
Outback Steakhouse Roasted Filet Sandwich						
1 serving	877.2	36.2	88.2	3334.1	48	4.4
Outback Steakhouse Roasted Filet Tenderloin with Port Wine Sauce						
1 serving	373.5	11.6	8.4	1640.7	52.9	1.5
Outback Steakhouse Savory Pepper Mill Steak						
1 serving	763.2	52.1	17	316.4	52.6	5.6
Outback Steakhouse Shrimp Caesar Salad						
1 serving	606.3	51.6	25.5	1405.7	13.3	6
Outback Steakhouse Shrimp en Fuego						
1 serving	888.8	72.6	24.6	1899.5	36.3	4.8
Outback Steakhouse Sweet Adventure Sampler Trio Dessert						
¼ plate	630.3	36.1	76.6	266.3	7.5	2.7
Outback Steakhouse Sweet Glazed Roasted Pork Tenderloin						
1 serving	349.3	8.1	32	425.5	37.3	1.2
Outback Steakhouse Teriyaki Marinated Sirloin Steak						
9 oz	418.3	11.7	17.2	1832.2	57.1	0.4
Outback Steakhouse The Bloomin' Burger						
1 serving	1156.1	63.9	75.6	2822.3	69.3	7.3
Outback Steakhouse The Melbourne Steak						
20 oz	1009.6	58.2	0.9	807.5	113.8	0.3

RESTAURANT/ FOOD ITEM	SERVING SIZE	CALORIES	FAT	CARBS	SODIUM	PROTEIN	FIBER
Outback Steakhouse The Outbacker Burger							
	1 serving	743.4	37.2	43.2	1282.2	56.8	3.7
Outback Steakhouse The Outbacker Burger with American Cheese							
	1 serving	743.4	37.2	43.2	1282.2	56.8	3.7
Outback Steakhouse The Outbacker Burger with Swiss Cheese							
	1 serving	793	41.2	42.6	1501	60.7	3.5
Outback Steakhouse Victoria's Filet Steak							
	7 oz	587.1	46.6	0.7	564.6	39.1	0.2
Outback Steakhouse Victoria's Filet Steak with Blue Cheese Crust							
	7 oz	810.9	68.1	5.2	798.3	42.9	0.5
Outback Steakhouse Victoria's Filet Steak with Horseradish Crumb Crust							
	7 oz	809.4	68	7.9	810.7	40.6	1.2
Panera Asiago Cheese							
	4 oz	330	6	55	570	13	2
Panera Asiago Cheese Demi							
	2 oz	160	4	22	320	7	1
Panera Asiago Cheese Loaf							
	2 oz	160	4	22	320	7	1
Panera Asiago Roast Beef on Asiago Cheese Sandwich							
	1 sandwich	710	32	57	1280	47	3
Panera Asian Sesame Chicken Salad							
	11.5 oz	410	19	31	900	32	5
Panera Bacon, Egg & Cheese Sandwich							
	6.75 oz	510	24	44	1060	28	2
Panera Bacon Turkey Bravo on Tomato Basil Sandwich							
	1 sandwich	840	32	87	2930	51	4
Panera Baked Potato Soup							
	12 oz	370	22	33	1140	8	3
Panera Blueberry Bagel							
	4.25 oz	330	1.5	67	490	10	2
Panera Broccoli Cheddar Soup							
	12 oz	290	16	24	1540	12	7
Panera Caesar Salad							
	9.75 oz	390	27	25	610	12	3
Panera Caffe Latte							
	8.5 oz	110	4.5	11	95	7	0
Panera Caffe Mocha							
	11.5 oz	380	17	48	160	11	2
Panera Cappuccino							
	8.5 oz	110	4.5	11	95	7	0
Panera Caramel							
	Grande/16 oz	580	25	83	170	6	1
Panera Caramel							
	Largo/20.5 oz	710	30	105	220	7	1
Panera Caramel Latte							
	11.5 oz	410	18	54	190	9	0

RESTAURANT/ FOOD ITEM SERVING SIZE	CALORIES	FAT	CARBS	SODIUM	PROTEIN	FIBER
Panera Caramel Pecan Brownie						
4 oz	490	25	64	170	5	2
Panera Carrot Walnut Muffin						
5 oz	430	19	61	380	8	2
Panera Chai Tea Latte						
10 oz	190	4	31	85	7	0
Panera Challah Bread						
2 oz	180	2.5	34	290	6	1
Panera Cheese Pastries						
3.75 oz	400	23	41	340	8	1
Panera Cherry Pastries						
5 oz	450	22	55	340	8	2
Panera Chicken Bacon Dijon on Country Hot Panini						
1 sandwich						
	940	36	96	2020	59	4
Panera Chicken Bacon Dijon on French Hot Panini						
1 sandwich						
	780	36	63	1540	53	2
Panera Chicken Caesar on Focaccia Sandwich						
1 sandwich						
	860	39	82	1640	43	4
Panera Chicken Caesar on Three Cheese Sandwich						
1 sandwich						
	800	33	83	1650	45	4
Panera Chicken Salad on Sesame Semolina Sandwich						
1 sandwich						
	710	25	101	1950	31	13
Panera Chicken Salad on Whole Grain Sandwich						
1 sandwich						
	620	26	77	1490	31	16
Panera Chipotle Chicken on Artisan French Sandwich						
1 sandwich						
	1070	55	87	2570	54	4
Panera Chipotle Chicken on French Sandwich						
1 sandwich						
	900	56	53	2090	49	3
Panera Chocolate Chip Bagel						
4.25 oz	370	6	69	480	10	2
Panera Chocolate Chip Muffin						
2.75 oz	270	12	40	140	4	1
Panera Chocolate Chipper Cookies						
3.25 oz	440	23	59	320	5	2
Panera Chocolate Duet with Walnut Cookies						
3.25 oz	450	24	55	330	6	3
Panera Chocolate Pastries						
3.5 oz	340	20	37	230	6	2
Panera Chopped Chicken Cobb Salad						
15.5 oz	490	35	9	1300	36	3
Panera Ciabatta						
6.25 oz	460	5	84	760	16	3

RESTAURANT/ FOOD ITEM	SERVING SIZE	CALORIES	FAT	CARBS	SODIUM	PROTEIN	FIBER
Panera Cinnamon Chip Scones							
	4.75 oz	530	27	67	310	8	2
Panera Cinnamon Crunch Bagel							
	4.5 oz	430	8	81	430	9	3
Panera Cinnamon Raisin Loaf							
	2 oz	180	3	34	135	5	1
Panera Cinnamon Swirl Bagel							
	3.75 oz	320	2.5	65	460	10	3
Panera Classic Café Salad							
	10 oz	170	11	19	270	3	4
Panera Country Loaf							
	2 oz	140	0.5	27	310	5	1
Panera Country Miche							
	3 oz	140	0.5	28	330	5	1
Panera Cream of Chicken & Wild Rice Soup							
	12 oz	300	17	29	1450	7	1
Panera Creamy Tomato Soup							
	12 oz	290	20	28	1040	4	3
Panera Creamy Tomato Soup with Croutons							
	12.75 oz	370	23	39	740	4	5
Panera Dutch Apple & Raisin Bagel							
	4.75 oz	360	3	77	620	8	2
Panera Egg & Cheese Sandwich							
	5.75 oz	380	14	43	620	18	2
Panera Everything Bagel							
	4 oz	300	2.5	59	630	10	2
Panera Focaccia							
	4 oz	160	2	29	330	5	1
Panera Focaccia with Asiago Cheese							
	2 oz	160	5	23	230	5	1
Panera Forest Mushroom Soup							
	12 oz	250	18	21	1150	4	2
Panera Four Cheese Baked Egg Souffle							
	5.75 oz	480	31	34	700	16	2
Panera French Baguette							
	2 oz	150	0.5	30	370	5	1
Panera French Loaf							
	2 oz	150	2	29	310	5	1
Panera French Miche							
	2 oz	140	0.5	28	360	5	1
Panera French Onion Soup (with Cheese & Croutons)							
	13.25 oz	250	11	30	2370	10	3
Panera French Onion Soup (without Cheese & Croutons)							
	12 oz	130	4.5	20	2340	3	2
Panera French Roll							
	2.25 oz	180	2	35	370	6	1
Panera French Toast Bagel							
	4 oz	350	5	67	610	9	2

RESTAURANT/ FOOD ITEM SERVING SIZE	CALORIES	FAT	CARBS	SODIUM	PROTEIN	FIBER
Panera French XL Loaf						
2 oz	150	2	29	300	5	1
Panera Fresh Apple Pastries						
4.5 oz	380	19	44	320	7	1
Panera Fresh Fruit Cup						
Large	150	0	37	30	2	2
Panera Fresh Fruit Cup						
Small	70	0	19	15	1	1
Panera Frontega Chicken on Focaccia Hot Panini						
1 sandwich						
	860	39	80	2150	46	4
Panera Frozen Lemonade						
Grande/16 oz						
	90	0	21	10	0	0
Panera Frozen Lemonade						
Largo/20.5 oz						
	120	0	29	15	1	0
Panera Gooey Butter Pastries						
3.75 oz	350	19	39	250	7	1
Panera Greek Salad						
13.75 oz	440	39	15	1370	10	6
Panera Grilled Chicken Caesar Salad						
13.25 oz	500	28	26	1000	35	3
Panera Honey Wheat Loaf						
2 oz	160	3	30	240	5	2
Panera Hot Chocolate						
11.5 oz	390	17	49	170	11	2
Panera Iced Chai Tea Latte						
16 oz	150	3.5	25	75	6	0
Panera Iced Green Tea						
Largo/20 fl oz						
	110	0	28	10	0	0
Panera Iced Green Tea						
Grande/16 fl oz						
	90	0	23	10	0	0
Panera Italian Combo on Ciabatta Sandwich						
1 sandwich						
	1040	45	94	3020	61	5
Panera Lemonade						
Grande/16 oz						
	90	0	22	10	0	0
Panera Lemonade						
Largo/20.5 oz						
	130	0	31	10	1	0
Panera Low-Fat Chicken Noodle Soup						
12 oz	140	2.5	20	1350	9	1
Panera Low-Fat Vegetarian Black Bean Soup						
12 oz	170	4	29	1590	10	5
Panera Low-Fat Vegetarian Garden Vegetable Soup						
12 oz	120	1	24	1970	4	7

RESTAURANT/ FOOD ITEM SERVING SIZE	CALORIES	FAT	CARBS	SODIUM	PROTEIN	FIBER
Panera Mango Smoothie						
Grande/18 oz						
	330	10	61	30	2	3
Panera Mango Smoothie						
Largo/21.5 oz						
	370	10	71	35	2	3
Panera Mediterranean Veggie on Tomato Basil Sandwich						
1 sandwich						
	610	13	102	1450	22	9
Panera Mocha						
Grande/16 oz						
	550	25	78	140	7	2
Panera Mocha						
Largo/20.5 oz						
	670	28	98	180	9	3
Panera New England Clam Chowder						
12 oz	450	34	29	1190	8	3
Panera Nutty Chocolate Chipper Cookies						
3.25 oz	460	27	54	300	5	3
Panera Oatmeal Raisin Cookies						
3.25 oz	370	14	57	310	5	2
Panera Orange Scones						
4.5 oz	460	20	65	290	8	1
Panera Pecan Braid Pastries						
4.25 oz	440	25	46	270	8	2
Panera Plain Bagel						
3.75 oz	290	1.5	59	450	10	2
Panera Plain Cream Cheese Spread						
1 oz	100	10	1	110	2	0
Panera Plain Cream Cheese Spread						
2 oz	180	18	2	210	3	0
Panera Pumpkin Muffin						
2.75 oz	250	10	39	200	3	1
Panera Pumpkin Muffin						
6 oz	530	20	81	430	6	2
Panera Reduced-Fat Hazelnut Cream Cheese Spread						
1 oz	80	6	3	110	2	0
Panera Reduced-Fat Hazelnut Cream Cheese Spread						
2 oz	140	11	6	210	5	1
Panera Reduced Fat Honey Walnut Cream Cheese Spread						
1 oz	80	6	4	105	2	0
Panera Reduced Fat Honey Walnut Cream Cheese Spread						
2 oz	150	11	8	200	5	1
Panera Reduced Fat Plain Cream Cheese Spread						
1 oz	70	6	1	120	3	0
Panera Reduced Fat Plain Cream Cheese Spread						
2 oz	130	12	2	230	5	1
Panera Reduced Fat Raspberry Cream Cheese Spread						
1 oz	70	5	4	105	2	1

RESTAURANT/ FOOD ITEM	SERVING SIZE	CALORIES	FAT	CARBS	SODIUM	PROTEIN	FIBER
Panera Reduced Fat Raspberry Cream Cheese Spread							
	2 oz	130	10	7	190	4	1
Panera Reduced Fat Sun-Dried Tomato Cream Cheese Spread							
	1 oz	70	6	2	115	3	1
Panera Reduced Fat Sun-Dried Tomato Cream Cheese Spread							
	2 oz	130	11	4	220	5	1
Panera Reduced Fat Veggie Cream Cheese Spread							
	1 oz	60	5	1	110	2	1
Panera Reduced Fat Veggie Cream Cheese Spread							
	2 oz	120	10	3	200	4	1
Panera Reduced Fat Wild Blueberry Muffin							
	4.5 oz	360	10	61	220	6	1
Panera Salt Bagel							
	4 oz	290	1.5	59	2790	10	2
Panera Sausage, Egg & Cheese Sandwich							
	7.5 oz	550	30	44	800	25	2
Panera Sesame Bagel							
	4 oz	310	3	59	450	10	2
Panera Sesame Semolina Loaf							
	2 oz	140	0.5	29	350	4	1
Panera Sesame Semolina Miche							
	2 oz	140	1	30	360	5	1
Panera Sierra Turkey on Focaccia with Asiago Cheese							
	1 sandwich						
		970	54	80	1970	39	4
Panera Smoked Ham & Swiss on Rye							
	1 sandwich						
		700	35	55	1890	40	4
Panera Smoked Ham & Swiss on Stone-Milled Rye							
	1 sandwich						
		780	29	82	2580	49	7
Panera Smoked Turkey Breast on Country							
	1 sandwich						
		730	23	92	2480	36	7
Panera Smoked Turkey Breast on Sourdough							
	1 sandwich						
		470	17	49	1680	30	3
Panera Smokehouse Turkey on Focaccia Hot Panini							
	1 sandwich						
		860	36	82	2620	52	4
Panera Smokehouse Turkey on Three Cheese Hot Panini							
	1 sandwich						
		810	30	83	2660	54	5
Panera Sourdough Baguette							
	2 oz	160	0.5	31	320	6	1
Panera Sourdough Loaf							
	2 oz	140	0.5	28	290	5	1
Panera Sourdough Roll							
	2.25 oz	200	1	39	400	7	1

RESTAURANT/ FOOD ITEM	SERVING SIZE	CALORIES	FAT	CARBS	SODIUM	PROTEIN	FIBER
Panera Sourdough Soup Bowl							
	8 oz	590	2.5	117	1210	22	4
Panera Sourdough XL Loaf							
	2 oz	140	0.5	28	290	5	1
Panera Spinach & Artichoke Baked Egg Souffle							
	6.25 oz	500	32	35	830	19	2
Panera Spinach & Bacon Baked Egg Souffle							
	6.5 oz	570	37	36	990	21	2
Panera Stone-Milled Rye Loaf							
	2 oz	140	0.5	28	380	5	2
Panera Stone-Milled Rye Miche							
	2 oz	140	0.5	27	410	5	2
Panera Strawberry Granola Parfait							
	8.25 oz	310	12	41	100	3	4
Panera Strawberry Poppyseed Salad							
	13 oz	170	6	27	200	3	5
Panera Strawberry Poppyseed with Chicken Salad							
	16.5 oz	290	9	29	470	26	5
Panera Strawberry Smoothie Grande/18 oz							
		240	1.5	51	190	5	3
Panera Strawberry Smoothie Largo/21.5 oz							
		290	1.5	62	230	6	5
Panera Summer Corn Chowder							
	12 oz	260	14	28	730	5	6
Panera Three Seed Demi							
	2 oz	160	3.5	27	300	6	2
Panera Toffee Nut Cookies							
	3.25 oz	460	19	59	330	5	1
Panera Tomato & Mozzarella on Ciabatta 1 sandwich							
		770	29	96	1290	30	6
Panera Tomato & Mozzarella Salad							
	18.75 oz	890	47	83	1660	36	6
Panera Tomato Basil Loaf							
	2 oz	140	0.5	27	330	5	1
Panera Tuna Salad on Honey Wheat 1 sandwich							
		750	47	65	1130	20	6
Panera Turkey Artichoke on Focaccia Hot Panini 1 sandwich							
		750	27	89	2340	40	7
Panera Turkey Sausage & Potato Baked Egg Souffle							
	5.75 oz	460	28	35	600	15	2
Panera Very Chocolate Brownie							
	4 oz	460	22	61	180	5	2
Panera White Whole Grain Loaf							
	2 oz	140	2.5	27	310	5	2

RESTAURANT/ FOOD ITEM SERVING SIZE	CALORIES	FAT	CARBS	SODIUM	PROTEIN	FIBER
Panera Whole Grain Bagel						
4.5 oz	370	3.5	70	420	13	6
Panera Whole Grain Baguette						
2 oz	140	1	28	320	6	3
Panera Whole Grain Loaf						
2 oz	130	1	26	240	6	3
Panera Whole Grain Miche						
2 oz	130	1	25	240	5	3
Panera Wild Blueberry Muffin						
4.5 oz	390	15	58	290	5	1
Papa John's Apple Pie						
4 sticks	480	10	90	520	8	2
Papa John's BBQ Wings						
2 wings	190	12	6	760	12	0
Papa John's Breadsticks						
2 sticks	290	4.5	54	540	8	2
Papa John's Buffalo Wings						
2 wings	170	13	3	1070	12	0
Papa John's Cheesesticks						
4 sticks	370	16	41	860	14	2
Papa John's Chickenstrips						
2 strips	130	4.5	10	430	12	0
Papa John's Chocolate Pastry Delights						
1 pastry	200	11	25	14	2	1
Papa John's Cinnamon Sweetsticks						
4 sticks	580	16	98	740	11	3
Papa John's Cinnapie						
4 sticks	560	19	90	540	8	2
Papa John's Garden Fresh Original Crust Pizza 10"						
1 slice	140	4.5	20	350	5	1
Papa John's Garden Fresh Original Crust Pizza 12"						
1 slice	200	7	27	500	8	2
Papa John's Garden Fresh Original Crust Pizza 14"						
1 slice	280	9	39	700	11	2
Papa John's Garden Fresh Original Crust Pizza 16"						
1 slice	300	10	42	740	11	2
Papa John's Garden Fresh Pan Crust Pizza 12"						
1 slice	380	20	38	710	11	2
Papa John's Garden Fresh Thin Crust Pizza 14"						
1 slice	210	11	22	490	8	2
Papa John's Garlic Parmesan Breadsticks						
2 sticks	340	10	54	720	9	2
Papa John's Hawaiian BBQ Chicken Original Crust Pizza 10"						
1 slice	240	8	31	680	10	1
Papa John's Hawaiian BBQ Chicken Original Crust Pizza 12"						
1 slice	250	8	33	730	11	1
Papa John's Hawaiian BBQ Chicken Original Crust Pizza 14"						
1 slice	350	12	46	1020	15	2
Papa John's Hawaiian BBQ Chicken Original Crust Pizza 16"						
1 slice	370	12	49	1080	16	2

RESTAURANT/ FOOD ITEM	SERVING SIZE	CALORIES	FAT	CARBS	SODIUM	PROTEIN	FIBER
Papa John's Hawaiian BBQ Chicken Pan Crust Pizza 12"							
	1 slice	440	22	45	1000	16	1
Papa John's Hawaiian BBQ Chicken Thin Crust Pizza 14"							
	1 slice	280	13	29	810	13	1
Papa John's Honey Chipotle Wings							
	2 wings	190	12	8	730	12	0
Papa John's Pepperoni Original Crust Pizza 10"							
	1 slice	220	9	25	580	8	1
Papa John's Pepperoni Original Crust Pizza 12"							
	1 slice	230	10	26	610	9	1
Papa John's Pepperoni Original Crust Pizza 14"							
	1 slice	330	14	37	870	13	2
Papa John's Pepperoni Original Crust Pizza 16"							
	1 slice	340	14	40	900	13	2
Papa John's Pepperoni Pan Crust Pizza 12"							
	1 slice	420	25	36	880	13	1
Papa John's Pepperoni Thin Crust Pizza 14"							
	1 slice	260	15	20	660	10	1
Papa John's Spinach Alfredo Original Crust Pizza 10"							
	1 slice	190	8	24	430	7	1
Papa John's Spinach Alfredo Original Crust Pizza 12"							
	1 slice	210	8	25	470	8	1
Papa John's Spinach Alfredo Original Crust Pizza 14"							
	1 slice	290	11	36	640	10	1
Papa John's Spinach Alfredo Original Crust Pizza 16"							
	1 slice	310	12	39	680	11	2
Papa John's Spinach Alfredo Pan Crust Pizza 12"							
	1 slice	380	22	34	630	11	1
Papa John's Spinach Alfredo Thin Crust Pizza 14"							
	1 slice	220	13	19	430	8	1
Papa John's The Meats Original Crust Pizza 10"							
	1 slice	250	12	25	700	10	1
Papa John's The Meats Original Crust Pizza 12"							
	1 slice	250	12	26	710	11	1
Papa John's The Meats Original Crust Pizza 14"							
	1 slice	370	17	38	1050	15	2
Papa John's The Meats Original Crust Pizza 16"							
	1 slice	400	19	40	1100	16	2
Papa John's The Meats Pan Crust Pizza 12"							
	1 slice	460	28	35	1040	15	2
Papa John's The Meats Thin Crust Pizza 14"							
	1 slice	300	19	20	840	13	1
Papa John's The Works Original Crust Pizza 10"							
	1 slice	220	9	26	620	9	1
Papa John's The Works Original Crust Pizza 12"							
	1 slice	230	9	27	650	9	1
Papa John's The Works Original Crust Pizza 14"							
	1 slice	330	6	39	930	13	2
Papa John's The Works Original Crust Pizza 16"							
	1 slice	350	6	42	980	14	2

RESTAURANT/ FOOD ITEM SERVING SIZE	CALORIES	FAT	CARBS	SODIUM	PROTEIN	FIBER
Papa John's The Works Pan Crust Pizza 12"						
1 slice	420	24	38	920	13	2
Papa John's The Works Thin Crust Pizza 14"						
1 slice	260	15	21	720	11	2
Pizza Hut 12" Fit 'n Delicious Pizza All Natural Chicken, Mushroom & Jalapeño						
1 slice	180	4.5	22	710	12	1
Pizza Hut 12" Fit 'n Delicious Pizza All Natural Chicken, Red Onion & Green Pepper						
1 slice	180	4.5	24	500	11	1
Pizza Hut 12" Fit 'n Delicious Pizza Diced Red Tomato, Mushroom & Jalapeño						
1 slice	150	4	23	610	6	2
Pizza Hut 12" Fit 'n Delicious Pizza Green Pepper, Red Onion & Diced Red Tomato						
1 slice	150	4	24	400	6	2
Pizza Hut 12" Fit 'n Delicious Pizza Ham, Pineapple & Diced Red Tomato						
1 slice	160	4.5	24	560	7	1
Pizza Hut 12" Fit 'n Delicious Pizza Ham, Red Onion & Mushroom						
1 slice	160	4.5	23	550	8	1
Pizza Hut 12" Medium Hand-Tossed Style Pizza All Natural Italian Sausage & Red Onion						
1 slice	240	10	27	590	10	2
Pizza Hut 12" Medium Hand-Tossed Style Pizza All Natural Pepperoni						
1 slice	230	10	25	620	10	1
Pizza Hut 12" Medium Hand-Tossed Style Pizza All Natural Pepperoni & Mushroom						
1 slice	210	8	26	550	9	2
Pizza Hut 12" Medium Hand-Tossed Style Pizza Cheese						
1 slice	220	8	26	550	10	1
Pizza Hut 12" Medium Hand-Tossed Style Pizza Dan's Original						
1 slice	260	12	26	660	11	2
Pizza Hut 12" Medium Hand-Tossed Style Pizza Ham & Pineapple						
1 slice	200	6	27	550	9	1
Pizza Hut 12" Medium Hand-Tossed Style Pizza Hawaiian Luau						
1 slice	230	10	27	650	10	1
Pizza Hut 12" Medium Hand-Tossed Style Pizza Meat Lover's						
1 slice	310	17	26	860	14	2
Pizza Hut 12" Medium Hand-Tossed Style Pizza Spicy Sicilian						
1 slice	250	11	26	730	11	2
Pizza Hut 12" Medium Hand-Tossed Style Pizza Supreme						
1 slice	260	12	26	660	11	2
Pizza Hut 12" Medium Hand-Tossed Style Pizza Triple Meat Italiano						
1 slice	260	12	25	740	12	2
Pizza Hut 12" Medium Hand-Tossed Style Pizza Veggie Lover's						
1 slice	200	7	27	530	8	2
Pizza Hut 12" Medium Pan Pizza All Natural Italian Sausage & Red Onion						
1 slice	260	11	28	550	11	2
Pizza Hut 12" Medium Pan Pizza All Natural Pepperoni						
1 slice	250	11	26	590	10	1

RESTAURANT/ FOOD ITEM SERVING SIZE	CALORIES	FAT	CARBS	SODIUM	PROTEIN	FIBER
Pizza Hut 12" Medium Pan Pizza All Natural Pepperoni & Mushroom						
1 slice	230	9	27	510	10	1
Pizza Hut 12" Medium Pan Pizza Cheese						
1 slice	230	9	27	520	10	1
Pizza Hut 12" Medium Pan Pizza Dan's Original						
1 slice	270	13	27	630	12	2
Pizza Hut 12" Medium Pan Pizza Ham & Pineapple						
1 slice	220	8	28	520	9	1
Pizza Hut 12" Medium Pan Pizza Hawaiian Luau						
1 slice	250	10	28	600	11	1
Pizza Hut 12" Medium Pan Pizza Meat Lover's						
1 slice	330	18	27	820	15	1
Pizza Hut 12" Medium Pan Pizza Spicy Sicilian						
1 slice	270	12	27	680	11	2
Pizza Hut 12" Medium Pan Pizza Supreme						
1 slice	280	13	27	630	12	2
Pizza Hut 12" Medium Pan Pizza Triple Meat Italiano						
1 slice	280	13	27	700	12	1
Pizza Hut 12" Medium Pan Pizza Veggie Lover's						
1 slice	220	8	28	490	9	2
Pizza Hut 12" Medium Thin 'N Crispy Pizza All Natural Italian Sausage & Red Onion						
1 slice	220	10	23	570	9	1
Pizza Hut 12" Medium Thin 'N Crispy Pizza All Natural Pepperoni						
1 slice	200	9	21	610	9	1
Pizza Hut 12" Medium Thin 'N Crispy Pizza All Natural Pepperoni & Mushroom						
1 slice	190	7	22	530	8	1
Pizza Hut 12" Medium Thin 'N Crispy Pizza Cheese						
1 slice	190	8	22	540	9	1
Pizza Hut 12" Medium Thin 'N Crispy Pizza Dan's Original						
1 slice	230	11	22	650	10	1
Pizza Hut 12" Medium Thin 'N Crispy Pizza Ham & Pineapple						
1 slice	180	6	23	530	8	1
Pizza Hut 12" Medium Thin 'N Crispy Pizza Hawaiian Luau						
1 slice	220	10	23	650	10	1
Pizza Hut 12" Medium Thin 'N Crispy Pizza Meat Lover's						
1 slice	290	16	22	850	13	1
Pizza Hut 12" Medium Thin 'N Crispy Pizza Spicy Sicilian						
1 slice	230	11	22	730	10	1
Pizza Hut 12" Medium Thin 'N Crispy Pizza Supreme						
1 slice	230	11	23	650	10	1
Pizza Hut 12" Medium Thin 'N Crispy Pizza Triple Meat Italiano						
1 slice	230	12	22	720	11	1
Pizza Hut 12" Medium Thin 'N Crispy Pizza Veggie Lover's						
1 slice	180	6	23	520	7	1
Pizza Hut 12" Pizza Mia All Natural Pepperoni						
1 slice	200	8	24	510	8	1
Pizza Hut 12" Pizza Mia Cheese						
1 slice	200	7	24	480	9	1

RESTAURANT/ FOOD ITEM SERVING SIZE	CALORIES	FAT	CARBS	SODIUM	PROTEIN	FIBER
Pizza Hut 12" The Natural Pizza All Natural Pepperoni						
1 slice	230	9	26	530	10	2
Pizza Hut 12" The Natural Pizza Cheese						
1 slice	220	8	26	460	10	2
Pizza Hut 12" The Natural Pizza Classicana						
1 slice	260	11	27	570	11	2
Pizza Hut 12" The Natural Pizza Veggie Lover's (No Olives)						
1 slice	190	6	27	380	9	2
Pizza Hut 14" Large Hand-Tossed Style Pizza All Natural Italian Sausage & Red Onion						
1 slice	350	15	39	860	15	3
Pizza Hut 14" Large Hand-Tossed Style Pizza All Natural Pepperoni						
1 slice	340	15	37	930	14	2
Pizza Hut 14" Large Hand-Tossed Style Pizza All Natural Pepperoni & Mushroom						
1 slice	310	12	38	820	14	2
Pizza Hut 14" Large Hand-Tossed Style Pizza Cheese						
1 slice	320	12	38	820	15	2
Pizza Hut 14" Large Hand-Tossed Style Pizza Dan's Original						
1 slice	370	17	38	970	17	2
Pizza Hut 14" Large Hand-Tossed Style Pizza Ham & Pineapple						
1 slice	300	10	39	820	13	2
Pizza Hut 14" Large Hand-Tossed Style Pizza Hawaiian Luau						
1 slice	340	14	40	940	15	2
Pizza Hut 14" Large Hand-Tossed Style Pizza Meat Lover's						
1 slice	450	24	38	1250	20	2
Pizza Hut 14" Large Hand-Tossed Style Pizza Spicy Sicilian						
1 slice	360	16	38	1040	16	3
Pizza Hut 14" Large Hand-Tossed Style Pizza Supreme						
1 slice	380	17	39	970	16	3
Pizza Hut 14" Large Hand-Tossed Style Pizza Triple Meat Italiano						
1 slice	380	18	38	1090	17	2
Pizza Hut 14" Large Hand-Tossed Style Pizza Veggie Lover's						
1 slice	290	10	39	770	12	3
Pizza Hut 14" Large Pan Pizza All Natural Italian Sausage & Red Onion						
1 slice	370	18	38	780	15	2
Pizza Hut 14" Large Pan Pizza All Natural Pepperoni						
1 slice	370	18	37	850	15	2
Pizza Hut 14" Large Pan Pizza All Natural Pepperoni & Mushroom						
1 slice	340	15	37	740	14	2
Pizza Hut 14" Large Pan Pizza Cheese						
1 slice	350	14	37	740	15	2
Pizza Hut 14" Large Pan Pizza Dan's Original						
1 slice	400	20	37	890	17	2
Pizza Hut 14" Large Pan Pizza Ham & Pineapple						
1 slice	320	13	38	740	14	2
Pizza Hut 14" Large Pan Pizza Hawaiian Luau						
1 slice	360	16	39	860	15	2
Pizza Hut 14" Large Pan Pizza Meat Lover's						
1 slice	470	27	37	1170	21	2

RESTAURANT/ FOOD ITEM	SERVING SIZE	CALORIES	FAT	CARBS	SODIUM	PROTEIN	FIBER
Pizza Hut 14" Large Pan Pizza Spicy Sicilian							
	1 slice	390	19	38	950	16	2
Pizza Hut 14" Large Pan Pizza Supreme							
	1 slice	400	20	38	890	17	2
Pizza Hut 14" Large Pan Pizza Triple Meat Italiano							
	1 slice	410	21	37	1010	18	2
Pizza Hut 14" Large Pan Pizza Veggie Lover's							
	1 slice	320	13	38	690	13	2
Pizza Hut 14" Large Stuffed Crust Pizza All Natural Italian Sausage & Red Onion							
	1 slice	390	18	40	980	17	2
Pizza Hut 14" Large Stuffed Crust Pizza All Natural Pepperoni							
	1 slice	380	18	39	1060	16	2
Pizza Hut 14" Large Stuffed Crust Pizza All Natural Pepperoni & Mushroom							
	1 slice	350	15	39	940	15	2
Pizza Hut 14" Large Stuffed Crust Pizza Cheese							
	1 slice	340	14	39	910	15	2
Pizza Hut 14" Large Stuffed Crust Pizza Dan's Original							
	1 slice	440	22	40	1170	20	2
Pizza Hut 14" Large Stuffed Crust Pizza Ham & Pineapple							
	1 slice	330	13	41	940	15	2
Pizza Hut 14" Large Stuffed Crust Pizza Hawaiian Luau							
	1 slice	360	14	41	1000	16	2
Pizza Hut 14" Large Stuffed Crust Pizza Meat Lover's							
	1 slice	480	26	39	1370	22	2
Pizza Hut 14" Large Stuffed Crust Pizza Spicy Sicilian							
	1 slice	430	21	40	1230	19	2
Pizza Hut 14" Large Stuffed Crust Pizza Supreme							
	1 slice	410	20	40	1090	18	3
Pizza Hut 14" Large Stuffed Crust Pizza Triple Meat Italiano							
	1 slice	440	23	40	1290	21	2
Pizza Hut 14" Large Stuffed Crust Pizza Veggie Lover's							
	1 slice	330	13	40	890	14	3
Pizza Hut 14" Large Thin 'N Crispy Pizza All Natural Italian Sausage & Red Onion							
	1 slice	290	14	30	780	13	2
Pizza Hut 14" Large Thin 'N Crispy Pizza All Natural Pepperoni							
	1 slice	290	14	28	860	12	1
Pizza Hut 14" Large Thin 'N Crispy Pizza All Natural Pepperoni & Mushroom							
	1 slice	260	11	29	740	12	1
Pizza Hut 14" Large Thin 'N Crispy Pizza Cheese							
	1 slice	260	11	29	740	12	1
Pizza Hut 14" Large Thin 'N Crispy Pizza Dan's Original							
	1 slice	320	16	29	900	15	2
Pizza Hut 14" Large Thin 'N Crispy Pizza Ham & Pineapple							
	1 slice	240	9	31	750	11	1
Pizza Hut 14" Large Thin 'N Crispy Pizza Hawaiian Luau							
	1 slice	300	14	31	900	13	1

RESTAURANT/ FOOD ITEM	SERVING SIZE	CALORIES	FAT	CARBS	SODIUM	PROTEIN	FIBER
Pizza Hut 14" Large Thin 'N Crispy Pizza Meat Lover's							
	1 slice	400	23	29	1190	19	1
Pizza Hut 14" Large Thin 'N Crispy Pizza Spicy Sicilian							
	1 slice	310	15	30	1010	14	2
Pizza Hut 14" Large Thin 'N Crispy Pizza Supreme							
	1 slice	320	16	30	900	14	2
Pizza Hut 14" Large Thin 'N Crispy Pizza Triple Meat Italiano							
	1 slice	320	17	28	1010	15	1
Pizza Hut 14" Large Thin 'N Crispy Pizza Veggie Lover's							
	1 slice	240	9	30	710	10	2
Pizza Hut 6" Personal Pan Pizza All Natural Italian Sausage & Red Onion							
	1 pizza	680	31	71	1450	28	4
Pizza Hut 6" Personal Pan Pizza All Natural Pepperoni							
	1 pizza	610	27	68	1420	25	3
Pizza Hut 6" Personal Pan Pizza All Natural Pepperoni & Mushroom							
	1 pizza	570	23	68	1260	24	4
Pizza Hut 6" Personal Pan Pizza Cheese							
	1 pizza	590	24	69	1290	26	3
Pizza Hut 6" Personal Pan Pizza Dan's Original							
	1 pizza	720	35	69	1620	31	4
Pizza Hut 6" Personal Pan Pizza Ham & Pineapple							
	1 pizza	550	20	71	1260	23	3
Pizza Hut 6" Personal Pan Pizza Hawaiian Luau							
	1 pizza	620	25	71	1440	26	3
Pizza Hut 6" Personal Pan Pizza Meat Lover's							
	1 pizza	850	47	69	2080	38	4
Pizza Hut 6" Personal Pan Pizza Spicy Sicilian							
	1 pizza	700	34	69	1700	30	4
Pizza Hut 6" Personal Pan Pizza Supreme							
	1 pizza	720	35	70	1620	31	4
Pizza Hut 6" Personal Pan Pizza Triple Meat Italiano							
	1 pizza	730	36	69	1780	32	4
Pizza Hut 6" Personal Pan Pizza Veggie Lover's							
	1 pizza	550	20	70	1190	22	4
Pizza Hut 9" Personal PANormous Pizza All Natural Italian Sausage & Red Onion							
	1 pizza	1210	55	128	2570	50	7
Pizza Hut 9" Personal PANormous Pizza All Natural Pepperoni							
	1 pizza	1110	48	122	2550	46	6
Pizza Hut 9" Personal PANormous Pizza All Natural Pepperoni & Mushroom							
	1 pizza	1050	43	123	2290	45	7
Pizza Hut 9" Personal PANormous Pizza Cheese							
	1 pizza	1100	45	124	2400	48	6
Pizza Hut 9" Personal PANormous Pizza Dan's Original							
	1 pizza	1270	61	125	2830	55	7
Pizza Hut 9" Personal PANormous Pizza Ham & Pineapple							
	1 pizza	1020	37	128	2300	43	6
Pizza Hut 9" Personal PANormous Pizza Hawaiian Luau							
	1 pizza	1150	49	129	2670	49	6

RESTAURANT/ FOOD ITEM SERVING SIZE	CALORIES	FAT	CARBS	SODIUM	PROTEIN	FIBER
Pizza Hut 9" Personal PANormous Pizza Meat Lover's						
1 pizza	1500	82	124	3640	66	7
Pizza Hut 9" Personal PANormous Pizza Spicy Sicilian						
1 pizza	1250	59	125	3110	53	7
Pizza Hut 9" Personal PANormous Pizza Supreme						
1 pizza	1270	61	127	2830	54	8
Pizza Hut 9" Personal PANormous Pizza Triple Meat Italiano						
1 pizza	1270	62	123	3100	56	7
Pizza Hut 9" Personal PANormous Pizza Veggie Lover's						
1 pizza	1000	38	126	2230	41	8
Pizza Hut All Natural Chicken Alfredo						
¼ pan	640	33	56	1190	28	4
Pizza Hut Bacon Mac N Cheese						
¼ pan	520	22	54	1170	24	4
Pizza Hut Baked Hot Wings						
2 pieces	120	7	1	500	11	0
Pizza Hut Baked Mild Wings						
2 pieces	110	7	1	440	11	0
Pizza Hut Breadsticks						
1 stick	140	6	18	240	4	1
Pizza Hut Cheese Breadsticks						
1 stick	180	7	20	370	7	1
Pizza Hut Cinnamon Sticks						
2 pieces	170	6	26	200	4	1
Pizza Hut Hershey's Chocolate Dunkers						
2 pieces	200	9	26	210	5	1
Pizza Hut Hershey's Chocolate Sauce						
1.5 oz	120	2.5	24	75	1	1
Pizza Hut Lasagna						
¼ pan	570	30	45	1670	29	5
Pizza Hut Marinara Dipping Sauce						
3 oz	60	0	12	440	2	2
Pizza Hut Meaty Marinara						
¼ pan	510	24	48	1310	25	5
Pizza Hut P'Zone Pizza All Natural Pepperoni						
½ order	630	24	76	1580	28	2
Pizza Hut P'Zone Pizza Classic						
½ order	630	23	77	1480	28	3
Pizza Hut P'Zone Pizza Meaty						
½ order	740	33	76	1840	34	3
Pizza Hut Ranch Dipping Sauce						
1.5 oz	220	23	2	420	0	0
Pizza Hut Stuffed Pizza Rolls						
1 roll	230	11	24	590	9	1
Pizza Hut White Icing Dipping Cup						
2 oz	190	0	47	0	0	0
Pizza Hut Wing Blue Cheese Dipping Sauce						
1.5 oz	230	24	2	430	1	0

RESTAURANT/ FOOD ITEM	SERVING SIZE	CALORIES	FAT	CARBS	SODIUM	PROTEIN	FIBER
Pizza Hut Wing Ranch Dipping Sauce							
	1.5 oz	220	23	3	400	1	0
Quiznos* Alpine Chicken Sammies							
	1 sandwich						
		380	n/a	28	620	n/a	n/a
Quiznos* Baja Chicken Signature Sub							
	Small	480	n/a	43	1290	n/a	n/a
Quiznos* Baja Chicken Signature Sub							
	Regular	790	n/a	71	2170	n/a	n/a
Quiznos* Baja Chicken Signature Sub							
	Large	1080	n/a	98	3030	n/a	n/a
Quiznos* Beef, Bacon & Cheddar Toasty Bullets							
	1 sandwich						
		385	n/a	38	1325	n/a	n/a
Quiznos* Beef, Bacon & Cheddar Toasty Torpedo							
	1 sandwich						
		730	n/a	79	2550	n/a	n/a
Quiznos* Big Kahuna Tuna Toasty Bullets							
	1 sandwich						
		455	n/a	35	945	n/a	n/a
Quiznos* Big Kahuna Tuna Toasty Torpedo							
	1 sandwich						
		880	n/a	73	1690	n/a	n/a
Quiznos* Bistro Steak Melt Sammies							
	1 sandwich						
		390	n/a	30	1050	n/a	n/a
Quiznos* Bourbon Grille Steak Signature Subs							
	Small	560	n/a	52	1400	n/a	n/a
Quiznos* Bourbon Grille Steak Signature Subs							
	Regular	870	n/a	82	2180	n/a	n/a
Quiznos* Bourbon Grille Steak Signature Subs							
	Large	1190	n/a	113	2950	n/a	n/a
Quiznos* Broccoli Cheese Soup							
	1 cup	175	n/a	17	780	n/a	n/a
Quiznos* Broccoli Cheese Soup							
	1 bowl	305	n/a	26	1420	n/a	n/a
Quiznos* Cantina Chicken Sammies							
	1 sandwich						
		265	n/a	35	625	n/a	n/a
Quiznos* Chicken Caesar Salad							
	Small	500	n/a	20	1265	n/a	n/a
Quiznos* Chicken Caesar Salad							
	Medium	970	n/a	39	2160	n/a	n/a
Quiznos* Chicken Carbonara Signature Subs							
	Small	515	n/a	41	1180	n/a	n/a
Quiznos* Chicken Carbonara Signature Subs							
	Regular	850	n/a	67	1990	n/a	n/a
Quiznos* Chicken Carbonara Signature Subs							
	Large	1180	n/a	92	2870	n/a	n/a

*Quiznos does not supply information on total fat values. For saturated fat and trans-fat values, please see its website, www.quiznos.com.

RESTAURANT/ FOOD ITEM	SERVING SIZE	CALORIES	FAT	CARBS	SODIUM	PROTEIN	FIBER
Quiznos* Chicken Noodle Soup							
	1 cup	105	n/a	16	880	n/a	n/a
Quiznos* Chicken Noodle Soup							
	1 bowl	155	n/a	25	1610	n/a	n/a
Quiznos* Chili							
	1 cup	185	n/a	21	750	n/a	n/a
Quiznos* Chili							
	1 bowl	360	n/a	38	1420	n/a	n/a
Quiznos* Classic Club							
	Small	550	n/a	42	1340	n/a	n/a
Quiznos* Classic Club							
	Regular	870	n/a	70	2530	n/a	n/a
Quiznos* Classic Club							
	Large	1250	n/a	96	3310	n/a	n/a
Quiznos* Classic Cobb Salad							
	Small	420	n/a	20	1035	n/a	n/a
Quiznos* Classic Cobb Salad							
	Medium	830	n/a	40	1830	n/a	n/a
Quiznos* Classic Italian Classic Sub							
	Small	505	n/a	43	1530	n/a	n/a
Quiznos* Classic Italian Classic Sub							
	Regular	880	n/a	71	2780	n/a	n/a
Quiznos* Classic Italian Classic Sub							
	Large	1240	n/a	98	3930	n/a	n/a
Quiznos* Double Cheese Cheesesteak Signature Subs							
	Small	670	n/a	45	1345	n/a	n/a
Quiznos* Double Cheese Cheesesteak Signature Subs							
	Regular	1050	n/a	72	2165	n/a	n/a
Quiznos* Double Cheese Cheesesteak Signature Subs							
	Large	1410	n/a	99	2960	n/a	n/a
Quiznos* Ham & Swiss Deli Sub							
	Small	470	n/a	42	1040	n/a	n/a
Quiznos* Ham & Swiss Deli Sub							
	Regular	790	n/a	70	2215	n/a	n/a
Quiznos* Ham & Swiss Deli Sub							
	Large	1100	n/a	96	2665	n/a	n/a
Quiznos* Honey Bacon Club Classic Sub							
	Small	470	n/a	52	1440	n/a	n/a
Quiznos* Honey Bacon Club Classic Sub							
	Regular	780	n/a	84	2535	n/a	n/a
Quiznos* Honey Bacon Club Classic Sub							
	Large	1070	n/a	117	3615	n/a	n/a
Quiznos* Honey Bourbon Chicken Classic Sub							
	Small	310	n/a	50	870	n/a	n/a
Quiznos* Honey Bourbon Chicken Classic Sub							
	Regular	530	n/a	80	1520	n/a	n/a
Quiznos* Honey Bourbon Chicken Classic Sub							
	Large	740	n/a	111	2150	n/a	n/a

*Quiznos does not supply information on total fat values. For saturated fat and trans-fat values, please see its website, www.quiznos.com.

RESTAURANT/ FOOD ITEM SERVING SIZE	CALORIES	FAT	CARBS	SODIUM	PROTEIN	FIBER
Quiznos* Honey Mustard Chicken Salad						
Small	525	n/a	25	915	n/a	n/a
Quiznos* Honey Mustard Chicken Salad						
Medium	1090	n/a	47	1935	n/a	n/a
Quiznos* Honey Mustard Chicken Signature Sub						
Small	510	n/a	45	1045	n/a	n/a
Quiznos* Honey Mustard Chicken Signature Sub						
Regular	860	n/a	72	1755	n/a	n/a
Quiznos* Honey Mustard Chicken Signature Sub						
Large	1200	n/a	100	2465	n/a	n/a
Quiznos* Italian Toasty Bullets						
1 sandwich	435	n/a	36	1345	n/a	n/a
Quiznos* Italian Toasty Torpedo						
1 sandwich	835	n/a	75	2610	n/a	n/a
Quiznos* Italiano Sammies						
1 sandwich	410	n/a	28	1025	n/a	n/a
Quiznos* Mesquite Chicken Signature Sub						
Small	490	n/a	42	1140	n/a	n/a
Quiznos* Mesquite Chicken Signature Sub						
Regular	800	n/a	68	1900	n/a	n/a
Quiznos* Mesquite Chicken Signature Sub						
Large	1110	n/a	94	2670	n/a	n/a
Quiznos* Pesto Turkey Toasty Bullets						
1 sandwich	325	n/a	37	1125	n/a	n/a
Quiznos* Pesto Turkey Toasty Torpedo						
1 sandwich	615	n/a	78	2190	n/a	n/a
Quiznos* Prime Rib and Peppercorn Signature Sub						
Small	595	n/a	45	1360	n/a	n/a
Quiznos* Prime Rib and Peppercorn Signature Sub						
Regular	950	n/a	73	2140	n/a	n/a
Quiznos* Prime Rib and Peppercorn Signature Sub						
Large	1290	n/a	100	2880	n/a	n/a
Quiznos* Primo Meatball Deli Sub						
Small	445	n/a	47	1380	n/a	n/a
Quiznos* Primo Meatball Deli Sub						
Regular	780	n/a	78	2290	n/a	n/a
Quiznos* Primo Meatball Deli Sub						
Large	1020	n/a	106	3020	n/a	n/a
Quiznos* Raspberry Chipotle Salad						
Small	325	n/a	42	835	n/a	n/a
Quiznos* Raspberry Chipotle Salad						
Medium	730	n/a	74	1705	n/a	n/a

*Quiznos does not supply information on total fat values. For saturated fat and trans-fat values, please see its website, www.quiznos.com.

RESTAURANT/ FOOD ITEM SERVING SIZE	CALORIES	FAT	CARBS	SODIUM	PROTEIN	FIBER
Quiznos* Roadhouse Steak Sammies						
1 sandwich	250	n/a	38	980	n/a	n/a
Quiznos* Roast Beef & Cheddar Deli Sub						
Small	480	n/a	43	1190	n/a	n/a
Quiznos* Roast Beef & Cheddar Deli Sub						
Regular	790	n/a	71	2120	n/a	n/a
Quiznos* Roast Beef & Cheddar Deli Sub						
Large	1100	n/a	98	3040	n/a	n/a
Quiznos* Sonoma Turkey Sammies						
1 sandwich	380	n/a	29	1135	n/a	n/a
Quiznos* Steak & Bleu Salad						
Small	230	n/a	39	1705	n/a	n/a
Quiznos* Steak & Bleu Salad						
Medium	510	n/a	68	2860	n/a	n/a
Quiznos* Steakhouse Beef Dip Signature Subs						
Small	570	n/a	46	1900	n/a	n/a
Quiznos* Steakhouse Beef Dip Signature Subs						
Regular	880	n/a	72	2635	n/a	n/a
Quiznos* Steakhouse Beef Dip Signature Subs						
Large	1180	n/a	99	3365	n/a	n/a
Quiznos* The Traditional Classic Sub						
Small	420	n/a	44	1280	n/a	n/a
Quiznos* The Traditional Classic Sub						
Regular	690	n/a	72	2420	n/a	n/a
Quiznos* The Traditional Classic Sub						
Large	950	n/a	100	3240	n/a	n/a
Quiznos* Tomato Basil Soup						
1 cup	125	n/a	14	660	n/a	n/a
Quiznos* Tomato Basil Soup						
1 bowl	205	n/a	19	1180	n/a	n/a
Quiznos* Tuna Melt Deli Sub						
Small	750	n/a	41	930	n/a	n/a
Quiznos* Tuna Melt Deli Sub						
Regular	1230	n/a	67	1510	n/a	n/a
Quiznos* Tuna Melt Deli Sub						
Large	1760	n/a	92	2120	n/a	n/a
Quiznos* Turkey & Cheddar Deli Sub						
Small	480	n/a	42	1190	n/a	n/a
Quiznos* Turkey & Cheddar Deli Sub						
Regular	780	n/a	70	2120	n/a	n/a
Quiznos* Turkey & Cheddar Deli Sub						
Large	1090	n/a	97	3040	n/a	n/a
Quiznos* Turkey Bacon Guacamole Classic Sub						
Small	525	n/a	44	1550	n/a	n/a
Quiznos* Turkey Bacon Guacamole Classic Sub						
Regular	810	n/a	74	2700	n/a	n/a

*Quiznos does not supply information on total fat values. For saturated fat and trans-fat values, please see its website, www.quiznos.com.

RESTAURANT/ FOOD ITEM SERVING SIZE	CALORIES	FAT	CARBS	SODIUM	PROTEIN	FIBER
Quiznos* Turkey Bacon Guacamole Classic Sub						
Large	1170	n/a	102	3780	n/a	n/a
Quiznos* Turkey Club Toasty Bullets						
1 sandwich						
	415	n/a	37	1215	n/a	n/a
Quiznos* Turkey Club Toasty Torpedo						
1 sandwich						
	755	n/a	77	2370	n/a	n/a
Quiznos* Turkey Ranch & Swiss Classic Sub						
Small	400	n/a	45	1160	n/a	n/a
Quiznos* Turkey Ranch & Swiss Classic Sub						
Regular	660	n/a	74	2085	n/a	n/a
Quiznos* Turkey Ranch & Swiss Classic Sub						
Large	880	n/a	100	2465	n/a	n/a
Quiznos* Veggie Classic Sub						
Small	490	n/a	44	1280	n/a	n/a
Quiznos* Veggie Classic Sub						
Regular	770	n/a	71	2020	n/a	n/a
Quiznos* Veggie Classic Sub						
Large	1060	n/a	96	2740	n/a	n/a
Quiznos* Veggie Sammies						
1 sandwich						
	340	n/a	29	745	n/a	n/a
Starbucks Blueberry Scone						
1 scone	460	22	61	420	7	2
Starbucks Blueberry Streusel Muffin						
1 muffin	360	11	59	390	7	2
Starbucks Butter Croissant						
1 croissant	310	18	32	290	5	<1
Starbucks Caffe Americano						
Short/8 oz	5	0	1	0	0	0
Starbucks Caffe Americano						
Tall/12 oz	10	0	2	5	1	0
Starbucks Caffe Americano						
Grande/16 oz						
	15	0	3	10	1	0
Starbucks Caffe Americano						
Venti/20 oz						
	25	0	4	10	1	0
Starbucks Caffe Latte with 2% Milk						
Short/8 oz	100	3.5	9	75	6	0
Starbucks Caffe Latte with 2% Milk						
Tall/12 oz	150	6	14	115	10	0
Starbucks Caffe Latte with 2% Milk						
Grande/16 oz						
	190	7	18	150	12	0
Starbucks Caffe Latte with 2% Milk						
Venti/20 oz						
	240	9	24	190	16	0

*Quiznos does not supply information on total fat values. For saturated fat and trans-fat values, please see its website, www.quiznos.com.

RESTAURANT/ FOOD ITEM SERVING SIZE	CALORIES	FAT	CARBS	SODIUM	PROTEIN	FIBER
Starbucks Caffe Latte with Nonfat Milk						
Short/8 oz	70	0	10	75	6	0
Starbucks Caffe Latte with Nonfat Milk						
Tall/12 oz	100	0	15	120	10	0
Starbucks Caffe Latte with Nonfat Milk						
Grande/16 oz						
	130	0	19	150	13	0
Starbucks Caffe Latte with Nonfat Milk						
Venti/20 oz						
	170	0	25	190	16	0
Starbucks Caffe Misto/Café au Lait with 2% Milk						
Short/8 oz	50	2	6	45	4	0
Starbucks Caffe Misto/Café au Lait with 2% Milk						
Tall/12 oz	80	3	7	70	5	0
Starbucks Caffe Misto/Café au Lait with 2% Milk						
Grande/16 oz						
	110	4	10	90	7	0
Starbucks Caffe Misto/Café au Lait with 2% Milk						
Venti/20 oz						
	130	5	12	115	9	0
Starbucks Caffe Misto/Café au Lait with Nonfat Milk						
Short/8 oz	35	0	5	45	4	0
Starbucks Caffe Misto/Café au Lait with Nonfat Milk						
Tall/12 oz	60	0	8	70	6	0
Starbucks Caffe Misto/Café au Lait with Nonfat Milk						
Grande/16 oz						
	70	0	10	90	7	0
Starbucks Caffe Misto/Café au Lait with Nonfat Milk						
Venti/20 oz						
	90	0	13	115	9	0
Starbucks Cappuccino with 2% Milk						
Short/8 oz	80	3	8	60	5	0
Starbucks Cappuccino with 2% Milk						
Tall/12 oz	90	3.5	9	70	6	0
Starbucks Cappuccino with 2% Milk						
Grande/16 oz						
	120	4	12	85	8	0
Starbucks Cappuccino with 2% Milk						
Venti/20 oz						
	150	6	15	120	10	0
Starbucks Cappuccino with Nonfat Milk						
Short/8 oz	50	0	8	60	5	0
Starbucks Cappuccino with Nonfat Milk						
Tall/12 oz	60	0	9	70	6	0
Starbucks Cappuccino with Nonfat Milk						
Grande/16 oz						
	80	0	12	90	8	0
Starbucks Cappuccino with Nonfat Milk						
Venti/20 oz						
	110	0	16	120	10	0

RESTAURANT/ FOOD ITEM SERVING SIZE	CALORIES	FAT	CARBS	SODIUM	PROTEIN	FIBER
Starbucks Coffee Frappuccino Blended Coffee						
Tall/12 oz 180	180	2.5	37	170	4	0
Starbucks Coffee Frappuccino Blended Coffee						
Grande/16 oz						
240	240	3	48	220	5	0
Starbucks Coffee Frappuccino Blended Coffee						
Venti/20 oz						
340	340	4.5	67	320	7	0
Starbucks Espresso Frappuccino Blended Coffee						
Tall/12 oz 140	140	1.5	27	125	3	0
Starbucks Espresso Frappuccino Blended Coffee						
Grande/16 oz						
190	190	2.5	38	170	4	0
Starbucks Espresso Frappuccino Blended Coffee						
Venti/20 oz						
290	290	3.5	57	270	6	0
Starbucks Mocha Frappuccino Blended Coffee						
Tall/12 oz 200	200	3	41	170	4	0
Starbucks Mocha Frappuccino Blended Coffee						
Grande/16 oz						
260	260	3.5	54	230	6	0
Starbucks Mocha Frappuccino Blended Coffee						
Venti/20 oz						
380	380	5	78	320	8	1
Starbucks Strawberry Blueberry Yogurt Parfait						
1 parfait 350	350	4.5	66	199	10	4
Subway 6" Big Philly Cheesesteak						
311.2 g 520	520	18	53	1570	39	6
Subway 6" Black Forest Ham						
226 g 290	290	4.5	47	1200	18	5
Subway 6" BLT						
164 g 360	360	13	45	990	17	5
Subway 6" Chicken & Bacon Ranch						
299 g 570	570	28	49	1190	35	6
Subway 6" Cold Cut Combo						
252 g 410	410	16	48	1450	21	5
Subway 6" Italian B.M.T.						
245 g 450	450	20	48	1730	22	5
Subway 6" Meatball Marinara						
379 g 580	580	23	70	1530	24	9
Subway 6" Oven Roasted Chicken						
240 g 320	320	4.5	49	750	23	5
Subway 6" Roast Beef						
240 g 310	310	4.5	46	840	26	5
Subway 6" Spicy Italian						
240 g 520	520	28	47	1830	22	5
Subway 6" Subway Club						
257 g 320	320	5	47	1160	26	5
Subway 6" Subway Melt						
256 g 380	380	11	49	1530	25	5

RESTAURANT/ FOOD ITEM	SERVING SIZE	CALORIES	FAT	CARBS	SODIUM	PROTEIN	FIBER
Subway 6" Sweet Onion Chicken Teriyaki							
	283 g	380	4.5	60	1010	26	5
Subway 6" The Feast							
	331 g	540	22	50	2470	39	5
Subway 6" Tuna							
	252 g	530	30	46	930	21	5
Subway 6" Turkey Breast							
	226 g	280	3.5	47	920	18	5
Subway 6" Turkey Breast & Black Forest Ham							
	236 g	300	4	47	1140	19	5
Subway 6" Veggie Delite							
	169 g	230	2.5	45	410	8	5
Subway Apple Pie							
	71 g	250	10	37	290	0	1
Subway Apple Slices							
	71 g	35	0	9	0	0	2
Subway Black Forest Ham & Cheese English Muffin with Regular Egg							
	119 g	180	7	18	650	15	5
Subway Black Forest Ham & Cheese on Flatbread							
	233 g	480	22	46	1530	27	3
Subway Black Forest Ham on Flatbread							
	242 g	320	7	47	1270	18	3
Subway Black Forest Ham Salad							
	356 g	110	3	12	850	12	4
Subway Cheese & Veggies Pizza							
	8" pizza	740	25	100	1270	36	5
Subway Cheese English Muffin with Regular Egg							
	105 g	170	6	18	450	13	5
Subway Cheese Pizza							
	8" pizza	680	22	96	1070	32	4
Subway Chicken & Dumpling Soup							
	10 oz	170	5	23	810	8	2
Subway Chicken Tortilla Soup							
	10 oz	110	1.5	11	440	6	3
Subway Chili Con Carne Soup							
	10 oz	340	11	35	950	20	10
Subway Chipotle Chicken Corn Chowder Soup							
	10 oz	140	3	22	900	6	2
Subway Chocolate Chip Cookie							
	45 g	210	10	30	150	2	1
Subway Chocolate Chunk Cookie							
	45 g	220	10	30	100	2	1
Subway Club on Flatbread							
	272 g	350	8	47	1230	26	3
Subway Club Salad							
	387 g	140	3.5	12	810	20	4
Subway Cream of Potato with Bacon Soup							
	10 oz	240	13	26	870	5	3
Subway Double Bacon & Cheese English Muffin with Regular Egg							
	120 g	240	11	18	740	17	5

RESTAURANT/ FOOD ITEM SERVING SIZE	CALORIES	FAT	CARBS	SODIUM	PROTEIN	FIBER
Subway Double Bacon & Cheese on Flatbread						
223 g	560	28	46	1540	30	3
Subway Double Chocolate Chip Cookie						
45 g	209.6	10	30	170	2	1
Subway Egg & Cheese on Flatbread						
204 g	460	21	45	1170	23	3
Subway Fat Free Italian Dressing						
57 g	35	0	7	720	1	0
Subway Fire-Roasted Tomato Orzo Soup						
10 oz	130	1	24	410	6	2
Subway Footlong Black Forest Ham						
452 g	570	9	94	2400	35	10
Subway Footlong Oven Roasted Chicken						
481 g	640	9	97	1490	46	11
Subway Footlong Roast Beef						
481 g	630	9	91	1690	52	11
Subway Footlong Subway Club						
514 g	640	10	95	2320	52	11
Subway Footlong Sweet Onion Chicken Teriyaki						
566 g	760	9	120	2020	51	10
Subway Footlong Turkey Breast						
452 g	570	7	94	1830	35	10
Subway Footlong Turkey Breast & Black Forest Ham						
471 g	590	8	95	2280	38	10
Subway Footlong Veggie Delite						
339 g	460	4.5	90	830	17	10
Subway Golden Broccoli & Cheese Soup						
10 oz	180	11	16	990	5	4
Subway Hash Browns						
4 pieces	150	9	17	440	1	2
Subway M&M Cookie						
45 g	210	10	32	100	2	<1
Subway Mega English Muffin with Regular Egg						
138 g	310	20	18	710	18	5
Subway Mega on Flatbread						
270 g	750	48	46	1650	34	3
Subway Minestrone Soup						
10 oz	90	1	17	910	4	3
Subway New England Style Clam Chowder						
10 oz	150	5	20	990	6	4
Subway Oatmeal Raisin Cookie						
45 g	200	8	30	170	3	1
Subway Oven Roasted Chicken on Flatbread						
256 g	350	7	48	820	24	3
Subway Oven Roasted Chicken (Strips) Salad						
371 g	130	2.5	10	280	20	4
Subway Peanut Butter Cookie						
45 g	220	12	26	190	4	1
Subway Pepperoni Pizza						
8" pizza	790	32	96	1350	38	4

RESTAURANT/ FOOD ITEM	SERVING SIZE	CALORIES	FAT	CARBS	SODIUM	PROTEIN	FIBER
Subway Ranch Dressing	57 g	290	30	3	540	1	0
Subway Roast Beef on Flatbread	256 g	340	8	45	920	27	3
Subway Roast Beef Salad	371 g	140	3.5	10	500	21	4
Subway Roasted Chicken Noodle Soup	10 oz	80	2	12	950	6	1
Subway Rosemary Chicken and Dumpling Soup	10 oz	90	1.5	14	810	6	1
Subway Sausage & Cheese on Flatbread	261 g	700	44	46	1460	30	3
Subway Sausage English Muffin with Regular Egg	134 g	290	18	18	620	16	5
Subway Sausage Pizza	8" pizza	820	34	97	1420	39	4
Subway Spanish Style Chicken & Rice with Pork Soup	10 oz	110	2.5	16	980	6	1
Subway Steak & Cheese English Muffin with Regular Egg	122 g	190	7	19	600	16	6
Subway Steak & Cheese on Flatbread	247 g	521	23	48	1470	32	3
Subway Sugar Cookie	45 g	220	12	28	140	2	<1
Subway Sweet Onion Chicken Teriyaki on Flatbread	298 g	410	7	59	1080	26	3
Subway Sweet Onion Chicken Teriyaki Salad	413 g	200	3	25	660	20	4
Subway Tomato Garden Vegetable with Rotini Soup	10 oz	90	0.5	20	820	3	3
Subway Turkey Breast & Black Forest Ham on Flatbread	251 g	330	7	47	1220	20	3
Subway Turkey Breast & Ham Salad	366 g	120	3	12	790	14	4
Subway Turkey Breast on Flatbread	242 g	310	6	47	990	18	3
Subway Turkey Breast Salad	356 g	110	2	12	570	12	4
Subway Vegetable Beef Soup	10 oz	100	2	17	960	5	3
Subway Veggie Delite on Flatbread	185 g	260	5	44	490	9	3
Subway Veggie Delite Salad	300 g	50	1	10	65	3	4
Subway Western & Cheese on Flatbread	244 g	490	22	47	1560	28	3
Subway Western with Cheese English Muffin with Regular Egg	125 g	180	7	19	650	15	6
Subway White Chip Macadamia Nut Cookie	45 g	220	11	29	160	2	<1

RESTAURANT/ FOOD ITEM SERVING SIZE	CALORIES	FAT	CARBS	SODIUM	PROTEIN	FIBER
Subway Wild Rice with Chicken Soup						
10 oz bowl	230	11	26	900	6	1
Subway Yogurt Dannon Light & Fit						
170 g	80	0	16	80	5	0
Taco Bell ½ lb Cheesy Potato Burrito						
248 g	530	25	57	1690	19	7
Taco Bell ½ lb Combo Burrito						
241 g	450	17	51	1610	21	9
Taco Bell ½ lb Nacho Crunch Burrito						
234 g	520	25	54	1400	19	6
Taco Bell 7-Layer Burrito						
283 g	490	17	67	1360	17	10
Taco Bell Bean Burrito						
198 g	350	9	54	1220	13	9
Taco Bell Burrito Supreme, Beef						
248 g	410	15	52	1350	17	8
Taco Bell Burrito Supreme, Chicken						
248 g	390	12	51	1390	20	6
Taco Bell Burrito Supreme, Steak						
248 g	380	12	50	1320	17	6
Taco Bell Caramel Apple Empanada						
85 g	310	15	39	310	3	2
Taco Bell Chalupa Baja, Beef						
153 g	410	26	31	720	13	5
Taco Bell Chalupa Baja, Chicken						
153 g	390	23	29	760	16	3
Taco Bell Chalupa Baja, Steak						
153 g	380	23	29	690	13	3
Taco Bell Chalupa Nacho Cheese, Beef						
153 g	370	22	31	730	12	4
Taco Bell Chalupa Nacho Cheese, Chicken						
153 g	340	18	30	770	15	3
Taco Bell Chalupa Nacho Cheese, Steak						
153 g	330	19	30	700	12	3
Taco Bell Chalupa Supreme, Beef						
153 g	370	21	31	600	13	4
Taco Bell Chalupa Supreme, Chicken						
153 g	350	18	30	640	17	3
Taco Bell Chalupa Supreme, Steak						
153 g	340	18	29	560	14	3
Taco Bell Cheese Roll-Up						
64 g	200	10	19	530	9	2
Taco Bell Cheesy Bean & Rice Burrito						
227 g	470	21	60	1420	12	6
Taco Bell Cheesy Double Beef Burrito						
227 g	470	20	54	1580	18	6
Taco Bell Cheesy Fiesta Potatoes						
135 g	270	16	28	840	4	3

RESTAURANT/ FOOD ITEM	SERVING SIZE	CALORIES	FAT	CARBS	SODIUM	PROTEIN	FIBER
Taco Bell Chicken Burrito	177 g	440	20	48	1260	16	3
Taco Bell Chicken Ranch Taco Salad	488 g	960	57	78	1710	36	8
Taco Bell Chicken Soft Taco	99 g	200	8	19	640	12	1
Taco Bell Chipotle Steak Taco Salad	488 g	950	59	76	1760	29	8
Taco Bell Cinnamon Twists	35 g	170	7	26	200	1	1
Taco Bell Crispy Potato Soft Taco	106 g	260	13	31	690	6	3
Taco Bell Crunchy Taco	78 g	170	10	12	330	8	3
Taco Bell Crunchy Taco Supreme	113 g	200	12	15	350	9	3
Taco Bell Double Decker Taco	156 g	320	13	38	800	14	7
Taco Bell Double Decker Taco Supreme	191 g	350	15	40	820	14	7
Taco Bell Fiesta Taco Salad	544 g	820	43	81	1740	30	15
Taco Bell Fiesta Taco Salad without Shell	475 g	460	22	41	1470	24	13
Taco Bell Fresco Bean Burrito	213 g	330	7	55	1230	11	9
Taco Bell Fresco Burrito Supreme Chicken	241 g	340	8	49	1390	18	6
Taco Bell Fresco Burrito Supreme Steak	241 g	330	8	49	1310	15	6
Taco Bell Fresco Crunchy Taco	92 g	150	7	13	350	7	3
Taco Bell Fresco Grilled Steak Soft Taco	128 g	160	4.5	21	600	9	2
Taco Bell Fresco Ranchero Chicken Soft Taco	135 g	170	4	22	740	12	2
Taco Bell Fresco Soft Taco Beef	113 g	180	7	22	640	8	3
Taco Bell Gordita Baja Beef	153 g	340	18	30	710	13	4
Taco Bell Gordita Baja Chicken	153 g	320	15	29	750	16	3
Taco Bell Gordita Baja Steak	153 g	310	15	28	670	14	3
Taco Bell Gordita Nacho Cheese Beef	153 g	290	14	31	720	12	4
Taco Bell Gordita Nacho Cheese Chicken	153 g	270	10	30	760	15	2
Taco Bell Gordita Nacho Cheese Steak	153 g	260	11	29	690	12	2

RESTAURANT/ FOOD ITEM	SERVING SIZE	CALORIES	FAT	CARBS	SODIUM	PROTEIN	FIBER
Taco Bell Gordita Supreme Beef	153 g	300	13	31	590	13	4
Taco Bell Gordita Supreme Chicken	153 g	270	10	29	620	17	2
Taco Bell Gordita Supreme Steak	153 g	270	11	29	550	14	2
Taco Bell Grilled Steak Soft Taco	128 g	250	14	20	710	11	2
Taco Bell Grilled Stuft Burrito—Beef	325 g	690	30	79	2110	26	10
Taco Bell Grilled Stuft Burrito—Chicken	325 g	650	23	76	2180	33	7
Taco Bell Grilled Stuft Burrito—Steak	325 g	630	24	75	2040	28	7
Taco Bell Mexican Rice	85 g	130	3.5	21	410	2	1
Taco Bell Nachos	99 g	330	21	31	520	4	2
Taco Bell Nachos Bell Grande	305 g	760	42	77	1250	19	12
Taco Bell Nachos Supreme	191 g	430	24	41	780	13	7
Taco Bell Pintos 'n Cheese	128 g	170	6	18	670	9	7
Taco Bell Ranchero Chicken Soft Taco	135 g	270	14	21	840	14	2
Taco Bell Soft Taco, Beef	99 g	210	9	21	620	10	3
Taco Bell Soft Taco Supreme, Beef	135 g	240	11	24	650	11	3
Taco Bell Triple Layer Nachos	142 g	340	18	38	720	7	6
Taco Bell Volcano Burrito	303 g	800	42	81	2010	24	8
Taco Bell Volcano Nachos	354 g	990	61	88	1880	20	14
Taco Bell Volcano Taco	92 g	240	17	14	470	8	3
Wendy's Bacon Deluxe Double	1 serving	860	50	46	1880	56	2
Wendy's Bacon Deluxe Single	1 serving	640	35	46	1620	37	2
Wendy's Bacon Deluxe Triple	1 serving	1140	71	47	2470	79	2
Wendy's Baconator	1 serving	970	60	44	2260	62	2
Wendy's Barbecue Nugget Sauce	1 serving	45	0	11	160	1	0
Wendy's Bold Buffalo Boneless Wings	1 serving	520	18	58	2630	31	2

RESTAURANT/ FOOD ITEM	SERVING SIZE	CALORIES	FAT	CARBS	SODIUM	PROTEIN	FIBER
Wendy's Caesar Side Salad	1 serving	70	4	4	170	6	2
Wendy's Caesar Side Salad Add-On: Homestyle Garlic Croutons	1 serving	70	2.5	9	125	2	0
Wendy's Caesar Side Salad Add-On: Supreme Caesar Dressing	1 serving	120	13	1	200	1	0
Wendy's Chicken BLT Salad	1 serving	470	27	23	1210	35	3
Wendy's Chicken BLT Salad Add-On: Homestyle Garlic Croutons	1 serving	70	2.5	9	125	2	0
Wendy's Chicken BLT Salad Add-On: Honey Dijon Dressing	1 serving	250	24	9	330	1	0
Wendy's Chicken Caesar Salad	1 serving	180	4	8	690	28	3
Wendy's Chicken Caesar Salad Add-On: Homestyle Garlic Croutons	1 serving	70	2.5	9	125	2	0
Wendy's Chicken Caesar Salad Add-On: Supreme Caesar Dressing	1 serving	120	13	1	200	1	0
Wendy's Chicken Club Sandwich	1 serving	620	29	55	1490	37	2
Wendy's Chicken Nuggets	10 pieces	470	32	21	960	23	0
Wendy's Chicken Nuggets	5 pieces	230	16	11	480	12	0
Wendy's Chicken Nuggets, Kids' Meal	4 pieces	190	13	9	380	9	0
Wendy's Chili	Large	280	9	29	1240	21	7
Wendy's Chili	Small	190	6	19	830	14	5
Wendy's Chili Topping: Cheddar Cheese, Shredded	1 serving	70	6	1	105	4	0
Wendy's Chocolate Frosty	Small	320	8	52	150	9	0
Wendy's Chocolate Fudge Frosty Shake	Large	530	13	94	310	11	1
Wendy's Chocolate Fudge Frosty Shake	Small	400	11	69	220	9	1
Wendy's Classic Ranch Dressing	1 serving	200	20	3	340	1	0
Wendy's Coffee Toffee Twisted Frosty, Chocolate	1 serving	540	20	83	240	9	1
Wendy's Coffee Toffee Twisted Frosty, Vanilla	1 serving	540	20	83	270	9	1
Wendy's Crispy Chicken Sandwich	1 serving	360	18	36	710	15	2
Wendy's Double Stack	1 serving	360	18	26	810	23	1
Wendy's Double with Everything and Cheese	1 serving	750	42	44	1520	50	3

RESTAURANT/ FOOD ITEM SERVING SIZE	CALORIES	FAT	CARBS	SODIUM	PROTEIN	FIBER
Wendy's Fat Free French Dressing						
1 serving	70	0	17	170	0	1
Wendy's French Fries						
Large	540	26	71	500	7	7
Wendy's French Fries						
Small	330	16	44	300	4	4
Wendy's Frosty-Cino						
Large	510	13	86	220	9	0
Wendy's Frosty-Cino						
Small	380	11	63	170	7	0
Wendy's Grilled Chicken Go Wrap						
1 serving	250	10	24	730	17	1
Wendy's Heartland Ranch Dipping Sauce						
1 serving	160	17	1	220	0	0
Wendy's Homestyle Chicken Fillet Sandwich						
1 serving	470	17	53	1100	27	2
Wendy's Homestyle Chicken Go Wrap						
1 serving	310	15	30	800	15	1
Wendy's Honey BBQ Boneless Wings						
1 serving	580	18	75	1990	32	2
Wendy's Honey Mustard Nugget Sauce						
1 serving	130	12	6	220	0	0
Wendy's Hot Chili Seasoning Packet						
1 serving	5	0	1	270	0	0
Wendy's Italian Vinaigrette Dressing						
1 serving	130	11	8	320	0	0
Wendy's Jr. Bacon Cheeseburger						
1 serving	310	16	25	670	17	1
Wendy's Jr. Cheeseburger						
1 serving	270	11	26	700	15	1
Wendy's Jr. Cheeseburger Deluxe						
1 serving	300	14	28	740	15	2
Wendy's Jr. Hamburger						
1 serving	230	8	26	500	13	1
Wendy's Ketchup						
1 packet	10	0	3	115	0	0
Wendy's Light Classic Ranch Dressing						
1 serving	90	8	4	360	1	0
Wendy's M&Ms Twisted Frosty, Chocolate						
1 serving	560	19	86	180	10	1
Wendy's M&Ms Twisted Frosty, Vanilla						
1 serving	550	19	86	210	10	1
Wendy's Mandarin Chicken Salad						
1 serving	180	2	16	630	24	2
Wendy's Mandarin Chicken Salad Add-On: Crispy Noodles						
1 serving	70	2.5	10	190	1	0
Wendy's Mandarin Chicken Salad Add-On: Oriental Sesame Dressing						
1 serving	170	10	19	360	1	0
Wendy's Mandarin Chicken Salad Add-On: Roasted Almonds						
1 serving	130	11	4	70	5	2

RESTAURANT/ FOOD ITEM SERVING SIZE	CALORIES	FAT	CARBS	SODIUM	PROTEIN	FIBER
Wendy's Mandarin Orange Cup						
1 serving	80	0	19	15	1	1
Wendy's Medium French Fries						
1 serving	420	20	55	380	5	5
Wendy's Nestlé Toll House Cookie Dough Twisted Frosty, Chocolate						
1 serving	480	16	77	220	10	1
Wendy's Nestlé Toll House Cookie Dough Twisted Frosty, Vanilla						
1 serving	480	16	77	240	9	1
Wendy's OreoTwisted Frosty, Chocolate						
1 serving	450	14	72	300	10	1
Wendy's OreoTwisted Frosty, Vanilla						
1 serving	440	14	72	320	9	1
Wendy's Plain Baked Potato						
10 oz	270	0	61	25	7	7
Wendy's Saltine Crackers						
1 serving	25	0.5	5	80	1	0
Wendy's Side Salad						
1 serving	35	0	8	25	1	2
Wendy's Single with Everything						
1 serving	470	21	43	940	27	3
Wendy's Sour Cream & Chives Baked Potato						
1 serving	320	3.5	63	50	8	7
Wendy's Sour Cream & Chives Baked Potato Buttery Best Spread						
1 serving	50	5	0	95	0	0
Wendy's Southwest Taco Salad						
1 serving	400	22	26	1140	27	7
Wendy's Southwest Taco Salad Add-On: Ancho Chipotle Ranch Dressing						
1 serving	90	8	3	240	1	0
Wendy's Southwest Taco Salad Add-On: Reduced Fat Acidified Sour Cream						
1 serving	45	3.5	2	25	1	0
Wendy's Southwest Taco Salad Add-On: Seasoned Tortilla Strips						
1 serving	110	5	13	160	2	1
Wendy's Spicy Chicken Fillet Sandwich						
1 serving	470	16	55	1250	27	2
Wendy's Spicy Chicken Go Wrap						
1 serving	320	15	30	880	16	1
Wendy's Strawberry Frosty Shake						
Large	510	13	89	210	9	1
Wendy's Strawberry Frosty Shake						
Small	390	11	66	170	7	0
Wendy's Sweet & Sour Nugget Sauce						
1 serving	50	0	12	120	0	0
Wendy's Sweet & Spicy Asian Boneless Wings						
1 serving	550	18	67	2530	31	3
Wendy's Thousand Island Dressing						
1 serving	290	28	9	530	1	0
Wendy's Triple with Everything and Cheese						
1 serving	1030	62	45	2110	73	3

RESTAURANT/ FOOD ITEM	SERVING SIZE	CALORIES	FAT	CARBS	SODIUM	PROTEIN	FIBER
Wendy's Ultimate Chicken Grill Sandwich							
	1 serving	350	7	41	1000	29	2
Wendy's Vanilla Bean Frosty Shake							
	Large	500	12	88	220	9	0
Wendy's Vanilla Bean Frosty Shake							
	Small	380	10	65	170	7	0
Wendy's Vanilla Frosty							
	Small	310	8	52	180	8	0
Wendy's Vanilla Frosty Float with Coca-Cola							
	1 serving	380	7	75	160	7	0

Afterword

....

USE IT TO LOSE IT

You now have all the information you need to take control of both the quantity and the quality of every bite that goes into your mouth. Keep yourself accountable—take this book along with you everywhere, and make it a habit to check, check, check that nutrition information, especially when you are in chain restaurants. (How about some of those calorie tabs? Pretty revolting, eh?) I want this book to be thumbed-through and used until it's falling apart—that'll be one of the best signs you're keeping your eating plan together!

And remember—you aren't in this alone.

The ULTIMATE weight-loss
machine JUST GOT BETTER.
LIVE
INTERACTIVE
FITNESS,
NUTRITION &
Motivational Support.
ifit
LIVE
NordicTrack
Incline training burns 5x the calories.
Add iFit® Live and you get the most
powerful fitness technology in the world.
JILLIAN MICHAELS
OFFICIAL PRODUCT
NordicTrack
Incline Trainer X7i Interactive
Order yours at
www.jillianmichaels.com

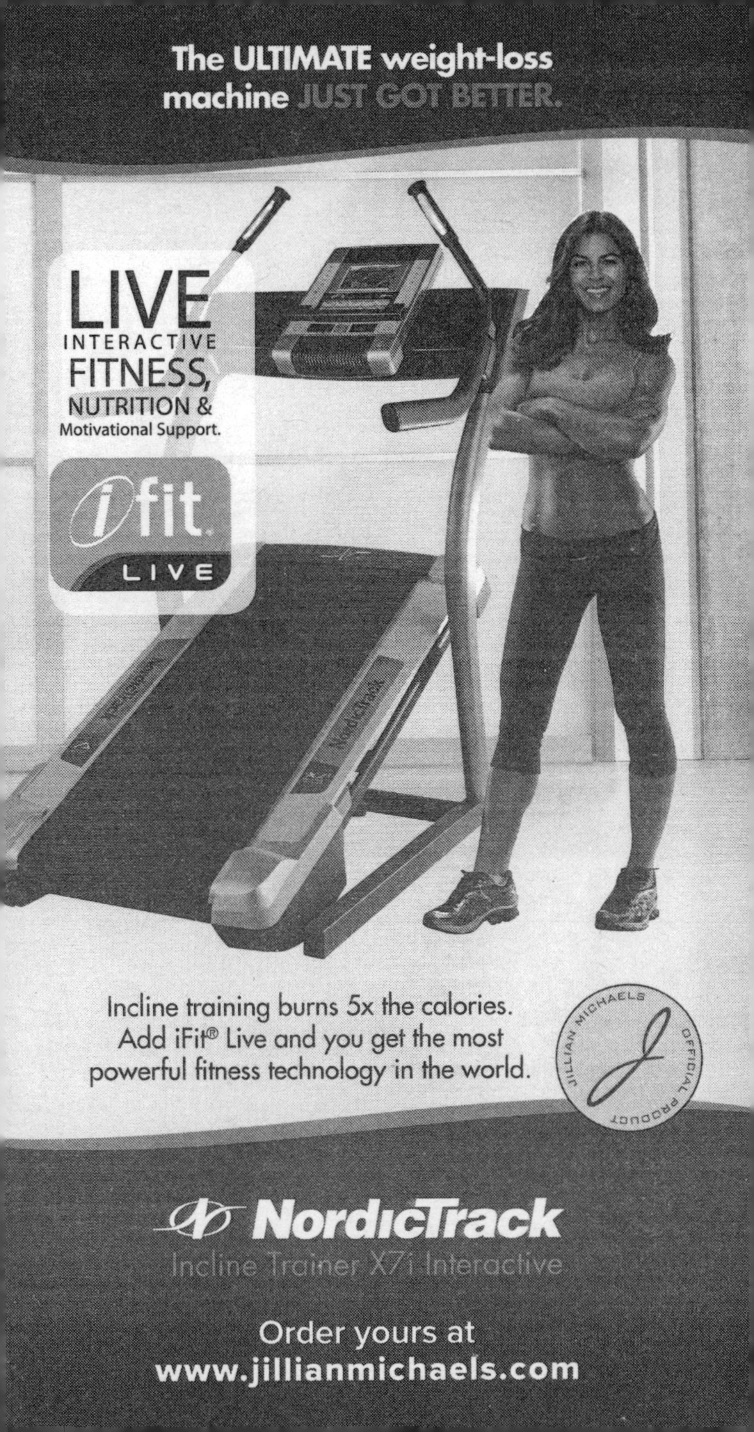

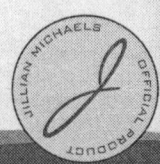

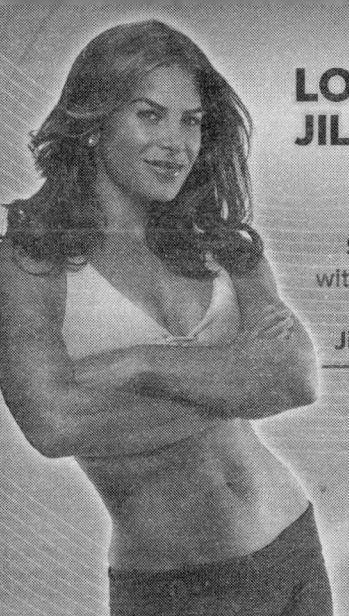